T0291642

The Clinical Use of Antipsychotic Plasma Levels

As personalized medicine in the field of psychopharmacology is turning from hope to hype, the need for precision tools in clinical practice is constantly growing. Among currently available precision tools, measuring antipsychotic plasma levels in patients prescribed antipsychotic medications, a method also known as therapeutic drug monitoring (TDM), is old, but a well-established method to account for the unique characteristics of each patient to aid in appropriate dose selection. With this readily comprehensible book, Dr. Meyer provides a comprehensive overview of the theoretical and practical framework for the effective use of TDM in clinical routine to improve the efficacy and safety of antipsychotic medications. Integrating TDM evidence for use in common clinical challenges in the practice of psychopharmacology, this book comprises an essential practical guide for routine TDM practice, a must-read work for all mental health professionals prescribing antipsychotic medications.

Georgios Schoretsanitis, MD, PhD, The Zucker Hillside Hospital, Psychiatry Research, Northwell Health, Glen Oaks, New York, USA, University Hospital of Psychiatry Zurich, Zurich, Switzerland

As we redouble our efforts to achieve the goals of personalized medicine, therapeutic drug monitoring (TDM) can play a critical role. Individuals vary enormously in how they absorb and metabolize different medications and which impactful environmental factors or co-occurring conditions they might encounter. In my view, the potential value of the knowledge that can be provided by TDM has been given less attention than it deserves. Meyer and Stahl have done an excellent job of reviewing this topic. They address all necessary perspectives, from optimizing response and tolerability to better monitoring of adherence and help to explain idiosyncratic or unexpected medication effects, as well as the timing and interpretation of plasma levels. This is an extremely useful text for anyone involved in the use of antipsychotic drugs.

John M. Kane, MD, Professor and Chairman, Department of Psychiatry, Donald and Barbara Zucker School of Medicine at Hofstra/Northwell, NY, USA

Dr. Meyer and Stahl have succeeded again in providing a well-written and evidence-based handbook with a focus on the use of antipsychotic plasma levels. This book offers so much more than a comprehensive review on the topic and provides us with important clinical pearls and helpful summarized recommendations. Most importantly, we walk away with having a good understanding and solid rationale for when and why plasma levels are important, but also having a reference we can revisit time and time again.

Deanna L. Kelly, PharmD., BCPP, Professor of Psychiatry, Director, Treatment Research Program (TRP) Maryland Psychiatric Research Center (MPRC), University of Maryland School of Medicine, MD, USA

The Clinical Use of Antipsychotic Plasma Levels

Stahl's Handbooks

Jonathan M. M

Clinical Professor of Psychiatry, Un San Diego

St

Clinical Pr uroscience,
University of Ca Adjunct Professor
of Psychiatry, ifornia, San Diego

With illustrations by

Nancy Muntner

Neuroscience Education Institute

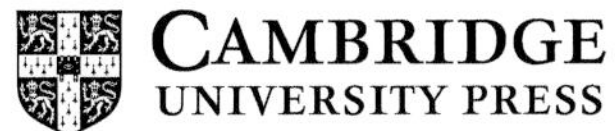

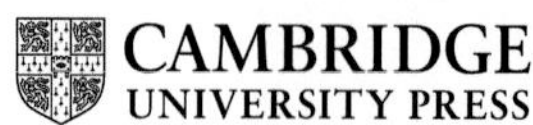

Shaftesbury Road, Cambridge CB2 8EA, United Kingdom

One Liberty Plaza, 20th Floor, New York, NY 10006, USA

477 Williamstown Road, Port Melbourne, VIC 3207, Australia

314–321, 3rd Floor, Plot 3, Splendor Forum, Jasola District Centre, New Delhi – 110025, India

103 Penang Road, #05–06/07, Visioncrest Commercial, Singapore 238467

Cambridge University Press is part of Cambridge University Press & Assessment, a department of the University of Cambridge.

We share the University's mission to contribute to society through the pursuit of education, learning and research at the highest international levels of excellence.

www.cambridge.org
Information on this title: www.cambridge.org/9781009009898

DOI: 10.1017/9781009002103

First published 2021

A catalogue record for this publication is available from the British Library

Library of Congress Cataloging-in-Publication data
Names: Meyer, Jonathan M., 1962– author. | Stahl, Stephen M., 1951– author.
Title: The clinical use of antipsychotic plasma levels / Jonathan M Meyer, Stephen M Stahl ; with illustrations by Nancy Munter.
Other titles: Stahl's handbooks.
Description: Cambridge ; New York, NY : Cambridge University Press, 2021. | Series: Stahl's handbooks | Includes bibliographical references and index.
Identifiers: LCCN 2021012648 (print) | LCCN 2021012649 (ebook) | ISBN 9781009009898 (paperback) | ISBN 9781009002103 (ebook)
Subjects: MESH: Antipsychotic Agents – blood | Dose-Response Relationship, Drug | Antipsychotic Agents – therapeutic use | Dose-Response Relationship, Drug | Psychotic Disorders – drug therapy | Schizophrenia – drug therapy | BISAC: MEDICAL / Mental Health | MEDICAL / Mental Health
Classification: LCC RM333.5 (print) | LCC RM333.5 (ebook) | NLM QV 77.9 | DDC 615.7/882–dc23
LC record available at https://lccn.loc.gov/2021012648
LC ebook record available at https://lccn.loc.gov/2021012649

ISBN 978-1-009-00989-8 Paperback

....

Jonathan M. Meyer, MD is Clinical Professor of Psychiatry at the University of California, San Diego, and a psychopharmacology consultant to the California Department of State Hospitals. Over the past 36 months, Dr. Meyer reports having served as a consultant to Acadia Pharmaceuticals, Alkermes, Allergan, Intra-Cellular Therapies, and Neurocrine; he has served on the speakers bureaus for Acadia Pharmaceuticals, AbbVie, Alkermes, Intra-Cellular Therapies, Neurocrine, Noven Pharmaceuticals, Inc., Otsuka America Inc., Sunovion Pharmaceuticals, and Teva Pharmaceutical Industries.

Stephen M. Stahl, MD, Ph.D., D.Sc. (Hon.) is Clinical Professor of Psychiatry and Neuroscience at the University of California, Riverside; Adjunct Professor of Psychiatry at the University of California, San Diego; Honorary Visiting Senior Fellow in Psychiatry at the University of Cambridge, UK; and Director of Psychopharmacology and Senior Academic Advisor to the California Department of State Hospitals. Over the past 36 months, Dr. Stahl has served as a consultant to AbbVie, Acadia, Adamas, Alkermes, Allergan, Arbor Pharmaceuticals, AstraZeneca, Avanir, Axovant, Axsome, Biogen, Biomarin, Biopharma, Celgene, ClearView, Concert, DepoMed, Eisai Pharmaceuticals, EMD Serono, EnVivo, Ferring, Forest, Forum, Genomind, Impel, Innovative Science Solutions, Intra-Cellular Therapies, Ironshore Pharmaceuticals, Janssen, Jazz, Karuna, Lilly, Lundbeck, Merck, Neos, NeuroPharma, Novartis, Noveida, Otsuka, Perrigo, Pfizer, Pierre Fabre, Relmada, Reviva, Sage Therapeutics, Servier, Shire, Sprout, Sunovion, Takeda, Taliaz, Teva, Tonix, Tris Pharma, Trius, Vanda, Vertex, and Viforpharma; he has been a board member of RCT Logic and Genomind; he has served on speakers bureaus for Acadia, Forum, Genentech, Janssen, Lundbeck, Merck, Otsuka, Servier, Sunovion, Takeda, and Teva, and he has received research and/or grant support from Acadia, Alkermes, AssureX, Astra Zeneca, Arbor Pharmaceuticals, Avanir, Axovant, Biogen, Braeburn Pharmaceuticals, BristolMyer Squibb, Celgene, CeNeRx, Cephalon, Dey, Eli Lilly, EnVivo, Forest, Forum, GenOmind, Glaxo Smith Kline, Intra-Cellular Therapies, ISSWSH, Janssen, JayMac, Jazz, Lundbeck, Merck, Neurocrine, Neuronetics, Novartis, Otsuka, Pfizer, Reviva, Roche, Servier, Shire, Sprout, Sunovion, Takeda, Teva, TMS NeuroHealth Centers, Tonix, and Vanda.

Contents

Foreword

In 1993, John Davis, Phil Janicak, and I co-edited a book titled *Clinical Use of Neuroleptic Plasma Levels* [1]. The publication pre-dated the introduction of most of the antipsychotics that are currently in clinical use. Among the guiding principles was the conviction that the available antipsychotics had a relatively narrow therapeutic index and that plasma concentrations could be useful for making everyday clinical decisions. The most important concern at that time was focused on extrapyramidal side effects (EPS) and the challenge was to find a "therapeutic window" that was associated with clinical effectiveness and minimal discomfort. The introduction of another generation of antipsychotics – led by risperidone, olanzapine, and quetiapine – led many prescribers to believe that these medications were better tolerated and that the search for a therapeutic window was unnecessary. Unfortunately, this belief was naïve and research in the clinical use of antipsychotic plasma levels decreased substantially.

Experience with the newer drugs demonstrated that, although many patients appeared comfortable on higher doses of medications such as olanzapine, all of these medications had dose-related side effects, including metabolic effects for some and EPS for others. In other words, the use of plasma concentrations or therapeutic drug monitoring (TDM) for making clinical decisions has great promise and this volume by Jonathan Meyer in Stephen Stahl's Handbook series is very welcome. An important strength of their approach is that it provides a thoughtful framework for interpreting plasma level information under different circumstances, and for differentiating nonadherence from kinetic issues when lower-than-expected levels are encountered. In most cases, patients will benefit when they are managed with drug doses within the recommended range, so there is not always a need to search for a plasma level window. On the other hand, TDM can be helpful for providing information when there are important clinical questions, as defined in a recent expert consensus [2]. The most obvious use is when clinicians are monitoring medication adherence on an ongoing basis, or in order to determine why an individual fails to respond to what appears to be an adequate drug dose. TDM may also be helpful when patients are being treated with medications with a high side burden at doses that are clinically effective. This is commonly the case with clozapine where there is evidence for a threshold below which patients are unlikely to respond [3]. For higher doses, this Handbook also introduces the concept of the point of futility, or a level above which there is a very low likelihood that patients will show additional improvement. Finally, TDM may also have a valuable role during long-term treatment when patients have minimal or few active symptoms and the goal is to prevent a psychotic relapse. Under these circumstances, symptoms cannot guide an assessment as to whether or not a patient is on an adequate amount of medication.

This volume addresses each of these clinical situations and others. It is also important to note that these situations are common and following the guidance provided by this volume has the potential for enhancing clinical care.

Stephen R. Marder, MD

Professor of Psychiatry and Director of the Section on Psychosis

UCLA Semel Institute for Neuroscience and Human Behavior

Director – VISN 22 Mental Illness Research, Education Clinical Center (MIRECC) for the Department of Veterans Affairs

References

1. **Marder, S. R., Davis, J. M., and Janicak, P. G., eds. (1993).** *Clinical Use of Neuroleptic Plasma Levels.* Washington, DC: American Psychiatric Press Inc.
2. **Schoretsanitis, G., Kane, J. M., Correll, C. U., *et al.* (2020).** Blood levels to optimize antipsychotic treatment in clinical practice: A joint consensus statement of the American Society of Clinical Psychopharmacology (ASCP) and the Therapeutic Drug Monitoring (TDM) Task Force of the Arbeitsgemeinschaft für Neuropsychopharmakologie und Pharmakopsychiatrie (AGNP). *J Clin Psychiatry*, 81, https://doi.org/10.4088/JCP.4019cs13169.
3. **Hiemke, C., Bergemann, N., Clement, H. W., *et al.* (2018).** Consensus guidelines for therapeutic drug monitoring in neuropsychopharmacology: Update 2017. *Pharmacopsychiatry*, 51, 9–62.

Preface: How to Use This Handbook and Useful Tables for Handy Reference

To best apply the information in this handbook, chapters 1-5 are worth reading initially, as they lay out some clinically important ideas such as coefficient of variation, time to steady state, the therapeutic threshold, and point of futility. One need not be an expert in antipsychotic kinetics to treat schizophrenia patients, but questions regarding oral medication adherence, when to obtain plasma levels, how to differentiate ultrarapid metabolizers from nonadherent patients, and the point at which further titration is unlikely to yield significant improvement are basic clinical decisions made every day. The sections covering specific antipsychotics builds on concepts explained in chapters 1–5 of the handbook. Reading the first five chapters will hopefully be enlightening, and provide the reader with the necessary tools to use plasma antipsychotic levels effectively. Those five chapters cover the following topics:

1. Sampling times for oral and long-acting injectable agents
2. The therapeutic threshold and the point of futility
3. Level interpretation including laboratory reporting issues, responding to high plasma levels, and special situations (hepatic dysfunction, renal dysfunction and hemodialysis, bariatric surgery)
4. Tracking oral antipsychotic adherence; differentiating treatment resistance from kinetic failure due to genetic variation or concurrent medications / environmental exposures, or adherence failure; use of pharmacogenomics
5. What is an adequate antipsychotic trial? Using plasma levels to optimize psychiatric response and tolerability (and when to use high-dose antipsychotics)

For easy reference, the following tables discussed elsewhere in this handbook are presented here:

Table P1 – Oral dose equivalency of commonly used first- and second-generation antipsychotics in acute schizophrenia

Table P2 – Antipsychotic nmol/l to ng/ml unit conversion

Table P3 – Mean half-life of commonly used oral antipsychotics and important metabolites

Table P4 – Mean half-life and kinetic properties of commonly used long-acting injectable antipsychotics

For easy access, the Appendix contains a single table that summarizes the therapeutic threshold, point of futility, and oral antipsychotic concentration–dose relationships.

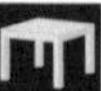

Table P1 Oral dose equivalency of commonly used first- and second-generation antipsychotics in acute schizophrenia [1, 2]

Medication	Oral equivalent (mg)
First generation	
Haloperidol	1.00
Fluphenazine	1.25
Trifluoperazine	2.50
Perphenazine	3.75
Thiothixene	3.75
Zuclopenthixol	3.75
Loxapine	12.5
Chlorpromazine	37.5
Second generation	
Amisulpride	82.4
Aripiprazole	1.82
Brexpiprazole	0.53
Cariprazine	1.21
Lurasidone	23.2
Risperidone	1.00
Olanzapine	2.15
Ziprasidone	29.5

Comments

[a] Clozapine dose equivalencies are not provided as the primary use is for treatment-resistant schizophrenia and there are no equivalent medications [3].

[b] Quetiapine dose equivalents are not provided as both naturalistic and clinical trials data raise concerns about efficacy as monotherapy for schizophrenia [4, 5]. When used at doses > 400 mg/d for schizophrenia treatment, quetiapine also has substantial metabolic adverse effects [6, 7].

Note: Other antipsychotic dose equivalencies for antipsychotics not listed here can be calculated using a spreadsheet developed by Professor Stefan Leucht and colleagues [2]. The results are reported based on a variety of methods (e.g. minimum effective dose, 95% effective dose, etc.) and the spreadsheet can be downloaded from their website:

www.cfdm.de/media/doc/Antipsychotic%20dose%20conversion%20calculator.xls

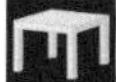

Table P2 Antipsychotic nmol/l to ng/ml unit conversion

Antipsychotic	To obtain plasma levels in ng/ml divide levels in nmol/l by the value below:
Amisulpride	2.71
Aripiprazole	2.23
Asenapine	3.50
Brexpiprazole	2.31
Cariprazine	2.34
Chlorpromazine	3.14
Clozapine	3.06
Flupenthixol	2.30
Fluphenazine	2.29
Haloperidol	2.66
Loxapine	3.05
Lurasidone	2.03
Olanzapine	3.20
Paliperidone	2.34
Perphenazine	2.48
Risperidone	2.44
Thiothixene	2.25
Trifluoperazine	2.45
Zuclopenthixol	2.49

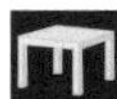

Table P3 Mean half-life of commonly used oral antipsychotics and important metabolites [8–18, 3, 19, 20]

Drug	$T_{1/2}$ (hours)
First-generation antipsychotics	
Chlorpromazine	11.05–15
Fluphenazine	13
Haloperidol	24
Loxapine 7-OH loxapine	4 ??[a]
Molindone	2[b]

Drug	$T_{1/2}$ (hours)
Perphenazine	9–12
Zuclopenthixol	17.6
Newer antipsychotics	
Amisulpride	12
Aripiprazole	75
Asenapine sublingual Asenapine transdermal patch	24 30[c]
Brexpiprazole	91
Cariprazine Desmethylcariprazine (DCAR) Didesmethylcariprazine (DDCAR)	31.6–68.4 29.7–39.5 (DCAR) 314–446 (DDCAR)
Clozapine Norclozapine	9–17 20
Iloperidone	15–22
Lumateperone	18
Lurasidone	28.8–37.4[d]
Olanzapine	30
Paliperidone (9-OH risperidone)[e]	23
Quetiapine Norquetiapine	7 12
Risperidone Paliperidone (9-OH risperidone)[f]	3 21
Sertindole	60–73
Ziprasidone	7

Comment

Half-lives may be markedly prolonged in individuals receiving metabolic inhibitors or who have lower-functioning polymorphisms of cytochrome P450 enzymes, other relevant enzymes, or transporters involved in drug disposition. Conversely, half-lives may be significantly shorter than the mean in individuals exposed to inducers, or who have higher-functioning polymorphisms of cytochrome P450 enzymes, other relevant enzymes, or transporters involved in drug disposition.

[a] Based on studies of inhaled loxapine, the half-life of 7-OH loxapine is likely to be substantially longer [21].

[b] The therapeutic effects persist for 24–36 hours despite the absence of active metabolites [18].

[c] After patch removal.

[d] Repeated dosing in adult schizophrenia patients. Single dose half-life in volunteers is 18 hours [22].

[e] When administered as oral paliperidone.

[f] When derived from orally administered risperidone.

Table P4 Mean half-life and kinetic properties of commonly used long-acting injectable (LAI) antipsychotics [23–26]

Drug	Vehicle	Dosage	T_{max}	$T_{1/2}$ multiple dosing	Able to be loaded
First-generation antipsychotics					
Fluphenazine decanoate	Sesame oil	12.5–75 mg/2 weeks **Max:** 75 mg/week	0.3–1.5 days	14 days	Yes
Haloperidol decanoate	Sesame oil	25–300 mg/4 weeks **Max:** 300 mg/2 weeks	3–9 days	21 days	Yes
Perphenazine decanoate	Sesame oil	27–216 mg/3–4 weeks	7 days	27 days	Yes
Flupenthixol decanoate	Coconut oil	20–40 mg/2–4 weeks **Max:** 100 mg/2 weeks	4–7 days	17 days	Yes
Zuclopenthixol decanoate	Coconut oil	25–100 mg/2–4 weeks **Max:** 400 mg/2 weeks	3–7 days	19 days	Yes
Newer antipsychotics					
Risperidone subcutaneous **(Perseris®)**	Water	90–120 mg/4 weeks	7–8 days	9–11 days	Not needed
Risperidone microspheres **(Risperdal Consta®)**	Water	12.5–50 mg/2 weeks	21 days	See note [a]	**No** (21–28 days oral overlap)
Paliperidone palmitate **(Invega Sustenna®)**	Water	39–234 mg/4 weeks	13 days	25–49 days	Yes
Paliperidone palmitate (3 mo) **(Invega Trinza®)**[b]	Water	273–819 mg/12 weeks	84–95 days (deltoid) 118–139 days (gluteal)	30–33 days	No

Drug	Vehicle	Dosage	T_{max}	$T_{1/2}$ multiple dosing	Able to be loaded
Olanzapine pamoate **(Zyprexa Relprevv®)**	Water	150–300 mg/2 weeks 300–405 mg/4 weeks	7 days	30 days	Yes
Aripiprazole monohydrate **(Abilify Maintena®)**	Water	300–400 mg/4 weeks	6.5–7.1 days	29.9–46.5 days	**No** (14 days oral overlap)
Aripiprazole lauroxil **(Aristada®)**[c]	Water	441 mg, 662 mg, 882 mg/4 wks 882 mg/6 weeks 1064 mg/8 weeks	41 days (single dose) [27] 24.4–35.2 days (repeated dosing) [28]	53.9–57.2 days	**No** (Start with AL_{NC} 675 mg IM + 30 mg oral ***OR*** 21 days oral overlap)
Aripiprazole lauroxil nanocrystal **(Aristada Initio®)**[d]	Water	675 mg once	27 days (range: 16 to 35 days)	15–18 days (single dose)	–

[a] Steady state plasma levels after 5 biweekly injections are maintained for 4–5 weeks, but decrease rapidly at that point with a mean half-life of 4–6 days [29].

[b] Only for those on paliperidone palmitate monthly for 4 months. Cannot be converted from oral medication.

[c] Requires 21 days oral overlap unless starting with aripiprazole lauroxil nanocrystal (AL_{NC}) + a single 30 mg oral dose.

[d] Aripiprazole lauroxil nanocrystal (AL_{NC}) is only used for initiation of treatment with aripiprazole lauroxil, or for resumption of treatment. It is always administered together with the clinician-determined dose of aripiprazole lauroxil, although the latter can be given up to 10 days after the aripiprazole lauroxil nanocrystal (AL_{NC}) injection.

For further reading about use of LAI antipsychotics, please see the comprehensive edited book ***Antipsychotic Long-Acting Injections***, now in its 2nd edition [30].

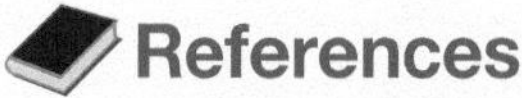

References

1. **Leucht, S., Samara, M., Heres, S., *et al.* (2016).** Dose equivalents for antipsychotic drugs: The DDD method. *Schizophr Bull*, 42 Suppl 1, S90–94.
2. **Leucht, S., Crippa, A., Siafis, S., *et al.* (2020).** Dose-response meta-analysis of antipsychotic drugs for acute schizophrenia. *Am J Psychiatry*, 177, 342–353.
3. **Meyer, J. M. and Stahl, S. M. (2019).** *The Clozapine Handbook*. Cambridge: Cambridge University Press.
4. **Asmal, L., Flegar, S. J., Wang, J., *et al.* (2013).** Quetiapine versus other atypical antipsychotics for schizophrenia. *Cochrane Database Syst Rev*, CD006625.
5. **Vanasse, A., Blais, L., Courteau, J., *et al.* (2016).** Comparative effectiveness and safety of antipsychotic drugs in schizophrenia treatment: A real-world observational study. *Acta Psychiatr Scand*, 134, 374–384.
6. **Meyer, J. M., Davis, V. G., Goff, D. C., *et al.* (2008).** Change in metabolic syndrome parameters with antipsychotic treatment in the CATIE Schizophrenia Trial: Prospective data from phase 1. *Schizophr Res*, 101, 273–286.
7. **Meyer, J. M. (2010).** Antipsychotics and metabolics in the post-CATIE era. *Curr Top Behav Neurosci*, 4, 23–42.
8. **Simpson, G. M., Cooper, T. B., Lee, J. H., *et al.* (1978).** Clinical and plasma level characteristics of intramuscular and oral loxapine. *Psychopharmacology (Berl)*, 56, 225–232.
9. **Zetin, M., Cramer, M., Garber, D., *et al.* (1985).** Bioavailability of oral and intramuscular molindone hydrochloride in schizophrenic patients. *Clin Ther*, 7, 169–175.
10. **Midha, K. K., Hawes, E. M., Hubbard, J. W., *et al.* (1988).** Variation in the single dose pharmacokinetics of fluphenazine in psychiatric patients. *Psychopharmacology (Berl)*, 96, 206–211.
11. **Dahl, M. L., Ekqvist, B., Widén, J., *et al.* (1991).** Disposition of the neuroleptic zuclopenthixol cosegregates with the polymorphic hydroxylation of debrisoquine in humans. *Acta Psychiatr Scand*, 84, 99–102.
12. **Midha, K. K., Hubbard, J. W., McKay, G., *et al.* (1993).** The role of metabolites in a bioequivalence study I: Loxapine, 7-hydroxyloxapine and 8-hydroxyloxapine. *Int J Clin Pharmacol Ther Toxicol*, 31, 177–183.
13. **Yeung, P. K., Hubbard, J. W., Korchinski, E. D., *et al.* (1993).** Pharmacokinetics of chlorpromazine and key metabolites. *Eur J Clin Pharmacol*, 45, 563–569.
14. **Wong, S. L. and Granneman, G. R. (1998).** Modeling of sertindole pharmacokinetic disposition in healthy volunteers in short term dose-escalation studies. *J Pharm Sci*, 87, 1629–1631.
15. **Kudo, S. and Ishizaki, T. (1999).** Pharmacokinetics of haloperidol: An update. *Clin Pharmacokinet*, 37, 435–456.
16. **Mauri, M. C., Volonteri, L. S., Colasanti, A., *et al.* (2007).** Clinical pharmacokinetics of atypical antipsychotics: A critical review of the relationship between plasma concentrations and clinical response. *Clin Pharmacokinet*, 46, 359–388.
17. **Meyer, J. M. (2018).** Pharmacotherapy of psychosis and mania. In L. L. Brunton, R. Hilal-Dandan, and B. C. Knollmann, eds., *Goodman & Gilman's The Pharmacological Basis of Therapeutics*, 13th edn. Chicago, IL: McGraw-Hill, pp. 279–302.
18. **Yu, C. and Gopalakrishnan, G. (2018).** In vitro pharmacological characterization of SPN-810 M (molindone). *J Exp Pharmacol*, 10, 65–73.
19. **Meyer, J. M. (2020).** Lumateperone for schizophrenia. *Curr Psychiatr*, 19, 33–39.
20. **Schoretsanitis, G., Kane, J. M., Correll, C. U., *et al.* (2020).** Blood levels to optimize antipsychotic treatment in clinical practice: A joint consensus statement of the American Society of Clinical Psychopharmacology (ASCP) and the Therapeutic Drug Monitoring (TDM) Task Force of

the Arbeitsgemeinschaft für Neuropsychopharmakologie und Pharmakopsychiatrie (AGNP). *J Clin Psychiatry*, 81, https://doi.org/10.4088/JCP.4019cs13169.

21. **Spyker, D. A., Voloshko, P., Heyman, E. R., *et al.* (2014).** Loxapine delivered as a thermally generated aerosol does not prolong QTc in a thorough QT/QTc study in healthy subjects. *J Clin Pharmacol*, 54, 665–674.
22. **Meyer, J. M., Loebel, A. D., and Schweizer, E. (2009).** Lurasidone: A new drug in development for schizophrenia. *Expert Opin Investig Drugs*, 18, 1715–1726.
23. **Larsen, N. E. and Hansen, L. B. (1989).** Prediction of the optimal perphenazine decanoate dose based on blood samples drawn within the first three weeks. *Ther Drug Monit*, 11, 642–646.
24. **Altamura, A. C., Sassella, F., Santini, A., *et al.* (2003).** Intramuscular preparations of antipsychotics: Uses and relevance in clinical practice. *Drugs*, 63, 493–512.
25. **Spanarello, S. and La Ferla, T. (2014).** The pharmacokinetics of long-acting antipsychotic medications. *Curr Clin Pharamacol*, 9, 310–317.
26. **Meyer, J. M. (2020).** Monitoring and improving antipsychotic adherence in outpatient forensic diversion programs. *CNS Spectr*, 25, 136–144.
27. **Hard, M. L., Mills, R. J., Sadler, B. M., *et al.* (2017).** Aripiprazole lauroxil: Pharmacokinetic profile of this long-acting injectable antipsychotic in persons with schizophrenia. *J Clin Psychopharmacol*, 37, 289–295.
28. **Hard, M. L., Mills, R. J., Sadler, B. M., *et al.* (2017).** Pharmacokinetic profile of a 2-month dose regimen of aripiprazole lauroxil: A phase I study and a population pharmacokinetic model. *CNS Drugs*, 31, 617–624.
29. **Gefvert, O., Eriksson, B., Persson, P., *et al.* (2005).** Pharmacokinetics and D2 receptor occupancy of long-acting injectable risperidone (Risperdal Consta) in patients with schizophrenia. *Int J Neuropsychopharmacol*, 8, 27–36.
30. **Haddad, P., Lambert, T., and Lauriello, J., eds. (2016).** *Antipsychotic Long-Acting Injections*, 2nd edn. New York: Oxford University Press.

Introduction

Antipsychotics have numerous evidence-based uses in the twenty-first century, including schizophrenia spectrum and other psychotic disorders, bipolar disorder, unipolar major depression, behavioral disturbances of autism, tic disorders, and obsessive compulsive disorder [1]. The application of antipsychotic therapy in many of these conditions is adjunctive, and it may be withdrawn during less active phases of the illness. For patients with schizophrenia spectrum disorders, antipsychotics are the foundation of treatment without which the patient is at risk for relapse, and the attendant psychiatric, social, and legal consequences [2, 3]. Given the level of disability often encountered with the onset of illness, the care and management of individuals with schizophrenia exerts a significant economic toll on society [4–6]; moreover, this burden accrues most directly to families and direct caregivers in the form of financial loss compounded by stress and decreased quality of life [7, 8]. Of particular concern are the disproportionate direct and indirect costs associated with treatment-resistant schizophrenia (TRS) [4] (see Figure 0.1).

That the care costs for TRS are 3–11 times higher than for other schizophrenia patients is not surprising, but the disturbing clinical reality is that, aside from treatment resistance, there are many reasons patients fail to respond adequately to an antipsychotic, with nonadherence, underdosing, and kinetic issues playing significant roles [9]. To emphasize this point, a study of 99 schizophrenia patients deemed treatment resistant in the South London and Maudsley National Health Service (NHS) foundation clinic found that 35% had subtherapeutic plasma antipsychotic levels [10]. Real-world data such as these encapsulate the basic arguments for monitoring of antipsychotic plasma levels: antipsychotic nonadherence is common in schizophrenia patients [11]; clinicians are poor estimators of medication nonadherence [12–14]; kinetic variations or underdosing contribute to inadequate response [10]; plasma level, and not prescribed dose, is the best proxy for central nervous system antipsychotic effects [15, 16].

Figure 0.1 Healthcare costs per patient-year for schizophrenia patients from studies published 1996–2012 worldwide, for US schizophrenia patients, and for treatment-resistant schizophrenia patients (2012 USD)[4]

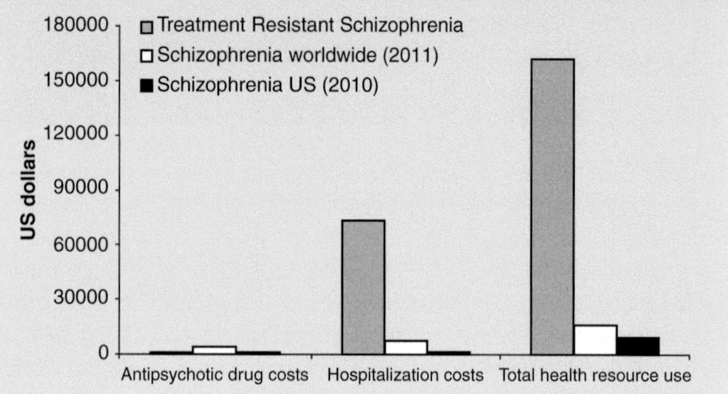

(Adapted from: J. L. Kennedy, C. A. Altar, D. L. Taylor, *et al*. [2014]. The social and economic burden of treatment-resistant schizophrenia: A systematic literature review. *Int Clin Psychopharmacol*, 29, 63–76.)

Deterrents to Clinical Use of Plasma Level Monitoring

Despite multiple evidence-based reasons for therapeutic drug monitoring (TDM) of antipsychotic treatment (see Box 0.1) [17], a certain degree of nihilism exists among clinicians regarding implementation in routine care. A 2014 UK survey study of 105 London consultant psychiatrists found that most based their choice of optimum antipsychotic dose on past clinical experience with similar patients (80%) and their subjective impression of dose equivalence between antipsychotics (70%) [18]. While the majority routinely used plasma levels for clozapine (82.9%), 32.4% did not agree that TDM would improve clinical outcomes for all antipsychotics [18].

Box 0.1 Reasons to Consider Antipsychotic Plasma Level Monitoring [17]

1. Uncertain adherence to antipsychotics
2. No clinical response within established therapeutic dose ranges
3. Symptom recurrence or relapse during maintenance treatment
4. Adverse drug reactions
5. Combination treatment with medication(s) with inducing or inhibiting properties

6. Genetic peculiarities for the pathways involved in the metabolism of antipsychotics (the prevalence of specific genetic variants affecting drug metabolism may vary highly in different ethnic groups, e.g., Caucasian versus Asian, middle Eastern versus the rest of the world)
7. Patients with abnormally high or low body weight or body mass index
8. Pregnant or lactating patients
9. Child or adolescent patients
10. Elderly patients
11. Patients with intellectual disabilities
12. Forensic patients or court-mandated individuals, as the treatment of this patient subgroup presents special challenges that underscore the need for tracking and mitigating nonadherence
13. Patients with pharmacokinetically relevant comorbidities, such as hepatic or renal dysfunction and severe cardiovascular disease (affecting hepatic and renal blood flow)
14. Patients with acute or chronic inflammatory conditions and infections
15. Postoperative care for patients undergoing restrictive gastrointestinal resection or bariatric surgery
16. Switching between the original preparation and generic forms of antipsychotics due to potential therapeutic equivalence differences, as well as related adherence aspects
17. Switching between oral antipsychotics and LAIs
18. Pharmacovigilance programs
19. Research

As alluded to above, and to be discussed extensively in Chapter 4, antipsychotic nonadherence has been recognized as inherent to schizophrenia for over 50 years [19, 20], yet clinicians have difficulty estimating the extent of this problem. The magnitude of nonadherence with oral antipsychotic therapy is illustrated in Figure 0.2. These data are derived from a study of 52 outpatients with a schizophrenia spectrum disorder, stabilized on the current oral antipsychotic dose for 3 or more months, who were enrolled in an adherence study [21]. Although these subjects knew they were being scrutinized as part of a study, only 48% managed to take 80% or more of their oral doses over 4 weeks, contrary to what one might assume for a stable group of schizophrenia outpatients. The data from the South London and Maudsley NHS foundation sample of 99 supposedly treatment-resistant patients being proposed for clozapine treatment represents one of many publications documenting the disconnect between clinician assessment of oral antipsychotic adherence and verified adherence using pill counts, plasma levels, or electronic devices such as the Medication Event

Monitoring System (MEMS): a medication bottle cap with a microprocessor that records each bottle opening [22].

Figure 0.2 Rates of adherence in stable schizophrenia patients monitored over four weeks [21]

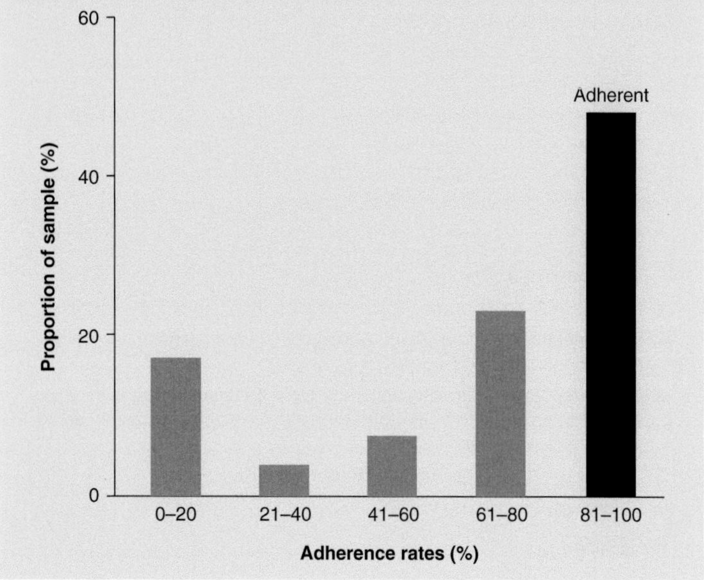

(Adapted from: G. Remington, C. Teo, S. Mann, *et al.* [2013]. Examining levels of antipsychotic adherence to better understand nonadherence. *J Clin Psychopharmacol*, 33, 261–263.)

Another impediment to routine use of antipsychotic TDM has been the paucity of information succinctly summarizing dose and plasma level correlations for most antipsychotics, aside from clozapine [23]. The motivated clinician who orders a plasma haloperidol level for a patient on 10 mg at bedtime (QHS) is left to scour the literature for a method of interpreting the result. (Of note, the expected 12h trough plasma level for that haloperidol dose is 7.78 ng/ml [24, 25].) Until recently, principles for interpreting levels were not covered extensively in the literature; moreover, clinicians were often provided insufficient guidance on how to react when levels were higher or lower than expected, or the expected range of plasma level variation between sample determinations in adherent patients [26].

The published literature can also be confusing with respect to the use of antipsychotic TDM to guide treatment. Review papers often lament the limited correlation between antipsychotic plasma level and schizophrenia treatment response [27], but fail to note that many antipsychotics exhibit response thresholds based on fixed dose studies, imaging data, or both [26, 17]. Clozapine is a classic example where a consensus plasma level of 350 ng/ml has been suggested as a response threshold (also known as a lower limit of the therapeutic reference range), thereby guiding clinicians to pursue higher doses and levels in nonresponders with clozapine levels below that value [28]. While the clozapine response threshold is widely cited [26, 17], the comparable information for other antipsychotics is not given the emphasis it deserves, despite the existence of thoughtful papers aimed at elucidating TDM principles in neuropsychiatry. A leading organization spearheading these efforts has been the German Arbeitsgemeinschaft für Neuropsychopharmakologie und Pharmakopsychiatrie (AGNP), whose interdisciplinary TDM group published three exhaustive reviews in 2004, 2011, and 2018 summarizing information across various classes of psychiatric medications [29, 30, 26]. Although these reviews are scholarly and were published in an English-language journal (*Pharmacopsychiatry*), the journal impact factor was not in the top 200 as of 2018, and their heroic efforts may have not been viewed by a wider audience. The growing interest in this topic, and the advent of newer technology (see Section C below), spurred the 2020 publication of a joint consensus statement by the American Society of Clinical Psychopharmacology (ASCP) and AGNP, covering the latest thinking on antipsychotic blood monitoring [17]. That this review was published in the *Journal of Clinical Psychiatry* (top-50 impact factor) hopefully represents a turning point in the clinical perception of antipsychotic TDM from a niche subject applicable only to clozapine therapy to an accepted and necessary tool in the management of schizophrenia patients.

As acknowledged by the AGNP TDM group, defining an upper limit of the therapeutic reference range is relatively easy for drugs with narrow therapeutic indices (e.g. carbamazepine, lithium, valproate), but becomes problematic for less toxic agents [26]. When adverse effects become limiting, one can utilize mathematical models to find an optimal cutpoint which maximizes the trade-off between efficacy and tolerability. Such receiver operating characteristic (ROC) curves require sufficient systematically collected plasma level data at higher levels, data that are often lacking for many antipsychotics [31]. For the AGNP guidelines, the upper limits were mostly generated by calculating expected antipsychotic-level concentrations under approved maximal doses, but the clinical reality is that many antipsychotics have sufficient evidence for use at doses beyond the initial approval range [32, 33]. Fully one-third of schizophrenia patients respond inadequately to non-clozapine antipsychotics, yet the refusal of such individuals to start clozapine forces the clinician to consider ongoing titration of existing agents beyond their approved maximal dosages where the safety of this approach is supported by the literature, and when the patient is not exhibiting dose-limiting adverse effects. Such trials are often terminated due to tolerability, but there is a distinct subgroup of patients who tolerate higher antipsychotic doses and plasma levels without developing neurological adverse effects (e.g. parkinsonism, akathisia, dystonia) [34]. However, there is a point beyond which expectancy of response is virtually nil based on the plasma antipsychotic level, yet there is limited guidance on this point of clinical futility [35]. In certain countries, one is limited to the maximum licensed dose, so the AGNP upper limits can be implemented; however, outside of these jurisdictions, clinicians are often directed to local laboratory-reported ranges, although gross inconsistencies exist between laboratories in the methods for establishing maxima, and in the suggested maximal actual levels themselves for antipsychotics [36]. (The other major source of consternation related to laboratories, slow turnaround for plasma level results, is discussed in Section C below.)

In spite of these numerous frustrations, there is evidence that clinicians do perceive a possible benefit of antipsychotic TDM, providing hope that improved education about its use and increased availability of plasma antipsychotic level testing might meet a receptive audience. Although the survey study of 105 London consultants documented that 32.4% did not believe TDM would improve care, previous use of plasma levels during clozapine management not only predicted future TDM use ($p = 0.019$), the respondents agreed that TDM could help to minimize risk of dose-related adverse effects (77.1%), and 84.8% stated that they would use antipsychotic TDM if it were widely available [18]. A larger UK follow-up study ($n = 181$) was also optimistic regarding implementation of antipsychotic TDM: 83% of the 181 clinicians agreed that "if TDM for antipsychotics were readily available, I would use it," but prospects of future use decreased with potential barriers, negative attitudes, and negative expectations [37].

B The Economic Argument

Schizophrenia point prevalence remains relatively constant, with the global estimate of 0.28% remaining unchanged from 1990 to 2016; however, the number of individuals suffering from schizophrenia rose nearly 60% in that time due to population increases [38, 6]. While many sources traditionally cite schizophrenia prevalence rates of 1%, a 2018 analysis of 101 studies examined the variation in point prevalence, 12-month, and lifetime estimates of psychotic disorders, and the methodological issues resulting in such variability [39]. Among studies specifically examining schizophrenia prevalence (as opposed to schizophrenia and other psychotic disorders, or 'nonaffective psychosis'), the median point, 12-month, and lifetime prevalence values were 0.35%, 0.37%, and 0.64%, respectively. Studies conducted in the general population provided higher rates than those carried out in patients receiving general health or social services ($p = 0.006$); prevalence rates were also higher for broadly worded diagnostic categories such as probable psychotic disorder ($p = 0.022$) and non-affective psychosis ($p = 0.009$). Not surprisingly, higher study quality was associated with a lower estimated prevalence of psychotic disorders ($p < 0.001$) [39].

There are now close to 21 million persons worldwide with schizophrenia, most of whom require extensive supportive resources, as only 13.5% meet criteria for functional recovery [6]. Using the outcome of years lived with disability, schizophrenia has consistently ranked fifteenth overall among 328 conditions (i.e. diseases or injuries) in the 1990, 2006, and 2016 World Health Organization (WHO) Global Burden of Disease studies, yet it carried the highest disability weight among all disorders and contributed 13.4 million years of life lost due to disability. This represented 1.7% of the total in the 2016 WHO study, a value six-fold greater than the prevalence of schizophrenia [6], and its economic burden was estimated to range from 0.02% to 1.65% of the gross domestic product [40]. For the United States (US) alone, the combination of direct healthcare costs, direct non-healthcare costs (law enforcement, homeless shelters, healthcare training, and research), and indirect costs (productivity loss from disability, premature mortality, caregiving) was estimated at $155.7 billion for 2013 [5]. The largest components were excess costs associated with unemployment (38%), productivity loss due to caregiving (34%), and direct healthcare costs (24%).

It is with this vast economic toll in mind that one can begin to appreciate the value of antipsychotic TDM. If one assumes the US 12-month prevalence estimate is comparable to the higher value cited above (0.37%), there are at least 1 million persons with schizophrenia in the US. A model generated in 2015 estimated that improved antipsychotic adherence could yield $1580 in annual savings *per patient* to state programs related to reductions in direct healthcare and criminal justice costs (in 2013 dollars) [41]. Nationally, this would amount to over $1.5B. A 2018 review concluded: "Public payers that operate under strict annual budget constraints and have discretion over which services to cover, such as Medicaid programs and the Veterans Health Administration, may be particularly interested in incorporating plasma level measurement into the routine care of people who are either not responding to standard antipsychotic treatment or are exhibiting intolerable side effects" [42].

Antipsychotic plasma level assay costs vary widely. In the UK, a clozapine assay was £25 per sample in February 2020 at King's College Hospital KingsPath Clinical Diagnostic Pathology Service (approximately $33), while this might be $100 (or more) within the US. Even if an assay costs $150 per determination in the US, one could order 3 per year and still derive a net benefit of at least $1000 per patient annually, or $1B annually for the US as a whole. As emerging technologies reduce the assay cost, these savings will increase over time. Thus, any arguments that TDM for antipsychotics are overly expensive are not only short sighted, but wrong by any economic analysis of the value to a payer who must absorb expensive direct care costs, particularly those involving inpatient psychiatric services.

Emergence of Point-of-Care Testing

Among the greatest impediments to antipsychotic plasma level determination is the paucity of laboratories running these assays, and the need to ship specimens from the place of phlebotomy to the reference laboratory. When the distance is short to the reference lab, and the laboratory volume great, assay results might be available within 2 days of sample receipt (e.g. KingsPath lab), but in common practice the entire process may take much longer due to several stumbling blocks [43]. The foremost of these is the need to send a patient for phlebotomy when such services are not available in the mental health clinic setting. If and when the patient goes to the lab, and whether the timing of the draw can yield an interpretable result are enormous problems that delay obtaining not only a result, but a result that can actually be used. When a supposed 12h trough is obtained 19 hours after the evening dose, the clinician is left to their own devices to decide what this result means. Added to the clinician's frustration is shipping time – as the local lab may batch samples sent to the outside reference lab – and the time to run the assay and report a result back to the referring source. The possibility of making urgent decisions using antipsychotic levels in a manner performed routinely with lithium or valproate becomes practically impossible. A clinician who strongly suspects nonadherence with oral antipsychotic therapy in a symptomatic outpatient may possibly obtain a level for future use, but in the short term will be forced to employ the same options as clinicians in the 1950s: make an educated guess whether nonadherence is at play for the current episode, and plan a course of action [43].

There are, however, emerging solutions in the form of point-of-care (POC) devices employing novel technology, with the goal of improving precision application of medical information with real-time results. One such device was approved in the US on November 5, 2018 (US Food and Drug Administration [FDA] 510(k)

Number K181288) for total white blood cell and absolute neutrophil counts, and includes a system created by the manufacturer to facilitate use in clozapine-treated patients (www.athelas.com). Using a finger stick rated less painful than traditional venipuncture, this device can be operated by any trained clinical personnel and provides results within 6 minutes [28, 44]. In March 2018, the first POC device was approved in the European Union (EU) for determination of an antipsychotic plasma level (www.saladax.com). The results of the test can be available as early as 1 hour from blood draw in certain settings, and within 48 hours in many others. This approval represented the culmination of many years of research into POC devices for antipsychotic TDM, starting initially with scientists at Janssen Pharmaceutica [43], and later continued by Saladax Biomedical, Inc. who completed final testing. The initial EU approval covered tests for total risperidone and paliperidone (9-OH risperidone) levels, but the platform will eventually include clozapine, olanzapine, and aripiprazole, and possibly others. As of this writing (April 2021), the company is working with the US FDA toward initial approval for total clozapine levels, with a plan to expand the suite of testing to the analytes noted above. That two POC technologies with direct application to psychiatry have been pursued in such a short time speaks not only to innovations that may significantly transform healthcare, but also to the specific technology need within the psychiatric space to improve care of the severely mentally ill. Schizophrenia management presents unique challenges, and any devices that remove barriers to treatment or improve a clinician's ability to effectively monitor and tailor antipsychotic therapy benefit all stakeholders involved in helping this patient population attain their functional goals. Precision dosing is the future of medical practice – the use of plasma levels is an important tool to add precision in the use of antipsychotic therapy [45, 46].

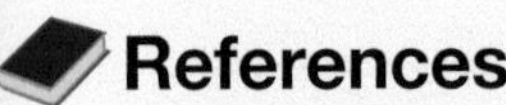

References

1. **Meyer, J. M. (2018).** Pharmacotherapy of psychosis and mania. In L. L. Brunton, R. Hilal-Dandan, and B. C. Knollmann, eds., *Goodman & Gilman's The Pharmacological Basis of Therapeutics*, 13th edn. Chicago, IL: McGraw-Hill, pp. 279–302.
2. **Rezansoff, S. N., Moniruzzaman, A., Fazel, S., *et al.* (2017).** Adherence to antipsychotic medication and criminal recidivism in a Canadian provincial offender population. *Schizophr Bull*, 43, 1002–1010.
3. **Takeuchi, H., Siu, C., Remington, G., *et al.* (2019).** Does relapse contribute to treatment resistance? Antipsychotic response in first- vs. second-episode schizophrenia. *Neuropsychopharmacology*, 44, 1036–1042.
4. **Kennedy, J. L., Altar, C. A., Taylor, D. L., *et al.* (2014).** The social and economic burden of treatment-resistant schizophrenia: A systematic literature review. *Int Clin Psychopharmacol*, 29, 63–76.
5. **Cloutier, M., Aigbogun, M. S., Guerin, A., *et al.* (2016).** The economic burden of schizophrenia in the United States in 2013. *J Clin Psychiatry*, 77, 764–771.
6. **Charlson, F. J., Ferrari, A. J., Santomauro, D. F., *et al.* (2018).** Global epidemiology and burden of schizophrenia: Findings from the Global Burden of Disease Study 2016. *Schizophr Bull*, 44, 1195–1203.
7. **Nuttall, A. K., Thakkar, K. N., Luo, X., *et al.* (2019).** Longitudinal associations of family burden and patient quality of life in the context of first-episode schizophrenia in the RAISE-ETP study. *Psychiatry Res*, 276, 60–68.
8. **Wan, K. F. and Wong, M. M. C. (2019).** Stress and burden faced by family caregivers of people with schizophrenia and early psychosis in Hong Kong. *Intern Med J*, 49 Suppl 1, 9–15.
9. **McCutcheon, R., Beck, K., Bloomfield, M. A., *et al.* (2015).** Treatment resistant or resistant to treatment? Antipsychotic plasma levels in patients with poorly controlled psychotic symptoms. *J Psychopharmacol*, 29, 892–897.
10. **McCutcheon, R., Beck, K., D'Ambrosio, E., *et al.* (2018).** Antipsychotic plasma levels in the assessment of poor treatment response in schizophrenia. *Acta Psychiatr Scand*, 137, 39–46.
11. **Dufort, A. and Zipursky, R. B. (2019).** Understanding and managing treatment adherence in schizophrenia. *Clin Schizophr Relat Psychoses*, https://doi.org/10.3371/CSRP.ADRZ.121218.
12. **Byerly, M. J., Thompson, A., Carmody, T., *et al.* (2007).** Validity of electronically monitored medication adherence and conventional adherence measures in schizophrenia. *Psychiatr Serv*, 58, 844–847.
13. **Brain, C., Sameby, B., Allerby, K., *et al.* (2014).** Twelve months of electronic monitoring (MEMS) in the Swedish COAST-study: A comparison of methods for the measurement of adherence in schizophrenia. *Eur Neuropsychopharmacol*, 24, 215–222.
14. **Lopez, V. L., Shaikh, A., Merson, J., *et al.* (2017).** Accuracy of clinician assessments of medication status in the emergency setting – a comparison of clinician assessment of antipsychotic usage and plasma level determination. *J Clin Psychopharmocol*, 37, 310–314.
15. **Correll, C. U., Jain, R., Meyer, J. M., *et al.* (2019).** Relationship between the timing of relapse and plasma drug levels following discontinuation of cariprazine treatment in patients with schizophrenia: indirect comparison with other second-generation antipsychotics after treatment discontinuation. *Neuropsychiatr Dis Treat*, 15, 2537–2550.
16. **Veselinovic, T., Scharpenberg, M., Heinze, M., *et al.* (2019).** Dopamine D2 receptor occupancy estimated from plasma concentrations of four different antipsychotics and the subjective experience of physical and mental well-being in schizophrenia: Results from the randomized NeSSy Trial. *J Clin Psychopharmacol*, 39, 550–560.

17. **Schoretsanitis, G., Kane, J. M., Correll, C. U., *et al.* (2020).** Blood levels to optimize antipsychotic treatment in clinical practice: A joint consensus statement of the American Society of Clinical Psychopharmacology (ASCP) and the Therapeutic Drug Monitoring (TDM) Task Force of the Arbeitsgemeinschaft für Neuropsychopharmakologie und Pharmakopsychiatrie (AGNP). *J Clin Psychiatry*, 81, https://doi.org/10.4088/JCP.4019cs13169.
18. **Best-Shaw, L., Gudbrandsen, M., Nagar, J., *et al.* (2014).** Psychiatrists' perspectives on antipsychotic dose and the role of plasma concentration therapeutic drug monitoring. *Ther Drug Monit*, 36, 486–493.
19. **Renton, C. A., Affleck, J. W., Carstairs, G. M., *et al.* (1963).** A follow-up of schizophrenic patients in Edinburgh. *Acta Psychiatr Scand*, 39, 548–600.
20. **Willcox, D. R., Gillan, R., and Hare, E. H. (1965).** Do psychiatric out-patients take their drugs? *BMJ*, 2, 790–792.
21. **Remington, G., Teo, C., Mann, S., *et al.* (2013).** Examining levels of antipsychotic adherence to better understand nonadherence. *J Clin Psychopharmacol*, 33, 261–263.
22. **Velligan, D. I., Wang, M., Diamond, P., *et al.* (2007).** Relationships among subjective and objective measures of adherence to oral antipsychotic medications. *Psychiatr Serv*, 58, 1187–1192.
23. **Rostami-Hodjegan, A., Amin, A. M., Spencer, E. P., *et al.* (2004).** Influence of dose, cigarette smoking, age, sex, and metabolic activity on plasma clozapine concentrations: A predictive model and nomograms to aid clozapine dose adjustment and to assess compliance in individual patients. *J Clin Psychopharmacol*, 24, 70–78.
24. **Van Putten, T., Marder, S. R., Wirshing, W. C., *et al.* (1991).** Neuroleptic plasma levels. *Schizophr Bull*, 17, 197–216.
25. **Wei, F. C., Jann, M. W., Lin, H. N., *et al.* (1996).** A practical loading dose method for converting schizophrenic patients from oral to depot haloperidol therapy. *J Clin Psychiatry*, 57, 298–302.
26. **Hiemke, C., Bergemann, N., Clement, H. W., *et al.* (2018).** Consensus guidelines for therapeutic drug monitoring in neuropsychopharmacology: Update 2017. *Pharmacopsychiatry*, 51, 9–62.
27. **Lopez, L. V. and Kane, J. M. (2013).** Plasma levels of second-generation antipsychotics and clinical response in acute psychosis: A review of the literature. *Schizophr Res*, 147, 368–374.
28. **Meyer, J. M. and Stahl, S. M. (2019).** *The Clozapine Handbook*. Cambridge: Cambridge University Press.
29. **Baumann, P., Hiemke, C., Ulrich, S., *et al.* (2004).** The AGNP-TDM expert group consensus guidelines: Therapeutic drug monitoring in psychiatry. *Pharmacopsychiatry*, 37, 243–265.
30. **Hiemke, C., Baumann, P., Bergemann, N., *et al.* (2011).** AGNP consensus guidelines for therapeutic drug monitoring in psychiatry: Update 2011. *Pharmacopsychiatry*, 44, 195–235.
31. **Muller, M. J., Regenbogen, B., Hartter, S., *et al.* (2007).** Therapeutic drug monitoring for optimizing amisulpride therapy in patients with schizophrenia. *J Psychiatr Res*, 41, 673–679.
32. **Marder, S. R. and Meibach, R. C. (1994).** Risperidone in the treatment of schizophrenia. *Am J Psychiatry*, 151, 825–835.
33. **Kelly, D. L., Richardson, C. M., Yang, Y., *et al.* (2006).** Plasma concentrations of high-dose olanzapine in a double-blind crossover study. *Hum Psychopharmacol*, 21, 393–398.
34. **Simpson, G. M. and Kunz-Bartholini, E. (1968).** Relationship of individual tolerance, behavior and phenothiazine produced extrapyramidal system disturbance. *Dis Nerv System*, 29, 269–274.
35. **Meyer, J. M. (2014).** A rational approach to employing high plasma levels of antipsychotics for violence associated with schizophrenia: case vignettes. *CNS Spectr*, 19, 432–438.
36. **Meyer, J. M. (2020).** Monitoring and improving antipsychotic adherence in outpatient forensic diversion programs. *CNS Spectr*, 25, 136–144.
37. **Law, S., Haddad, P. M., Chaudhry, I. B., *et al.* (2015).** Antipsychotic therapeutic drug monitoring: psychiatrists' attitudes and factors predicting likely future use. *Ther Adv Psychopharmacol*, 5, 214–223.

38. **Vos, T., Abajobir, A. A., Abbafati, C., *et al.* (2017).** Global, regional, and national incidence, prevalence, and years lived with disability for 328 diseases and injuries for 195 countries, 1990–2016: A systematic analysis for the Global Burden of Disease Study 2016. *Lancet*, 390, 1211–1259.

39. **Moreno-Kustner, B., Martin, C., and Pastor, L. (2018).** Prevalence of psychotic disorders and its association with methodological issues: A systematic review and meta-analyses. *PLoS One*, 13, e0195687.

40. **Chong, H. Y., Teoh, S. L., Wu, D. B., *et al.* (2016).** Global economic burden of schizophrenia: a systematic review. *Neuropsychiatr Dis Treat*, 12, 357–373.

41. **Predmore, Z., Mattke, S., and Horvitz-Lennon, M. (2015).** Improving antipsychotic adherence among patients with schizophrenia: savings for states. *Psychiatr Serv*, 66, 343–345.

42. **Predmore, Z., Mattke, S., and Horvitz-Lennon, M. (2018).** Potential benefits to patients and payers from increased measurement of antipsychotic plasma levels in the management of schizophrenia. *Psychiatr Serv*, 69, 12–14.

43. **Green, B., Korell, J., Remmerie, B., *et al.* (2017).** Optimizing antipsychotic patient management using population pharmacokinetic models and point-of-care testing. *CPT Pharmacometrics Syst Pharmacol*, 6, 573–575.

44. **Kelly, D., Glassman, M., Mackowick, M., *et al.* (2020).** 09.1. Satisfaction with using a novel fingerstick for absolute neutrophil count (ANC) at the point of treatment in patients treated with clozapine. *Schizophr Bull*, 46, S20–S21.

45. **Maxfield, K. and Zineh, I. (2021).** Precision dosing: a clinical and public health imperative. *JAMA*, doi: 10.1001/jama.2021.1004. Online ahead of print.

46. **Passos, I. C., Ballester, P., Rabelo-da-Ponte, F. D., *et al.* (2021).** Precision psychiatry: the future is now. *Can J Psychiatry*, 24, doi: 10.1177/0706743721998044.

1 Sampling Times for Oral and Long-Acting Injectable Agents

QUICK CHECK

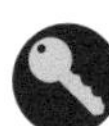

PRINCIPLES

- Although half-lives vary dramatically between antipsychotics, by convention levels for oral antipsychotics are obtained as 12h troughs at steady state (i.e. after five half-lives have passed for the drug of interest and a major active metabolite if also assayed). Future research may define the optimum time since last dose for each antipsychotic that best correlates with clinical outcomes.
- Half-lives also vary dramatically between long-acting injectable (LAI) antipsychotic preparations. The time to steady state may differ from that predicted by the half-life alone if the LAI is loaded at the beginning of treatment.
- By convention, levels for LAI antipsychotics are obtained at steady state 1h–72h prior to the next injection.
- Levels taken before steady state is reached or at nonstandard time intervals for oral antipsychotics (e.g. 16 hours, 24 hours) are difficult to interpret for purposes of examining drug metabolism or managing inadequate response.

INTRODUCTION

The use of antipsychotics to treat schizophrenia is fraught with many layers of complexity as prescribers try to tailor the pharmacodynamic properties of an agent to a specific patient based primarily on subjective response. Variations in drug metabolism related to genetic polymorphisms, or to medication or environmental exposures (e.g. smoking), and variable adherence with oral medications lead to scenarios that confound even seasoned clinicians. Excluding the realization that up to one-third of schizophrenia patients may not respond adequately to non-clozapine antipsychotics, 60 years of antipsychotic research has demonstrated that dose is a poor correlate of response likelihood, whereas plasma drug levels represent the best ***clinically available tool*** that quantifies the relationship between drug exposure and central nervous system (CNS) activity [1]. The classic equation by psychopharmacologist Sheldon Preskorn illustrates the variables involved in clinical drug response (Figure 1.1). The typical method of antipsychotic initiation starts with "usual" doses, followed by subsequent titration until one of two hard endpoints are met: adequate clinical response or intolerable adverse effects. Given the numerous permutations outlined by Preskorn, including the fact that a major limiting factor on absorption is failure to take the prescribed dose, the common clinical approach is inefficient at best, and can lead to erroneous conclusions when patients are outliers on a dose–response curve. In a sample of 99 schizophrenia patients deemed treatment-resistant and in need of clozapine at an academically affiliated London clinic, 35% had plasma antipsychotic levels that were subtherapeutic, and, of these, 34% were undetectable [2]. As will be covered extensively in this handbook, noting that inadequate responders have lower than expected antipsychotic levels is a crucial first step in optimizing treatment, followed by a determination of whether this is due to poor adherence or kinetic factors.

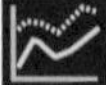

Figure 1.1 Preskorn's equation for clinical drug response [1]

Clinical response	=	Drug affinity for and activity at the site of action	X	Drug concentration at the site of action*	X	Underlying patient biology**

Variables

* Absorption, distribution, metabolism, elimination

** Genetics, age, disease, environment

(Adapted from: S. H. Preskorn [2010]. Outliers on the dose–response curve: How to minimize this problem using therapeutic drug monitoring, an underutilized tool in psychiatry. *J Psychiatr Pract*, 16, 177–182.)

Whether tracked via plasma levels, pill counts, or medication event monitoring system (MEMS) pill bottle caps that electronically record each opening, oral antipsychotic nonadherence in schizophrenia patients is greater than 50% for short periods (e.g. four weeks), and increases over time [3, 4]. Even in the ideal situation where highly motivated individuals are 100% adherent with an oral antipsychotic, the construction of models to correlate dose and systemic levels is exceedingly difficult. One study sought to create a model of olanzapine exposure based on data acquired from paid healthy volunteers [5]. The investigators found that the following variables were needed for the final model to robustly predict olanzapine trough levels: ethnicity, gender, age, height, weight, liver and kidney function, and cytochrome P450 1A2 phenotype (as determined by the ratio of caffeine metabolites to caffeine in saliva). This model did have a correlation coefficient of 0.833 compared with observed values, but serves as a powerful reminder that any assumptions about antipsychotic levels based on dose alone are unlikely to be accurate [5].

The ability to use plasma antipsychotic levels for treatment optimization requires that clinicians understand basic kinetic principles so samples are obtained at times that are interpretable for the purposes of assessing adherence and optimizing antipsychotic response [6, 7]. In addition to differing actions at CNS receptors, antipsychotics (and any active metabolites) also have a range of kinetic properties. The extent of drug exposure over a period of time (e.g. 24 hours) is referred to as the **area under the curve, or AUC,** and this totality of exposure as measured in plasma is highly correlated with that obtained in cerebrospinal fluid [8]. Calculation of AUC as performed in pharmacokinetic (PK) studies requires multiple specimens to be obtained at frequent intervals over the time frame in question (typically 24 hours) (Figure 1.2). While AUC is the best proxy for overall CNS drug exposure, determining this value for an individual patient is impractical. However, not only is determination of a trough antipsychotic plasma level feasible in routine clinical practice, PK models have shown that this single point estimate serves as a useful proxy for AUC, and thereby for the extent of CNS exposure [9].

Given the broad range of antipsychotic half-lives, the optimal approach to this problem would involve determining the ideal time point that a single plasma level should be drawn for a specific antipsychotic at steady state to predict AUC [9]. The US Clinical Antipsychotic Trials of Intervention Effectiveness (CATIE) schizophrenia study provided a large body of real-world plasma level data that investigators have mined to model optimal sampling times. The CATIE schizophrenia trial data set contains many

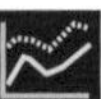

Figure 1.2 Illustrated example of area under the curve

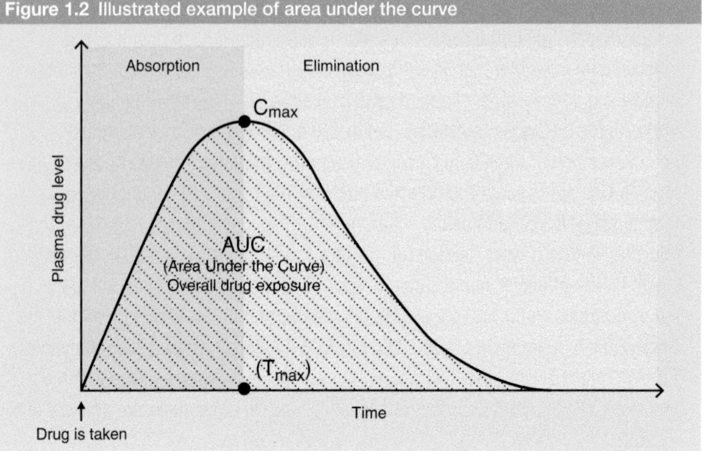

samples drawn at nonstandard times and is considered quite noisy for the purposes of data analysis, but to some extent it does represent the messiness of real-world antipsychotic usage. Figure 1.3 illustrates examples of the variations in drug levels over time for two medications with different half-lives approaching their respective steady state levels. Based on detailed analyses of the multiple antipsychotics used in CATIE, the authors concluded that collection of samples at ***three time points*** might be needed for optimal sampling of each antipsychotic medicine. The authors did acknowledge that this is a preliminary attempt to examine this problem, that the recommendation for three timed samples is not practical for clinical purposes, and that many antipsychotics contain active metabolites, so future studies must model both the parent compound and the principal active metabolites [9]. Until that time when research identifies practical methods for individual antipsychotic preparations that best correlate with AUC and CNS drug actions, the literature has focused on presenting data obtained at standard post-dose intervals for oral and long-acting injectable antipsychotics (LAIs) that represent a defined trough value at steady state: 12 hours for oral antipsychotics, and just prior to the next injection for LAIs.

When Is Steady State Achieved?

Steady state represents the period when equilibrium has been reached in the variables that govern drug absorption, distribution, metabolism, and elimination. While some oral antipsychotics have poor bioavailability as a consequence of extensive first-pass

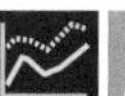

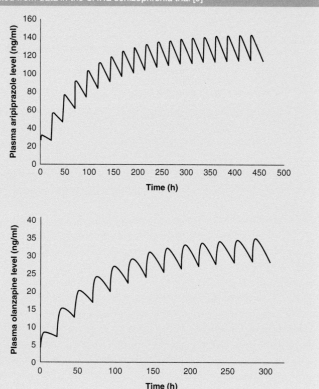

Figure 1.3 Time to steady for aripiprazole 30 mg/d and olanzapine 20 mg/d calculated from data in the CATIE schizophrenia trial [9]

(Adapted from: V. Perera, R. R. Bies, G. Mo, *et al.* [2014]. Optimal sampling of antipsychotic medicines: A pharmacometric approach for clinical practice. *Br J Clin Pharmacol*, 78, 800–814.)

metabolism, the portion of active drug reaching systemic circulation tends to appear quite rapidly, with the time to maximal blood levels (T_{max}) ranging from 1 to 2 hours for most agents [10]. The half-life of an oral antipsychotic (once absorbed) is mostly related to the rapidity of drug metabolism, and to a lesser extent excretion of active drug or active metabolites. The rise toward steady state can be predicted by the drug half-life, and is based on the mathematical calculation that repeated dosing allows an oral medication to reach 97% of steady state trough values after five half-lives (see Box 1.1).

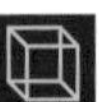

Box 1.1 Why Five Half-Lives Equates to Steady State

Example: Antipsychotic with a 24-hour half-life is dosed once daily. The accumulated medication levels and contribution from each dose are noted below. After five half-lives, the medication is at 97% of the steady state value.

	1st dose	2nd dose	3rd dose	4th dose	5th dose	Total
24 hours	50%	–	–	–	–	50%
48 hours	25%	50%	–	–	–	75%
72 hours	12.5%	25%	50%	–	–	87.5%
96 hours	6.25%	12.5%	25%	50%	–	93.75%
120 hours	3.125%	6.25%	12.5%	25%	50%	96.875%

Obtaining a plasma level before steady state is reached may lead to erroneous conclusions about adherence or drug metabolism, so clinicians should have a working knowledge of half-lives for commonly used antipsychotics, and for important active metabolites such as 9-OH risperidone and norclozapine, whose levels are typically provided along with the parent compound concentration (Table 1.1). The majority of antipsychotics have half-lives under 34 hours, meaning that steady state will be achieved within a week of drug initiation or a dose increase [7]. The important exceptions include sertindole (60–73 hours), aripiprazole (75 hours), brexpiprazole (91 hours), and cariprazine (31.6–68.4 hours, with active metabolites desmethylcariprazine [DCAR] 29.7–39.5 hours, and didesmethylcariprazine [DDCAR] 314–446 hours). As seen in Figure 1.4, the extremely long half-life of DDCAR means that steady state for the active moiety (i.e. the combination of drug levels for cariprazine and its active metabolites) may not be achieved for 30 days or longer [11]. As of this writing, no commercial laboratory is offering cariprazine assays, but should these be available they may be difficult to assess if DCAR and DDCAR levels are not provided, and if the level is obtained before all components of the active moiety are at steady state.

While there are antipsychotics with half-lives significantly less than 24 hours (e.g. clozapine, molindone, risperidone, ziprasidone), most appear effective in routine clinical practice with once daily dosing, with compelling evidence that tolerability across all antipsychotics is improved when that daily dose is administered at bedtime [13, 14]. For clozapine and risperidone, the formation of active metabolites with longer half-lives provides a rationale for efficacy with q 24 hour dosing, while molindone appears not to have active metabolites and remains a bit of a mystery since clinical trials indicate persistent effectiveness with once daily dosing [15]. The ziprasidone package insert advises twice daily (BID) dosing with 500 kcal food, but ziprasidone administered once

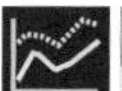

Figure 1.4 Oral cariprazine kinetics [12]

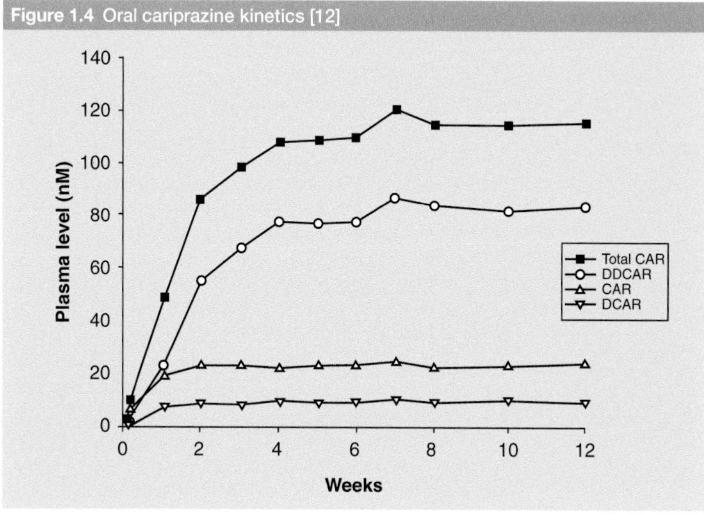

(Adapted from: Allergan USA Inc. [2019]. Vraylar package insert. Madison, NJ.)

daily has been studied. In a long-term double-blind randomized trial using haloperidol as an active comparator, ziprasidone 80–120 mg once daily appeared as efficacious as 40–80 mg given twice daily, based on discontinuation rates: 65% for ziprasidone BID vs. 58% for ziprasidone qD [16]. The proportion who attained at least one period of symptomatic remission (during the 40-week initial period and 156-week blinded continuation study) was 57% for ziprasidone in either the BID or qD group, compared to 45% for haloperidol, a difference that was not statistically significant. As will be discussed in Section B below, in those uncommon instances where BID dosing is necessary (e.g. a clozapine-treated patient who has reached their maximum tolerated bedtime [QHS] dose; a ziprasidone patient who does better with BID dosing), the bulk of the dose should be given as close to bedtime as possible so that the 12h trough level will not be distorted by having a large proportion of the medication (e.g. 50%) administered 24 hours previously.

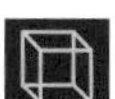

Box 1.2 Why Oral Antipsychotics Should Be Dosed Predominantly at Night

a It is difficult to interpret plasma levels drawn on samples obtained 24 hours after a dose (as seen with qam dosing, or with twice daily dosing where half of the dose will have been administered 24 hours before the plasma level is obtained)

Rationale:

i The majority of studies examining correlations between oral and trough plasma levels are based on 12h post-dose data.

ii The majority of data examining the correlation between plasma antipsychotic levels and response is based on 12h post-dose data.

b There is no therapeutic advantage to multiple daily dosing. In those uncommon instances where BID dosing is necessary (e.g. a clozapine-treated patient who has reached their maximum tolerated bedtime dose; a ziprasidone patient who does better with BID dosing), the bulk of the dose should be given as close to bedtime as possible so that the 12h trough level will not be distorted by having a large proportion of the medication (e.g. 50%) administered 24 hours previously.

Rationale:

i Despite short peripheral half-lives, most antipsychotics have central nervous system (CNS) half-lives and effects that persist ≥ 24 hours, so once daily dosing is sufficient. Clozapine is the best cited example, and exhibits no demonstrable loss of efficacy when dosed exclusively at bedtime [13, 17]. Molindone has a half-life of 2 hours, but is also effective with once daily dosing [18].

ii There is compelling evidence that evening dosing improves tolerability, as peak CNS levels that might exceed the tolerability threshold are achieved during sleep. The best illustration of this concept is seen in the clinical trials of lurasidone. Initial adult schizophrenia studies were performed with morning dosing: "Study medication was administered in the morning with a meal or within 30 minutes after eating" [19]. Later studies administered medication with an evening meal, and analyses of adverse effects found that somnolence and akathisia were markedly reduced with evening meal dosing. In particular, the 160 mg dose had an akathisia rate when dosed with an evening meal of 6.5%, less than one-third that seen with 120 mg when given in the morning (20.3%) [20, 14].

Table Morning-meal versus evening-meal dosing: placebo subtracted rates of somnolence and akathisia in short-term adult schizophrenia trials with lurasidone [14]

	40 mg	80 mg	120 mg	160 mg
Akathisia – AM meal	7.1%	9.1%	**20.3%**	Not studied
Akathisia – PM meal	2.3%*	8.7%	Not studied	**6.5%**
Somnolence – AM meal	3.6%	4.9%	**9.3%**	Not studied
Somnolence – PM meal	2.8%	0.2%*	Not studied	**5.8%**

* Not significantly different from placebo.

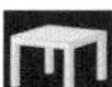

Table 1.1 Mean half-life of commonly used oral antipsychotics and important metabolites [21–29, 10, 15, 17, 30, 7]

Drug	$T_{1/2}$ (hours)
First-generation antipsychotics	
Chlorpromazine	11.05–15
Fluphenazine	13
Haloperidol	24
Loxapine	4
7-OH loxapine	??[a]
Molindone	2[b]
Perphenazine	9–12
Zuclopenthixol	17.6
Newer antipsychotics	
Amisulpride	12
Aripiprazole	75
Asenapine sublingual	24
Asenapine transdermal patch	30[c]
Brexpiprazole	91
Cariprazine	31.6–68.4
Desmethylcariprazine (DCAR)	29.7–39.5 (DCAR)
Didesmethylcariprazine (DDCAR)	314–446 (DDCAR)
Clozapine	9–17
Norclozapine	20
Iloperidone	15–22
Lumateperone	18
Lurasidone	28.8–37.4[d]
Olanzapine	30
Paliperidone (9-OH risperidone)[e]	23
Quetiapine	7
Norquetiapine	12
Risperidone	3
Paliperidone (9-OH risperidone)[f]	21

Drug	$T_{1/2}$ (hours)
Sertindole	60–73
Ziprasidone	7

Comment
Half-lives may be markedly prolonged in individuals receiving metabolic inhibitors or who have lower-functioning polymorphisms of cytochrome P450 enzymes, other relevant enzymes, or transporters involved in drug disposition. Conversely, half-lives may be significantly shorter than the mean in individuals exposed to inducers, or who have higher-functioning polymorphisms of cytochrome P450 enzymes, other relevant enzymes, or transporters involved in drug disposition.

[a] Based on studies of inhaled loxapine, the half-life of 7-OH loxapine is likely to be substantially longer [31].
[b] The therapeutic effects persist for 24–36 hours despite the absence of active metabolites [13].
[c] After patch removal.
[d] Repeated dosing in adult schizophrenia patients. Single dose half-life in volunteers is 18 hours [32].
[e] When administered as oral paliperidone.
[f] When derived from orally administered risperidone.

While the half-life of oral antipsychotics is based on how quickly one can eliminate the drug via metabolism and excretion, that for LAIs relates to the rate of drug absorption from the injection site.

To create an LAI medication, one must develop a prodrug or technology (e.g. embedded microspheres, polymer gel solution) that limits absorption into systemic circulation so delivery occurs in a slow, predictable manner [33, 34]. It is the time course of absorption, or absorption half-life, that becomes the determining factor of drug exposure following each injection, not the metabolism of the absorbed drug. For example, haloperidol has a half-life of 18 hours when administered intravenously [35], but the decanoate LAI preparation has a half-life of 21 days [36]. The term for this phenomenon is 'flip-flop kinetics' as the LAI half-life has been flipped on its head, so to speak, and no longer bears any relation to the drug itself but only that of the delivery system [36, 37]. Due to the systemic delivery, the antipsychotic enters tissue compartments more readily than with oral administration making the calculation of half-lives dependent on complex models of multicompartment kinetics, often with biphasic elimination curves [38, 39]. An underlying concept is that partitioning into tissue compartments eventually slows down as tissue sites reach a point of saturation. When that occurs, increased systemic drug levels are seen and a state of equilibrium is finally achieved [38].

Despite the more complicated kinetics of LAIs, clinicians can use half-life estimates to obtain an approximate calculation of when steady state might be achieved (Table 1.2), with the caveat that steady state might be achieved sooner than

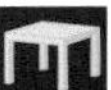

Table 1.2 Mean half-life and kinetic properties of commonly used long-acting injectable (LAI) antipsychotics [45–48]

Drug	Vehicle	Dosage	T_{max}	$T_{1/2}$ multiple dosing	Able to be loaded
First-generation antipsychotics					
Fluphenazine decanoate	Sesame Oil	12.5–75 mg/2 weeks **Max:** 75 mg/week	0.3–1.5 days	14 days	Yes
Haloperidol decanoate	Sesame Oil	25–300 mg/4 weeks **Max:** 300 mg/2 weeks	3–9 days	21 days	Yes
Perphenazine decanoate	Sesame Oil	27–216 mg/3–4 weeks **Max:** 216 mg/3 weeks	7 days	27 days	Yes
Flupenthixol decanoate	Coconut Oil	20–40 mg/2–4 weeks **Max:** 100 mg/2 weeks	4–7 days	17 days	Yes
Zuclopenthixol decanoate	Coconut Oil	25–100 mg/2–4 weeks **Max:** 400 mg/2 weeks	3–7 days	19 days	Yes
Newer antipsychotics					
Risperidone subcutaneous **(Perseris®)**	Water	90–120 mg/4 weeks **Max:** 120 mg/4 weeks	7–8 days	9–11 days	Not needed
Risperidone microspheres **(Risperdal Consta®)**	Water	12.5 – 50 mg/2 weeks **Max:** 50 mg/2 weeks	21 days	See note [a]	**No** (21–28 days oral overlap)
Paliperidone palmitate **(Invega Sustenna®)**[b]	Water	39–234 mg/4 weeks (25–150 mg/4 weeks) **Max:** 234 mg/4 weeks (150 mg/4 weeks)	13 days	25–49 days	Yes

Drug	Vehicle	Dosage	T_{max}	$T_{1/2}$ multiple dosing	Able to be loaded
Paliperidone palmitate (3 mo) **(Invega Trinza®)**[c]	Water	273–819 mg/12 weeks (175–525 mg/12 weeks) **Max:** 819 mg/12 weeks (525 mg/12 weeks)	84–95 days (deltoid) 118–139 days (gluteal)	30–33 days	**No**
Olanzapine pamoate **(Zyprexa Relprevv®)**	Water	150–300 mg/2 weeks 300–405 mg/4 weeks **Max:** 300 mg/2 weeks	7 days	30 days	Yes
Aripiprazole monohydrate **(Abilify Maintena®)**	Water	300–400 mg/4 weeks **Max:** 400 mg/4 weeks	6.5–7.1 days	29.9–46.5 days	**No** (14 days oral overlap)
Aripiprazole lauroxil **(Aristada®)**[d]	Water	441 mg, 662 mg, 882 mg/4 wks 882 mg/6 weeks 1064 mg/8 weeks **Max:** 882 mg/4 weeks	41 days (single dose) [49] 24.4–35.2 days (repeated dosing) [50]	53.9–57.2 days	No (Start with AL_{NC} 675 mg IM + 30 mg oral ***OR*** 21 days oral overlap)
Aripiprazole lauroxil nanocrystal **(Aristada Initio®)**[e]	Water	675 mg once	27 days (range: 16 to 35 days)	15–18 days (single dose)	–

[a] Steady state plasma levels after 5 biweekly injections are maintained for 4–5 weeks, but decrease rapidly at that point with a mean half-life of 4–6 days [51].

[b] The dosages in parentheses reflect those used outside the US, expressed as paliperidone equivalent doses.

[c] Only for those on paliperidone palmitate monthly for 4 months. Cannot be converted from oral medication.

[d] Requires 21 days oral overlap unless starting with aripiprazole lauroxil nanocrystal (AL_{NC}) + a single 30 mg oral dose.

[e] Aripiprazole lauroxil nanocrystal (AL_{NC}) is only used for initiation of treatment with aripiprazole lauroxil, or for resumption of treatment. It is always administered together with the clinician-determined dose of aripiprazole lauroxil, although the latter can be given ≤ 10 days after the aripiprazole lauroxil nanocrystal injection.

predicted if the LAI is loaded at the onset of treatment. Sadly, the data provided in LAI package inserts may not provide an accurate picture of the kinetic picture and time to steady state [40]. Visual illustrations of LAI plasma levels over time are very helpful in deciding when an LAI is at steady state and a trough plasma level can be obtained [41]. (Whenever possible, such graphic representations of LAI kinetics will be provided in this volume in the respective chapters covering a particular antipsychotic.) Figure 1.5 is one example of an expected slow rise to steady state plasma levels over 4–6 months, in this case for fluphenazine decanoate 25 mg administered every 2 weeks (q 14 d) [42]. Risperidone microspheres have an unusual kinetic profile and the package insert lists a half-life of 3–6 days for the active moiety (risperidone + 9-OH risperidone) mostly due to the delayed erosion of the microspheres and relatively sharp rise and decay in drug levels [43]. As noted in Figure 1.6, steady state levels, in practice, are not seen in the expected five half-lives predicted by the package insert (i.e. 15–30 days), but after 6 weeks of treatment with q 14 d injections [44, 40]. In general, the basic principle noted in Box 1.1 for oral antipsychotics holds for LAIs: with repeated dosing there is a steady accumulation of medication over time until an equilibrium level is reached. Figure 1.7 illustrates this concept from a kinetic modeling study of LAI olanzapine covering 1 year of treatment with monthly injections [37].

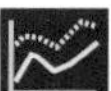

Figure 1.5 Time to steady state for fluphenazine decanoate 25 mg every 2 weeks when resuming treatment after holding injections for 4 weeks [42]

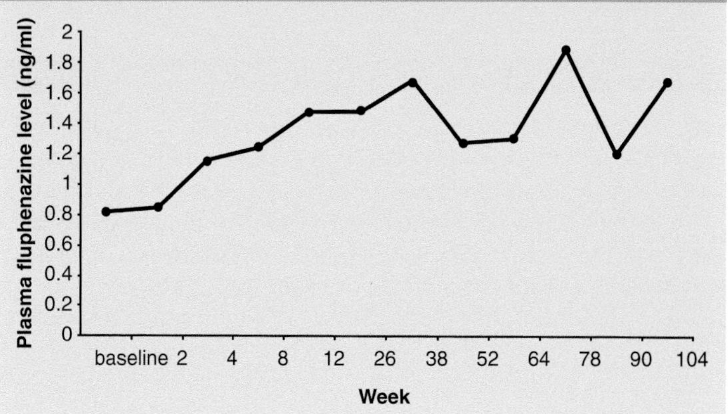

(Adapted from: S. R. Marder, K. K. Midha, T. Van Putten, *et al*. [1991]. Plasma levels of fluphenazine in patients receiving fluphenazine decanoate: Relationship to clinical response. *Br J Psychiatry*, 158, 658–665.)

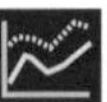

Figure 1.6 Model of active moiety levels (risperidone + 9-OH risperidone) from risperidone microsphere 25 mg IM every 2 weeks with no bridging oral therapy [44]

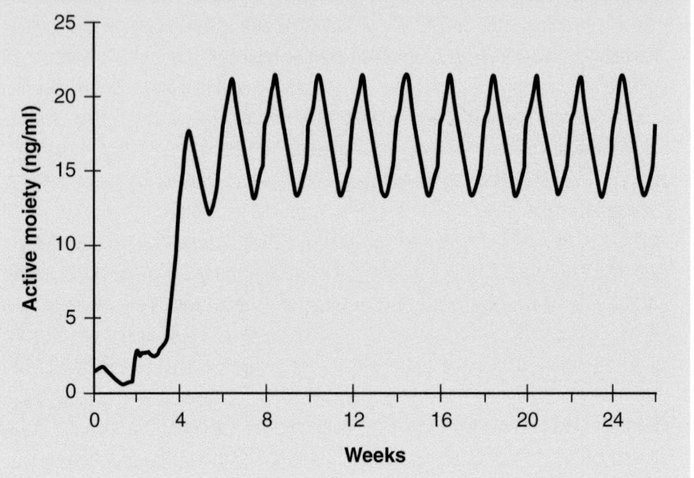

(Adapted from: W. H. Wilson [2004]. A visual guide to expected blood levels of long-acting injectable risperidone in clinical practice. *J Psychiatr Pract*, 10, 393–401.)

Sampling Times for Oral and Long-Acting Injectable Antipsychotics

Half-lives of oral antipsychotics can be estimated accurately for groups of individuals who are not taking medications that alter drug metabolism or excretion, or who lack genetic variants that influence these processes; however, there is marked interindividual variation from the mean half-life in real-world practice. Moreover, the early literature correlating use of plasma antipsychotic levels and clinical outcomes (efficacy and tolerability) reported data from a variety of time points from 2h to 24h post-dose, making comparisons between studies difficult [52, 53]. As the literature evolved through the late 1970s, investigators settled on the use of a 12h trough for oral antipsychotics and most other psychotropic medications [54]. This decision represents a compromise that favors feasibility. The nadir plasma level for any oral medication given once daily is 24h post-dose, but obtaining plasma levels at 9 PM or 10 PM for patients who take medication at bedtime is not possible for the majority of outpatients, and at times can be challenging on inpatient psychiatric units that do not have round-the-clock

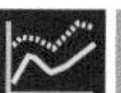

Figure 1.7 Contribution of individual injections to steady state levels for olanzapine LAI [37]

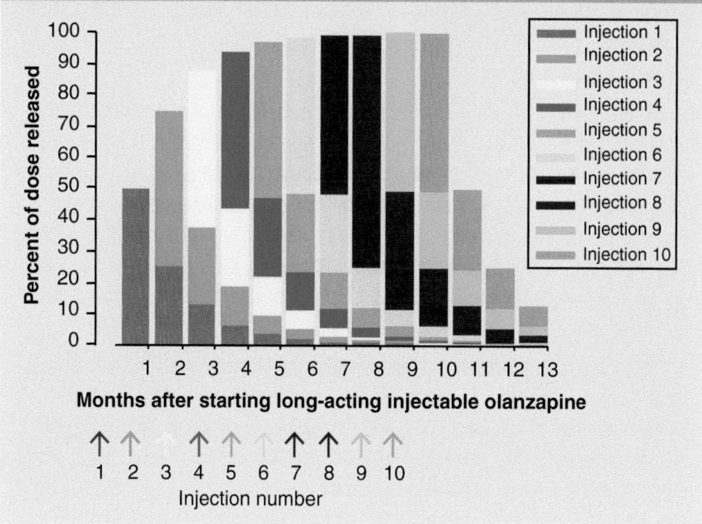

(Adapted from: S. Heres, S. Kraemer, R. F. Bergstrom, *et al.* [2014]. Pharmacokinetics of olanzapine long-acting injection: the clinical perspective. *Int Clin Psychopharmacol*, 29, 299–312.)

phlebotomy services. There are also no compelling data to suggest that plasma levels obtained at time points other than 12h are better at predicting outcomes [55]. The convergence of the literature toward measurement of 12h trough levels thus provides a time interval for a level between 8 AM and 10 AM that is practical for hospital settings, less inconvenient for outpatients, and easily reproduced across studies.

One important use of plasma antipsychotic levels is to optimize treatment efficacy and minimize adverse effect burden, but the other crucial value in level measurement is to track adherence and determine whether low levels are the product of ultrarapid metabolism [2]. The bulk of modern data correlates dose and plasma levels based on 12h trough values, so clinicians can readily find the expected level based on a given dose, assuming the level was drawn approximately 12±2h after the dose. When the level is obtained more than 2h from the 12h mark, interpretation becomes difficult as it may be impossible to find the expected level for an 8h or 16h trough. However, levels drawn at nonstandard times can be used to monitor adherence if the same time since last dose is observed. An example would be a patient who can only obtain levels as 16h troughs (e.g. at noon) as they do not wish to miss their part-time morning employment. In an adherent individual, the expectation is that the level would fluctuate no more than 30% between determinations [56]. (See Chapter 4 for further discussion on levels and adherence.)

As noted previously, there is no compelling evidence that antipsychotic efficacy is increased with BID dosing. Many medications with short peripheral half-lives, such as clozapine, are commonly dosed on a QHS schedule [13]. There will be instances when some portion of the antipsychotic dose cannot be given in the evening, but clinicians should keep the largest fraction of the dose at bedtime. As noted in Box 1.3, when a drug with a 24h half-life is evenly divided in BID doses, the level obtained the next day will be at least 20% lower than expected, as it represents a 12h trough for half of the drug dose, and a 24h trough for the other half.

For LAIs, the trough levels at steady state occur just prior to the next injection. Ideally, one would draw the plasma antipsychotic level in the clinic just prior to administering the next LAI injection; however, some clinics do not have an on-site phlebotomy service, and the level must be drawn at an outside laboratory. As a matter of practicality, a trough LAI level can be obtained any time from 1h to 72h before the next dose. The time to steady state for an LAI will depend on whether there is a loading or initiation regimen, so clinicians must know if the level obtained is indeed at steady state, or is drawn at other relevant time points (i.e. after a loading regimen) to ascertain the extent of systemic antipsychotic exposure [57]. It is crucial that one avoids obtaining steady state trough levels at times that are too close to the maximum

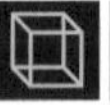

Box 1.3 How Trough Levels Are Influenced by Dosing Interval: An Example from Lithium

Like many antipsychotics, lithium has a 24-hour half-life, but older literature recommended split daily dosing [58]. Below are trough plasma levels obtained 12 hours after the evening dose at steady state in patients on identical daily doses administered one of two ways: all at bedtime (QHS) or twice daily (BID). The levels obtained on BID dosing are 22% lower than those with QHS dosing.

	Level on QHS dosing	BID dosing
Amdisen 1977 [59]	1.37 mEq/L	1.07 mEq/L
Greil 1981 [60]	1.04 mEq/L	0.81 mEq/L
Swartz [61]	0.90 mEq/L	0.70 mEq/L
Mean	**1.10** mEq/L	**0.86** mEq/L

plasma concentration (T_{max}) of the LAI preparation. In general, a plasma level drawn 1h–72h before the next LAI dose avoids these issues, even for agents with short injection intervals (e.g. fluphenazine decanoate, risperidone microspheres).

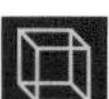

Box 1.4 Basic Guidelines for Obtaining Trough Antipsychotic Plasma Levels

a Oral antipsychotics

i Trough levels should be drawn at steady state. This is reached after five half-lives from initiation or after a dose increase, and should factor in the half-life of active metabolites that are often reported (e.g. 9-OH risperidone, norclozapine).

ii By convention, trough levels are drawn 12h post-dose [7]. There is no compelling efficacy reason to routinely divide antipsychotic doses throughout the day, and bedtime dosing improves tolerability [14]. Even clozapine is usually administered all at bedtime despite the short peripheral half-life [13]. In instances where the dose must be divided, the bulk of the dose should be given at bedtime. If evenly split into qam and QHS doses, the trough level drawn the next morning will be 20% lower for a medication with a 24h half-life, as half of the dose was administered 24h before the level was drawn.

iii Levels drawn at nonstandard times (e.g. 16h post-dose) may be difficult to interpret. If obtained consistently at that time, the level could be used to track adherence based on the assumption that it should not vary by more than ± 30% if drawn at the same time interval post-dose (± 2h) (see Chapter 4) [17].

b LAI antipsychotics

i Trough levels should be drawn at steady state. This may not be exactly after five half-lives from initiation due to the more complex kinetics of LAI preparations, and whether a loading regimen was used. Clinicians should be familiar with the kinetic profiles of LAIs that they use frequently, and the plasma level and kinetic profiles of LAIs that can be loaded or have an initiation regimen.

ii The trough level is typically obtained 1h–72h before the next injection. Levels drawn at earlier time points run the risk that the medication level is closer to the maximum concentration than to the nadir level.

Summary Points

a Whether the antipsychotic is taken orally or as a long-acting injection (LAI), trough levels must be obtained at appropriate time intervals since the last dose. By convention this is 12h after oral dosing, or 1h–72h before the next LAI dose.

b Clinicians should be familiar with the half-lives of commonly used oral antipsychotics and understand that steady state is reached after five half-lives of the medication, including those of active metabolites. Levels of two active metabolites are frequently reported by laboratories: 9-OH risperidone and norclozapine.

c Steady state for LAI preparations is governed by what is termed flip-flop kinetics: the half-life is primarily related to the rate of drug absorption (i.e. the delivery-system kinetics) and not to the molecule that is being delivered. The time to steady state may vary from the rule of five half-lives due to the complexities of systemically delivered drug distribution, and whether the LAI was loaded. Clinicians should be familiar with the kinetic profiles of commonly used LAI agents under both circumstances (loading and non-loading).

References

1. **Preskorn, S. H. (2010).** Outliers on the dose–response curve: How to minimize this problem using therapeutic drug monitoring, an underutilized tool in psychiatry. *J Psychiatr Pract*, 16, 177–182.
2. **McCutcheon, R., Beck, K., D'Ambrosio, E., *et al.* (2018).** Antipsychotic plasma levels in the assessment of poor treatment response in schizophrenia. *Acta Psychiatr Scand*, 137, 39–46.
3. **Velligan, D. I., Wang, M., Diamond, P., *et al.* (2007).** Relationships among subjective and objective measures of adherence to oral antipsychotic medications. *Psychiatr Serv*, 58, 1187–1192.
4. **Velligan, D. I., Maples, N. J., Pokorny, J. J., *et al.* (2020).** Assessment of adherence to oral antipsychotic medications: What has changed over the past decade? *Schizophr Res*, 215, 17–24.
5. **Polasek, T. M., Tucker, G. T., Sorich, M. J., *et al.* (2018).** Prediction of olanzapine exposure in individual patients using physiologically based pharmacokinetic modelling and simulation. *Br J Clin Pharmacol*, 84, 462–476.
6. **Hiemke, C., Bergemann, N., Clement, H. W., *et al.* (2018).** Consensus guidelines for therapeutic drug monitoring in neuropsychopharmacology: Update 2017. *Pharmacopsychiatry*, 51, 9–62.
7. **Schoretsanitis, G., Kane, J. M., Correll, C. U., *et al.* (2020).** Blood levels to optimize antipsychotic treatment in clinical practice: A joint consensus statement of the American Society of Clinical Psychopharmacology (ASCP) and the Therapeutic Drug Monitoring (TDM) Task Force of the Arbeitsgemeinschaft für Neuropsychopharmakologie und Pharmakopsychiatrie (AGNP). *J Clin Psychiatry*, 81, https://doi.org/10.4088/JCP.4019cs13169.
8. **Wode-Helgodt, B. and Alfredsson, G. (1981).** Concentrations of chlorpromazine and two of its active metabolites in plasma and cerebrospinal fluid of psychotic patients treated with fixed drug doses. *Psychopharmacology (Berl)*, 73, 55–62.
9. **Perera, V., Bies, R. R., Mo, G., *et al.* (2014).** Optimal sampling of antipsychotic medicines: A pharmacometric approach for clinical practice. *Br J Clin Pharmacol*, 78, 800–814.
10. **Meyer, J. M. (2018).** Pharmacotherapy of psychosis and mania. In L. L. Brunton, R. Hilal-Dandan, and B. C. Knollmann, eds., *Goodman & Gilman's The Pharmacological Basis of Therapeutics*, 13th edn. Chicago, IL: McGraw-Hill, pp. 279–302.
11. **Nakamura, T., Kubota, T., Iwakaji, A., *et al.* (2016).** Clinical pharmacology study of cariprazine (MP-214) in patients with schizophrenia (12-week treatment). *Drug Des Devel Ther*, 10, 327–338.
12. **Allergan USA Inc. (2019).** Vraylar package insert. Madison, NJ.
13. **Takeuchi, H., Powell, V., Geisler, S., *et al.* (2016).** Clozapine administration in clinical practice: Once-daily versus divided dosing. *Acta Psychiatr Scand*, 134, 234–240.
14. **Hagi, K., Tadashi, N. and Pikalov, A. (2020).** S5. Does the time of drug administration alter the adverse event risk of lurasidone? *Schizophr Bull*, 46, S31–32.
15. **Yu, C. and Gopalakrishnan, G. (2018).** In vitro pharmacological characterization of SPN-810 M (molindone). *J Exp Pharmacol*, 10, 65–73.
16. **Greenberg, W. M. and Citrome, L. (2007).** Ziprasidone for schizophrenia and bipolar disorder: A review of the clinical trials. *CNS Drug Rev*, 13, 137–177.
17. **Meyer, J. M. and Stahl, S. M. (2019).** *The Clozapine Handbook*. Cambridge: Cambridge University Press.
18. **Claghorn, J. L. (1985).** Review of clinical and laboratory experiences with molindone hydrochloride. *J Clin Psychiatry*, 46, 30–33.
19. **Meltzer, H. Y., Cucchiaro, J., Silva, R., *et al.* (2011).** Lurasidone in the treatment of schizophrenia: A randomized, double-blind, placebo- and olanzapine-controlled study. *Am J Psychiatry*, 168, 957–967.

20. **Loebel, A., Cucchiaro, J., Sarma, K., *et al.* (2013).** Efficacy and safety of lurasidone 80 mg/day and 160 mg/day in the treatment of schizophrenia: A randomized, double-blind, placebo- and active-controlled trial. *Schizophr Res*, 145, 101–109.
21. **Simpson, G. M., Cooper, T. B., Lee, J. H., *et al.* (1978).** Clinical and plasma level characteristics of intramuscular and oral loxapine. *Psychopharmacology (Berl)*, 56, 225–232.
22. **Zetin, M., Cramer, M., Garber, D., *et al.* (1985).** Bioavailability of oral and intramuscular molindone hydrochloride in schizophrenic patients. *Clin Ther*, 7, 169–175.
23. **Midha, K. K., Hawes, E. M., Hubbard, J. W., *et al.* (1988).** Variation in the single dose pharmacokinetics of fluphenazine in psychiatric patients. *Psychopharmacology (Berl)*, 96, 206–211.
24. **Dahl, M. L., Ekqvist, B., Widén, J., *et al.* (1991).** Disposition of the neuroleptic zuclopenthixol cosegregates with the polymorphic hydroxylation of debrisoquine in humans. *Acta Psychiatr Scand*, 84, 99–102.
25. **Midha, K. K., Hubbard, J. W., McKay, G., *et al.* (1993).** The role of metabolites in a bioequivalence study I: Loxapine, 7-hydroxyloxapine and 8-hydroxyloxapine. *Int J Clin Pharmacol Ther Toxicol*, 31, 177–183.
26. **Yeung, P. K., Hubbard, J. W., Korchinski, E. D., *et al.* (1993).** Pharmacokinetics of chlorpromazine and key metabolites. *Eur J Clin Pharmacol*, 45, 563–569.
27. **Wong, S. L. and Granneman, G. R. (1998).** Modeling of sertindole pharmacokinetic disposition in healthy volunteers in short term dose-escalation studies. *J Pharm Sci*, 87, 1629–1631.
28. **Kudo, S. and Ishizaki, T. (1999).** Pharmacokinetics of haloperidol: An update. *Clin Pharmacokinet*, 37, 435–456.
29. **Mauri, M. C., Volonteri, L. S., Colasanti, A., *et al.* (2007).** Clinical pharmacokinetics of atypical antipsychotics: A critical review of the relationship between plasma concentrations and clinical response. *Clin Pharmacokinet*, 46, 359–388.
30. **Meyer, J. M. (2020).** Lumateperone for schizophrenia. *Curr Psychiatr*, 19, 33–39.
31. **Spyker, D. A., Voloshko, P., Heyman, E. R., *et al.* (2014).** Loxapine delivered as a thermally generated aerosol does not prolong QTc in a thorough QT/QTc study in healthy subjects. *J Clin Pharmacol*, 54, 665–674.
32. **Meyer, J. M., Loebel, A. D., and Schweizer, E. (2009).** Lurasidone: A new drug in development for schizophrenia. *Expert Opin Investig Drugs*, 18, 1715–1726.
33. **Selmin, F., Blasi, P., and DeLuca, P. P. (2012).** Accelerated polymer biodegradation of risperidone poly(D, L-lactide-co-glycolide) microspheres. *AAPS PharmSciTech*, 13, 1465–1472.
34. **Ivaturi, V., Gopalakrishnan, M., Gobburu, J. V. S., *et al.* (2017).** Exposure–response analysis after subcutaneous administration of RBP-7000, a once-a-month long-acting Atrigel formulation of risperidone. *Br J Clin Pharmacol*, 83, 1476–1498.
35. **Cheng, Y. F., Paalzow, L. K., Bondesson, U., *et al.* (1987).** Pharmacokinetics of haloperidol in psychotic patients. *Psychopharmacology (Berl)*, 91, 410–414.
36. **Jann, M. W., Ereshefsky, L., and Saklad, S. R. (1985).** Clinical pharmacokinetics of the depot antipsychotics. *Clin Pharmacokinet*, 10, 315–333.
37. **Heres, S., Kraemer, S., Bergstrom, R. F., *et al.* (2014).** Pharmacokinetics of olanzapine long-acting injection: The clinical perspective. *Int Clin Psychopharmacol*, 29, 299–312.
38. **Ereshefsky, L., Saklad, S. R., Jann, M. W., *et al.* (1984).** Future of depot neuroleptic therapy: Pharmacokinetic and pharmacodynamic approaches. *J Clin Psychiatry*, 45, 50–59.
39. **Samtani, M. N., Vermeulen, A., and Stuyckens, K. (2009).** Population pharmacokinetics of intramuscular paliperidone palmitate in patients with schizophrenia: A novel once-monthly, long-acting formulation of an atypical antipsychotic. *Clin Pharmacokinet*, 48, 585–600.
40. **Lee, L. H., Choi, C., Collier, A. C., *et al.* (2015).** The pharmacokinetics of second-generation long-acting injectable antipsychotics: Limitations of monograph values. *CNS Drugs*, 29, 975–983.

41. **Meyer, J. M. (2013).** Understanding depot antipsychotics: An illustrated guide to kinetics. *CNS Spectr*, 18, 55–68.
42. **Marder, S. R., Midha, K. K., Van Putten, T., *et al.* (1991).** Plasma levels of fluphenazine in patients receiving fluphenazine decanoate: Relationship to clinical response. *Br J Psychiatry*, 158, 658–665.
43. **Janssen Pharmaceuticals Inc. (2020).** Risperdal Consta package insert. Titusville, NJ.
44. **Wilson, W. H. (2004).** A visual guide to expected blood levels of long-acting injectable risperidone in clinical practice. *J Psychiatr Pract*, 10, 393–401.
45. **Larsen, N. E. and Hansen, L. B. (1989).** Prediction of the optimal perphenazine decanoate dose based on blood samples drawn within the first three weeks. *Ther Drug Monit*, 11, 642–646.
46. **Altamura, A. C., Sassella, F., Santini, A., *et al.* (2003).** Intramuscular preparations of antipsychotics: Uses and relevance in clinical practice. *Drugs*, 63, 493–512.
47. **Spanarello, S. and La Ferla, T. (2014).** The pharmacokinetics of long-acting antipsychotic medications. *Curr Clin Pharamacol*, 9, 310–317.
48. **Meyer, J. M. (2020).** Monitoring and improving antipsychotic adherence in outpatient forensic diversion programs. *CNS Spectr*, 25, 136–144.
49. **Hard, M. L., Mills, R. J., Sadler, B. M., *et al.* (2017).** Aripiprazole lauroxil: Pharmacokinetic profile of this long-acting injectable antipsychotic in persons with schizophrenia. *J Clin Psychopharmacol*, 37, 289–295.
50. **Hard, M. L., Mills, R. J., Sadler, B. M., *et al.* (2017).** Pharmacokinetic profile of a 2-month dose regimen of aripiprazole lauroxil: A phase I study and a population pharmacokinetic model. *CNS Drugs*, 31, 617–624.
51. **Gefvert, O., Eriksson, B., Persson, P., *et al.* (2005).** Pharmacokinetics and D2 receptor occupancy of long-acting injectable risperidone (Risperdal Consta) in patients with schizophrenia. *Int J Neuropsychopharmacol*, 8, 27–36.
52. **Wiles, D. H., Kolakowska, T., McNeilly, A. S., *et al.* (1976).** Clinical significance of plasma chlorpromazine levels. I: Plasma levels of the drug, some of its metabolites and prolactin during acute treatment. *Psychol Med*, 6, 407–415.
53. **Kolakowska, T., Wiles, D. H., Gelder, M. G., *et al.* (1976).** Clinical significance of plasma chlorpromazine levels. II: Plasma levels of the drug, some of its metabolites and prolactin in patients receiving long-term phenothiazine treatment. *Psychopharmacology (Berl)*, 49, 101–107.
54. **Van Putten, T., Marder, S. R., Wirshing, W. C., *et al.* (1991).** Neuroleptic plasma levels. *Schizophr Bull*, 17, 197–216.
55. **Midha, K. K., Hubbard, J. W., Marder, S. R., *et al.* (1994).** Impact of clinical pharmacokinetics on neuroleptic therapy in patients with schizophrenia. *J Psychiatry Neurosci*, 19, 254–264.
56. **Lee, J., Bies, R., Takeuchi, H., *et al.* (2016).** Quantifying intraindividual variations in plasma clozapine levels: A population pharmacokinetic approach. *J Clin Psychiatry*, 77, 681–687.
57. **Wei, F. C., Jann, M. W., Lin, H. N., *et al.* (1996).** A practical loading dose method for converting schizophrenic patients from oral to depot haloperidol therapy. *J Clin Psychiatry*, 57, 298–302.
58. **Castro, V. M., Roberson, A. M., McCoy, T. H., *et al.* (2016).** Stratifying risk for renal insufficiency among lithium-treated patients: An electronic health record study. *Neuropsychopharmacology*, 41, 1138–1143.
59. **Amdisen, A. (1977).** Serum level monitoring and clinical pharmacokinetics of lithium. *Clin Pharmacokinet*, 2, 73–92.
60. **Greil, W. (1981).** [Pharmacokinetics and toxicology of lithium]. *Bibl Psychiatr*, 69–103.
61. **Swartz, C. M. (1987).** Correction of lithium levels for dose and blood sampling times. *J Clin Psychiatry*, 48, 60–64.

2 The Therapeutic Threshold and the Point of Futility

QUICK CHECK

PRINCIPLES

- The bulk of the data correlating plasma antipsychotic levels and psychiatric response relates to the treatment of schizophrenia spectrum disorders, with extremely limited information for other diagnoses. For that reason, the discussions within this handbook about symptomatic improvement pertain only to the management of schizophrenia. Antipsychotic plasma levels can be used for monitoring adherence regardless of the indication (see Chapter 4).
- The therapeutic threshold represents a value achieved by a synthesis of the available data to arrive at a plasma level that best discriminates true responders from nonresponders. This information comes primarily from clinical studies of oral antipsychotics, supported by imaging data on dopamine receptor occupancy. There are a range of numbers presented in the literature, but there is often a convergence among the more widely studied antipsychotics (e.g. haloperidol, fluphenazine, clozapine, olanzapine, risperidone, etc.).
- Some patients may respond adequately below the usual response threshold, and this may be more common with long-acting injectable agents. For clinical use, the therapeutic threshold represents an initial target plasma level for patients who are inadequate responders and who do not have dose-limiting adverse effects.

- **The definition of an upper limit is quite variable and confusing. What laboratories report as the upper limit varies dramatically between sources, and may represent a reference range based on doses instead of a therapeutic range. Consensus guidelines may also vary in their definitions, and at times will employ tolerability thresholds or plasma levels based on maximum approved dosages.**
- **The point of futility is a *term of art* utilized within the extensive California Department of State Hospitals to educate clinicians about two important concepts with regard to an upper limit for antipsychotic plasma levels: (1) a small proportion of patients may never exhibit dose-limiting adverse effects and will tolerate further titration; (2) ongoing titration beyond a certain plasma level (the point of futility) is fruitless as < 5% of patients may respond to these higher plasma levels.**

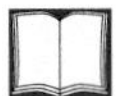

INTRODUCTION

Prior to our modern understanding of differences in drug metabolism, it was apparent that a wide range of response to antipsychotic dosages existed, with some schizophrenia patients responding minimally regardless of dose. Whether this variation was due to nonadherence or other biological factors [1, 2], the need to quantify antipsychotic exposure and clinical response spurred interest in development of reliable laboratory assays and improved psychiatric research instruments in the 1960s. The Brief Psychiatric Rating Scale (BPRS) was developed in 1962 to rate major symptom characteristics of acute psychosis, and represented an important advancement over older methods that lacked "efficiency, speed and economy" [3]. Papers discussing the measurement and the significance of plasma chlorpromazine levels appeared in 1968 [4, 5], followed by improved precision of laboratory drug assays, and the advent of newer rating scales for schizophrenia clinical trials (e.g. the Positive and Negative Syndrome Scale [PANSS] by Kay, Fiszbein, and Opler in 1987) [6]. The increased availability of antipsychotic plasma level data allowed schizophrenia investigators to explore fundamental questions about the relationships between antipsychotic exposure, clinical response, and tolerability [7]. By 1981, Dr. Theodore Van Putten, a professor at UCLA and an early proponent of this research, was able to define a therapeutic range for chlorpromazine (CPZ), and described one clinical scenario wherein a plasma level could inform treatment: "It is in the inaccessible patient whose illness is only minimally, or not at all, sensitive to CPZ that a plasma level might be especially useful" [8].

To arrive at therapeutic plasma level ranges, these early investigators used mathematical models for calculating the response threshold, but defining an upper limit relied less on computational analysis and more on agreeing to a point where the plasma level became intolerable for the vast majority of patients (e.g. 90%) [9]. Though overdose with certain first-generation antipsychotics could lead to fatal QT prolongation (e.g. chlorpromazine, pimozide, thioridazine) [10], antipsychotics as a class possessed a broader therapeutic index than other commonly used psychotropics in the 1960s–1980s (e.g. tricyclic antidepressants, lithium), so the upper limit definition was not primarily a safety issue, but a tolerability one [11]. As the initial studies utilized first-generation antipsychotics (FGAs), neurological adverse effects (e.g. parkinsonism, akathisia, dystonia) were the common dose-limiting issue (Figure 2.1) [9]. The development of atypical antipsychotics altered tolerability profiles, but the basic questions persist: whether this upper limit should be defined by a certain intolerability rate (e.g. 50%, 90%, etc.), or by other measures. Where to draw this upper limit remains a healthy source of debate, and one area where the field has not reached consensus [12–15].

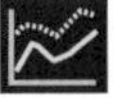

Figure 2.1 Plasma haloperidol levels and the proportion of patients with intolerable adverse effects [9, 16]

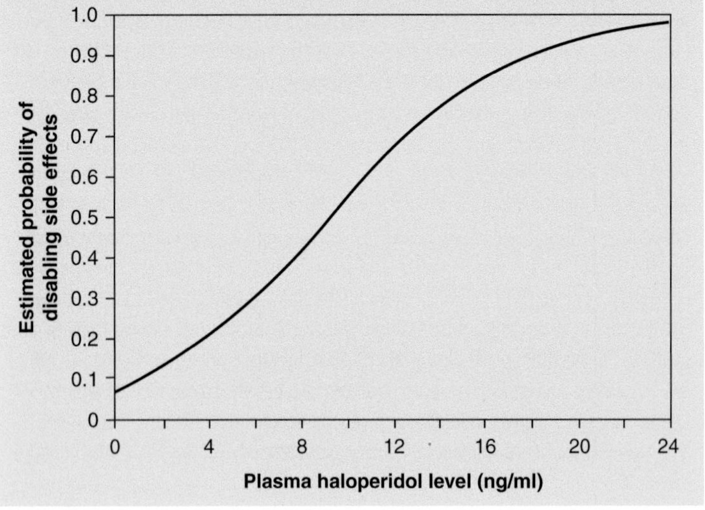

(Adapted from: K. K. Midha, J. W. Hubbard, S. Marder, *et al*. [1994]. Impact of clinical pharmacokinetics on neuroleptic therapy in patients with schizophrenia. *J Psychiatry Neurosci*, 19, 254–264.)

Over 25 years of research documents the clinical value of directly measuring antipsychotic exposure, yet routine use waned dramatically in the early 1990s despite the publication of Marder, Davis, and Janicak's edited 1993 book entitled ***Clinical Use of Neuroleptic Plasma Levels*** [17]. As noted in the Introduction, practical issues in obtaining rapid results can frustrate attempts to make clinical decisions within time frames achieved when ordering other drug levels (e.g. lithium). The 1993 Marder *et al.* volume is scholarly but contains discussions about mathematical concepts such as receiver operating characteristic (ROC) analyses that are pivotal to academic debates over response thresholds but have less appeal to a broader clinical audience. Importantly, there has been a paucity of discussion regarding the variable reporting of upper limit thresholds in the literature, and how clinicians should make sense of this literature [18]. In addition to the aforementioned, perhaps the biggest impediment to widespread use of antipsychotic plasma levels was the development of second-generation antipsychotics (SGAs). To arrive at robust correlations between a drug dose and a plasma level, or between a plasma level and clinical response, requires multiple fixed-dose studies. Unfortunately, this data is less available than with FGAs – clozapine being the notable exception [19]. A 2013 review covering SGAs (other than clozapine) available in the US (risperidone, olanzapine, quetiapine, aripiprazole, ziprasidone, paliperidone, iloperidone, asenapine, lurasidone) found 192 papers, of which only 11 provided data from prospective trials of acute psychosis that correlated levels with efficacy [20]. Moreover, of the nine antipsychotics involved in the search, only four had relevant articles, and only two medications were involved in multiple trials. Studies also varied widely in methodology, with only four employing a fixed-dose model. Based on the limited data for SGAs, the authors concluded: "The utility of therapeutic drug monitoring of SGAs (other than clozapine) remains an open question, although limited evidence from fixed-dose studies is encouraging" [20].

While the 2013 review might engender a certain degree of nihilism, there have been concerted attempts to refocus clinicians' attention on the significant value that measurement of antipsychotic levels can bring to clinical decision making, led by the Therapeutic Drug Monitoring (TDM) task force of the German Arbeitsgemeinschaft für Neuropsychopharmakologie und Pharmakopsychiatrie (AGNP). AGNP issued their first guidelines for TDM across all psychiatric medications in 2004, followed by updates in 2011 and 2018, and by a consensus statement in 2020 issued jointly with the American Society for Clinical Psychopharmacology (ASCP) that covered use of antipsychotic levels [13, 15]. In crafting the consensus paper, AGNP and ASCP sought to remind clinicians that levels are obtainable, that there are numerous clinical reasons to check levels, and that antipsychotic response is low below certain threshold levels, whether due to poor adherence or rapid drug metabolism [15]. The discussion below will assist all clinicians in developing a fuller understanding of how level recommendations are arrived at, and, importantly, how to make sense of the recommendations in this volume and other sources about the use of plasma level information to optimize likelihood of clinical response for schizophrenia patients.

Evidence Used to Define a Therapeutic Threshold

Astute clinicians will appreciate that therapeutic thresholds for psychotropic medications are consensus conclusions which attempt to provide clarity from a range of values [21, 22, 13]. For antipsychotics, the degree of certainty is based on the extent and quality of the data [15], and whether the estimate comes primarily from fixed-dose trials, is inferred from single photon (SPECT) or Positron (PET) Emission Tomography studies of dopamine D_2 receptor occupancy, or is calculated from minimum effective doses [23, 24]. Bearing in mind that these are all **monotherapy** studies and thus cannot be used for antipsychotic combination therapy or for uses other than schizophrenia, estimates of the therapeutic threshold derived from fixed-dose antipsychotic trials provide the most indisputable connection between plasma levels and response, and, unlike imaging, require no assumption that the therapeutic mechanism is primarily correlated with D_2 receptor occupancy [13, 15]. Regardless of the data source, the identification of correlation between response likelihood and a plasma level, dose, or imaging result comes from clinical studies that are typically performed in adult patients with an acute exacerbation of schizophrenia. Conclusions can also be gleaned from longer-term maintenance studies by examining the plasma level threshold below which higher relapse rates are experienced [25, 26].

For acute psychosis trials, response is based on a certain degree of symptom relief using a standard rating scale administered by trained research personnel (e.g. PANSS, BPRS). Varying response definitions are seen throughout the literature, but a 50% reduction in the primary outcome measure is most commonly employed, although lower values may be acceptable in more treatment-resistant populations [27]. Differences in study design, rating scales, and patient populations generate some of the mathematical 'noise' that results in differing plasma level values reported for the therapeutic threshold. Clinicians are sometimes frustrated that there is more than one value reported in the literature as various scientists choose to weigh certain types of data in different ways. However, as the body of information increases for a particular antipsychotic (e.g. clozapine, haloperidol), there is a much narrower range of suggested response thresholds (Box 2.1). Having an understanding of how the various data sources translate into a recommended response threshold is helpful for appreciating the currently available recommendations, and for understanding changes that might occur based on newer studies.

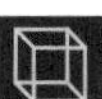

Box 2.1 Important Concepts in Using Response Thresholds for Schizophrenia Treatment

a. There is no one 'right' answer with respect to therapeutic threshold levels for any antipsychotic, but a range of values presented in the literature, whose degree of certainty is enhanced by the breadth of data. When the sample size is large across clinical studies, there is greater agreement (e.g. a clozapine response threshold of 350 ng/ml) [28]. The AGNP/ASCP consensus paper divides antipsychotics into four groups based on the extent of supporting data to justify therapeutic drug monitoring: Level 1 – strongly recommended; Level 2 – recommended; Level 3 – useful; Level 4 – potentially useful [15].

b. Throughout this volume, a justification will be provided for why a particular value is selected, but clinicians are free to settle on any evidence-based value for a response threshold within the range reported in the literature. For haloperidol, there are response thresholds of 1 ng/ml, 2 ng/ml, 3 ng/ml, and 5 ng/ml described in various papers [29, 9, 16, 12, 15]. The crucial issue is to decide on values for those antipsychotics one uses frequently, and modify these as newer literature dictates.

c. Some patients may respond adequately to levels below the response threshold. As discussed in Chapter 5, the therapeutic threshold is a guidepost to assist clinicians in maximizing the chances of converting an inadequate responder who is tolerating a medication into a responder.

d. Having a plasma level above the threshold is no guarantee of adequate response. Where in the therapeutic range a patient will respond, or whether the patient responds at all, relates to pharmacogenetic and other variables that cannot be estimated as of 2021. (See Chapter 5 for an extensive discussion on using plasma antipsychotic levels to maximize the likelihood of response.)

1 Receiver Operating Characteristic (ROC) Curve Analysis of Clinical Data

In World War II, radar engineers were motivated to develop methods that better discriminated between enemy objects and friendly forces on the battlefield. In doing so, these engineers sought to improve the signal detection ability of the receivers used by radar operators, and the plots created were termed *receiver operating characteristic* (ROC) curves. To use the appropriate statistical terminology, the goal was to maximize the chances of identifying all enemy objects (the true positive rate, or sensitivity, which is plotted on the y-axis), while minimizing the odds of incorrectly labeling a friendly force as an enemy (the false positive rate, calculated as 1-specificity and plotted on the x-axis). These concepts quickly moved from the battlefield to the scientific arena where the applications focused on optimizing diagnostic test results to find a value that might accurately distinguish true responders from nonresponders (false positives). An early ROC analysis for clozapine, published in 1991 from a trial of 29 treatment-resistant adult schizophrenia patients, suggested that a threshold of 350 ng/ml best identified true responders without sacrificing the extent of false positives [30]. A subsequent 1995 study of 45 treatment-resistant schizophrenia patients came to similar conclusions [31]. Figure 2.2 presents the graph achieved from the 1995 study with the corresponding percentage of responders and nonresponders plotted for each plasma clozapine level. Treatment response was defined as a 20% decrease in the BPRS score, and either a clinical global impression (CGI) severity rating of mildly ill (score of 3 or below) or a BPRS score of 35 or less.

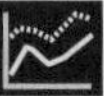

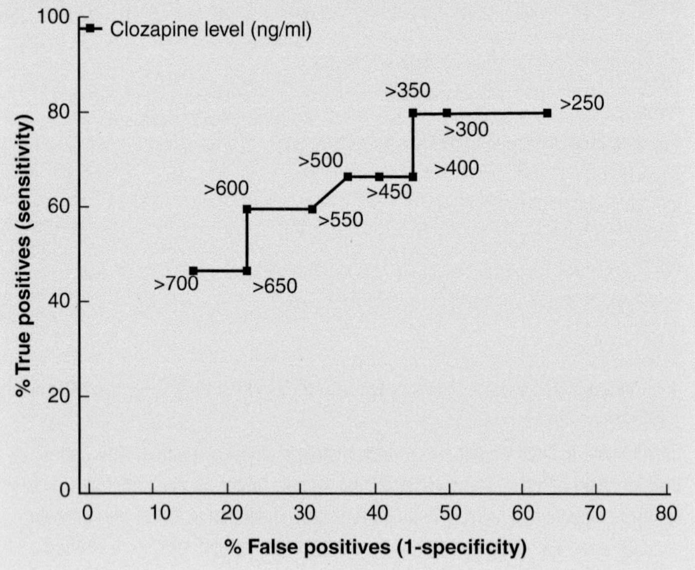

Figure 2.2 Receiver operating characteristic (ROC) curve from 1995 data on the proportion of clozapine responders and nonresponders for plasma clozapine levels in 50 ng/ml increments plotted from the data in Table 2.1 [31]

(Adapted from: M. H. Kronig, R. A. Munne, S. Szymanski, *et al.* [1995]. Plasma clozapine levels and clinical response for treatment-refractory schizophrenic patients. *Am J Psychiatry*, 152, 179–182.)

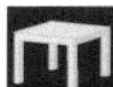

Table 2.1 Responders (sensitivity) and nonresponders (1-specificity) for plasma clozapine levels in 50 ng/ml increments [31]

Blood level (ng/ml)	% responders (sensitivity)	% nonresponders (1-specificity)	*p*
250	80.0	63.6	0.28
300	80.0	50.0	0.06
350	80.0	45.5	**<0.04**
400	66.7	45.5	0.20
450	66.7	40.9	0.12
500	66.7	36.4	0.07
550	60.0	31.8	0.09
600	60.0	22.7	**<0.03**
650	46.7	22.7	0.12
700	46.7	13.6	**<0.03**

Not surprisingly, the proportion of nonresponders increases with lower plasma levels on the x-axis, with 35% being classified as nonresponders with clozapine levels < 250 ng/ml. Conversely, the proportion of responders increases along with the plasma level; however, one can see by the shape of the curve that, for this data set, plasma clozapine levels > 350 ng/ml, > 600 ng/ml and > 700 ng/ml identify intervals with marked reduction in the proportion of nonresponders (i.e. lower false positive rate). Mathematically, one selects a cutoff that maximizes sensitivity (i.e. the distance from the x-axis is maximized), while false positives (calculated as 1-specificity) are minimized (i.e. distance from the y-axis is minimized) [31]. Statistical analysis found that the plasma clozapine level of 350 ng/ml best satisfied those criteria, and this value was chosen as the response threshold. Figure 2.3 represents data from a 2016 study of olanzapine response in 151 Taiwanese adult schizophrenia patients illustrating the cutoff of 22.77 ng/ml that was mathematically calculated to discriminate responders from nonresponders using a PANSS total score ≤ 58 as the criterion for response [32].

The differing definitions of treatment response represent one of many reasons why various threshold cutoffs are reported in the literature from ROC analyses. In some instances, investigators who want to increase the precision of an ROC analysis by combining results of several studies will use the original raw PANSS scoring data to look specifically at an outcome measure that can be calculated for all participants (e.g. a PANSS reduction of 50%). When there is a commonly used definition of

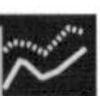

Figure 2.3 2016 ROC curve of the plasma olanzapine level required to be rated as mildly ill (PANSS score ≤ 58) from a cohort of Taiwanese schizophrenia patients (n = 151) [32]

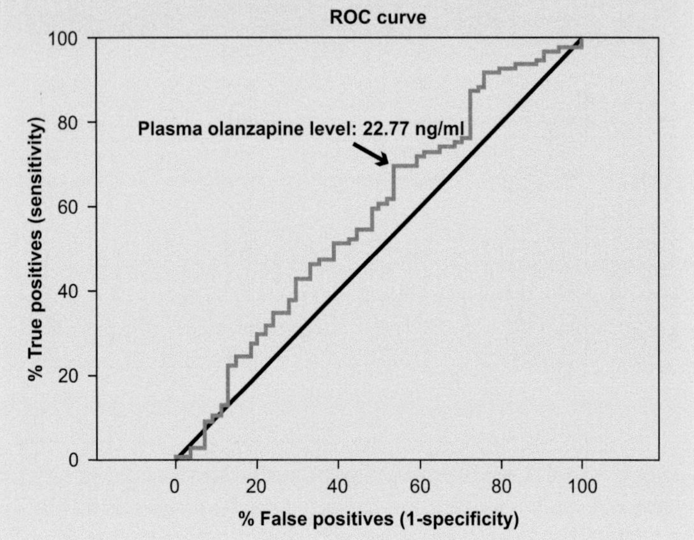

(Adapted from: M. L. Lu, Y. X. Wu, C. H. Chen, *et al.* [2016]. Application of plasma levels of olanzapine and N-desmethyl-olanzapine to monitor clinical efficacy in patients with schizophrenia. *PLoS One*, 11, e0148539.)

response, and sufficient data from multiple samples, ROC analysis is considered a gold standard method for arriving at response threshold plasma levels, and this method has been used in papers on antipsychotic response dating back to 1981 [17]. These ROC analyses have also confirmed that plasma antipsychotic threshold levels significantly correlate with clinical response, although conclusions for individual agents are often limited by the paucity of studies reporting the proportion of responders and nonresponders at various plasma levels.

2 Imaging of Dopamine D_2 Occupancy Relationships with Plasma Antipsychotic Levels

Based on the common mechanism of action for first-generation antipsychotics, the paradigm for drug development through the late 1980s rested on animal models designed to predict significant dopamine D_2 receptor antagonism [33]. The synthesis of ligands in the mid-1980s for imaging research allowed investigators to use SPECT and later PET scans to quantify D_2 receptor occupancy in human subjects, correlate occupancy with response and neurological adverse effects (e.g. parkinsonism, akathisia, dystonia), and infer expected plasma antipsychotic levels for the response threshold [34]. As with ROC analyses derived from plasma level data, varying definitions of response gave rise to slightly different conclusions using ROC curves or other methods to calculate the threshold D_2 occupancy for antipsychotic response. Moreover, there are technical aspects of imaging studies that introduce another layer of complexity (e.g. ligand choice, time since last antipsychotic dose), with PET data providing superior results compared to older SPECT studies. Moreover, PET studies typically have very small sample sizes (under 10 subjects), and often include normal volunteers or younger (nongeriatric) schizophrenia patients, possibly limiting the generalizability of findings [35]. Using antipsychotics whose presumed mechanism is D_2 antagonism, PET scans obtained at steady state, 12h post-dose, show a range of occupancy thresholds for antipsychotic response from 50% to 65% [23, 36]. While 60% or 65% are the more commonly cited numbers, lower figures have emerged from studies of first-episode schizophrenia patients, perhaps related to several differences compared to more chronic patients: younger age, limited (or absent) prior antipsychotic exposure, generally higher response rates, and sensitivity to D_2 antagonism (Figure 2.4) [37].

Imaging of D_2 occupancy provided the psychiatric community with *in vivo* data clearly establishing the link between peripherally obtained plasma antipsychotic levels and effects at a known central nervous system (CNS) receptor target. The consensus conclusion that 60%–65% 12h trough D_2 occupancy best predicts response from D_2 antagonists is drawn from a large body of data with chronic schizophrenia patients. Unfortunately, estimates of the plasma level thresholds needed to achieve 60%–65% D_2 occupancy are often obtained from studies using younger schizophrenia patients or normal volunteers. The use of younger patients or those without schizophrenia may be one factor giving rise to plasma levels required for 60% or 65% D_2 occupancy that are different from, and usually much lower than, those derived from ROC analyses of plasma level thresholds in a chronic schizophrenia population. For example, a 2011 review calculated the plasma concentration needed to achieve 60% D_2 occupancy for a range of antipsychotics: risperidone + 9-OH risperidone level: 10.5 ng/ml; olanzapine: 13.9 ng/ml; haloperidol: 0.8 ng/ml; and ziprasidone: 70.0 ng/ml [23]. The implied olanzapine level of 13.9 ng/ml derived from this analysis is well below values of 22.77 ng/ml (n = 151) [39] and 23.2 ng/ml (n = 84) [39] obtained by ROC analyses from clinical trials enrolling chronic schizophrenia patients with mean ages of 41.3 and 36.8 years, respectively.

Figure 2.4 Adverse effects and response based on fitted D_2 occupancy curves for D_2 antagonist antipsychotics [38]

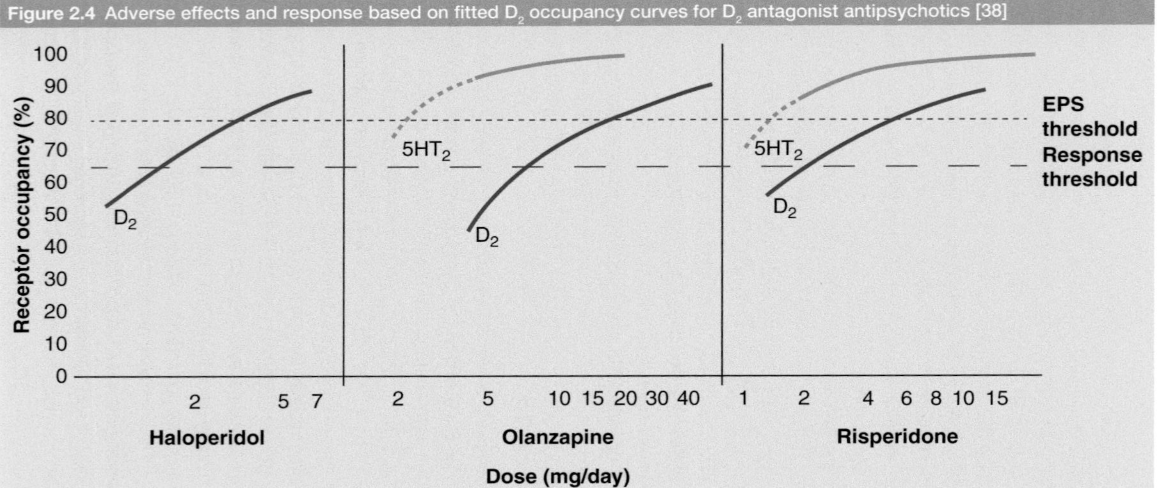

(Adapted from: S. Kapur and P. Seeman [2001]. Does fast dissociation from the dopamine d(2) receptor explain the action of atypical antipsychotics? A new hypothesis. *Am J Psychiatry*, 158, 360–369.)

The development of imaging techniques has been a boon to our understanding of D_2 antagonism, and helped to define ranges of D_2 occupancy best suited to antagonist antipsychotics for most patients with schizophrenia. The difficulty in translating thresholds averaged from numerous participants is the need to treat outliers on the dose and plasma level response curve [40, 12]. Unlike medications with very narrow therapeutic indices, there is an extremely broad range of plasma antipsychotic levels which some patients tolerate and where they respond. PET imaging has shown that the risk for neurological adverse effects is seen (on average) when one exceeds 78%–80% D_2 occupancy [41]; however, clinical studies clearly indicate that a substantial proportion may tolerate significantly higher levels of D_2 receptor blockade without experiencing neurological adverse effects. One example is seen in the 1994 pivotal risperidone trial results. The authors noted that 39% of subjects receiving risperidone 16 mg/d, and 47% receiving haloperidol 20 mg/d required antiparkinsonian medications despite exposure to doses associated with > 90% D_2 blockade [42]. Many schizophrenia patients do not benefit from very high plasma antipsychotic levels, and, in routine usage, this is often discouraged by practice guidelines or by local prescribing regulations that restrict maximum dosages to the licensed dosage range [13, 14]. Nonetheless, there are certain outpatients or inpatients in specialized forensic settings who require and tolerate > 80% D_2 antagonism for optimal positive symptom control [12]. Using antipsychotics in this manner for these patients is not inherently unsafe, but must be pursued with careful documentation of plasma levels and other safety monitoring as appropriate, and with a full understanding that the benefit to most schizophrenia patients from high plasma levels that exceed 80% D_2 occupancy is limited, even when tolerated [14].

The 'ideal' range of 65%–80% D_2 occupancy may not apply to certain outliers, and also does not apply to antipsychotics whose primary therapeutic mechanism is not D_2 antagonism. Since 2002, three partial agonist antipsychotics have been approved in the US (aripiprazole, brexpiprazole, cariprazine), all of which have intrinsic activity at D_2 receptors estimated in the range 18%–24% [43, 44]. To achieve clinical response in schizophrenia, the partial agonists not only have very high *in vitro* affinity for the D_2 receptor, they generally require a minimum of 80% D_2 occupancy. For aripiprazole and cariprazine, the expected D_2 occupancy threshold for response is close to 80%, and the upper end of the range is essentially 100% (Figure 2.5) [45–47]. Brexpiprazole is also a partial agonist, but appears to have a slightly lower threshold for response of 65% to 80% as seen with D_2 antagonists. The recommended brexpiprazole dose range for schizophrenia is 2–4 mg/d, and a PET study of schizophrenia patients (mean age 42 ± 8 years) found that the subtherapeutic dose of 1 mg yielded 65% D_2 receptor occupancy, while 4 mg averaged 80% [48].

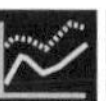

Figure 2.5 Fitted D_2 occupancy curve for aripiprazole in the dosage range of 10–30 mg/d [49]

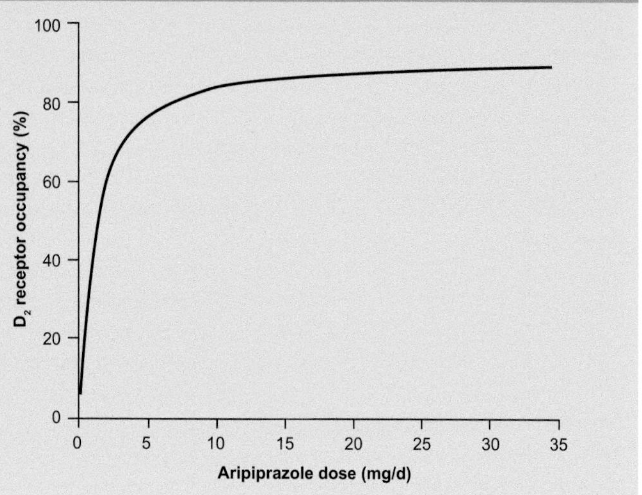

(Adapted from: D. Mamo, A. Graff, R. Mizrahi, *et al.* [2007]. Differential effects of aripiprazole on D(2), 5-HT(2), and 5-HT(1A) receptor occupancy in patients with schizophrenia: a triple tracer PET study. *Am J Psychiatry*, 164, 1411–1417.)

Dopamine D_2 occupancy thresholds also do not apply to agents whose mechanism is not highly dependent on D_2 antagonism. Clozapine was the first example of an antipsychotic for which trough levels of D_2 occupancy were well under 65%, and even at peak plasma levels only transiently exceeded this occupancy threshold [50]. This same finding is also seen with the weak D_2 antagonist quetiapine [51], and the newly approved antipsychotic lumateperone [52]. Perhaps the most extreme example is the antipsychotic pimavanserin, a medication approved for Parkinson's disease psychosis with positive data for dementia-related psychosis. Pimavanserin is a highly selective inverse agonist at serotonin $5HT_{2A}$ (Ki 0.087 nM) and $5HT_{2C}$ (Ki 0.44 nM) receptors, and lacks affinity for any other monoamine receptor [53, 54]. While pimavanserin is not approved for the treatment of schizophrenia, there are agents in development for schizophrenia which lack any D_2 binding: the muscarinic M_1 and M_4 agonist xanomeline, and the trace amine associated receptor-1 (TAAR1) agonist SEP-363856 [55–58]. A range of D_2 occupancy is thus associated with antipsychotic response depending on the molecule (Figure 2.6), but for medications whose mechanism is not fully understood

Figure 2.6 Range of D_2 occupancy for antipsychotics

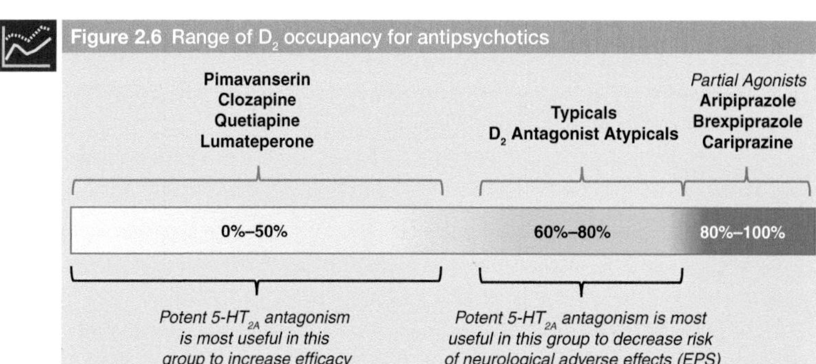

(e.g. TAAR1 agonists), or that have limited or no D_2 binding (e.g. clozapine, lumateperone, pimavanserin, xanomeline, SEP-363856), PET imaging will not be the primary means to decide on a plasma level cutoff for response. For these agents, one can still create ROC analyses from clinical trials to calculate a plasma level response threshold. ROC analyses are based solely on the proportion of responders/nonresponders at various plasma levels, and are thus agnostic with regards to the presumed mechanism of action.

3 Inference from Minimum Effective Dose

Since the fortuitous discovery of chlorpromazine's antipsychotic property, it has become apparent that the extremely high antipsychotic doses routinely used in the 1950s–1980s are not necessary for most patients [24]. PET studies find that a haloperidol dose of 2–5 mg/d generates roughly 65%–80% D_2 occupancy (Figure 2.4), yet starting doses of 40 mg/d or more were not uncommon in the 1970s [59]. The large NIMH-sponsored Clinical Antipsychotic Trials of Intervention Effectiveness (CATIE) schizophrenia study used perphenazine as the first-generation comparator to the second-generation antipsychotics for that study [60]. In this group of chronic schizophrenia patients (n = 1493), the mean modal dose of perphenazine was 20.8 mg/d, equivalent to only 5.55 mg/d of haloperidol [33]. Based on analyses of clinical trials outcomes, investigators have sought to find the minimum effective dose (MED) for antipsychotics as a means of expressing relative equivalent doses [61]. The leading author of these studies is Stefan Leucht, a professor of psychiatry at Technische Universität in Munich, and his many papers examine a variety of means to express antipsychotic equivalent dosages, including the World Health Organization defined daily dose (DDD) method, and consensus guidelines [61–63, 24]. MED is clinically useful as it is the lowest dose that significantly differs from placebo in a double-blind randomized trial. MED thus serves as a point of reference for an initial dose, and can be used to guide dosing based on an international consensus study which recommended that an antipsychotic dose for acute schizophrenia should be in the range of 2–3 times the MED [64]. From MED estimates, one can calculate the corresponding plasma level for any antipsychotic dose from known data on plasma concentration–dose relationships.

MED estimates have a significant amount of clinical value, but the approach is quite different than ROC analyses of responder and nonresponders drawn directly from the plasma level data. Any method which uses dosing cannot account for low rates of adherence with oral antipsychotics, and population variations in drug metabolism due to genetic or environmental exposures (e.g. inhibitors/inducers, smoking, etc.). However, plasma levels for certain antipsychotics are often not available due to the lack of qualified laboratories performing the assay locally, or the fact that the medication is very new (e.g. cariprazine, lumateperone), and there is not as yet widespread demand to develop a commercial laboratory assay. In those instances, the MED is extremely helpful and clinicians can read the publications employing this method to arrive at clinically relevant doses for oral and long-acting injectable antipsychotics [63, 65].

B Evidence Used to Define an Upper Limit

Increased systemic antipsychotic exposure not only increases the likelihood of adverse effects, this often comes with little promise of increased efficacy [14]. It is due to the compelling need to balance efficacy and tolerability that the British Association for Psychopharmacology (BAP) 2020 guidelines suggest aiming for doses that are effective in 50% of the population [14]. The BAP guidelines also note that: "There is little evidence to support exceeding British National Formulary (BNF) maximum recommended doses or even maximum effective doses identified in reviews and meta-analyses of trials, and certainly not unless blood concentrations are unexpectedly low on testing." Yet the BAP also acknowledges that outliers do exist, and comments that for cases where the risk of continuing illness is high, clinicians might consider doses effective in 90% of the population. The question confronting societies and clinicians is where to draw a line based on plasma levels that acknowledges that the spectrum of tolerability and response might necessarily need to incorporate outliers. ROC analyses performed to estimate a response threshold only demand that one come to a definition of response (e.g. 50% symptom reduction) – from this response definition, the ROC result is immediately understandable [27]. Depending on how one wishes to weight tolerability or prioritize the inclusion of outliers on the response curve, a myriad of possible cutoffs can be generated to justify an upper limit.

Unfortunately, the numerous suggested upper limits for antipsychotic levels are at times confusing, and often do not make explicit the reasoning regarding trade-offs between decreasing tolerability and incremental response. (What laboratories choose to report as their upper limit is even more problematic, and is discussed extensively in Chapter 3). There are also varying rationales about the weighting of imaging data in this process, and whether the upper limit is based on regulations that preclude exceeding licensed dose maxima. The difficulties encountered by experts in this area reflect these issues. As noted previously, the AGNP/ASCP consensus paper represents the most current well-reasoned source on use of plasma antipsychotic levels, drawing heavily on prior extensive work from AGNP [13, 15]. The suggested upper limit for haloperidol is 10 ng/ml, a level where slightly more than 50% might experience intolerable adverse effects [9], yet the recommended upper limit for fluphenazine, another potent D_2 antagonist, is 10 ng/ml, a level that presumably would be intolerable to > 95% of patients if one extrapolates from available data (Figure 2.7) [16]. That thoughtful investigators struggle with defining plasma level upper limits reflects the

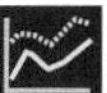

Figure 2.7 Plasma fluphenazine levels and proportion of patients with response (dotted line) or intolerable adverse effects (solid line) [16]

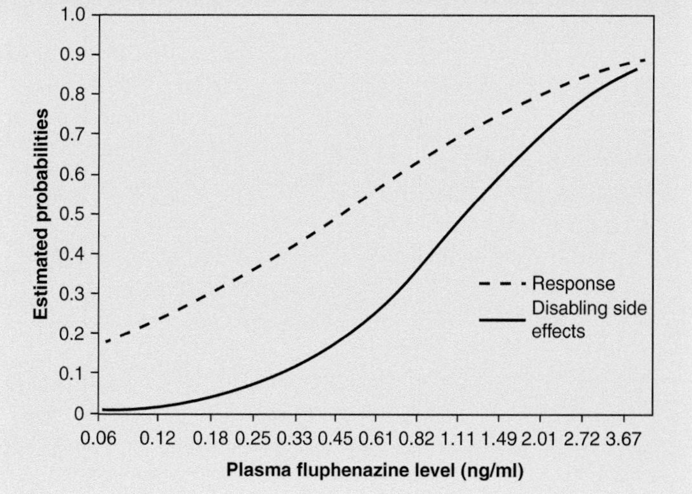

(Adapted from: K. K. Midha, J. W. Hubbard, S. R. Marder, *et al.* [1994]. Impact of clinical pharmacokinetics on neuroleptic therapy in patients with schizophrenia. *J Psychiatry Neurosci*, 19, 254–264.)

myriad of inputs involved, and the limitations of existing clinical data. Clinicians should appreciate the sources of information that go into these decisions, and the evolution of a concept elaborated for treatment of more severely ill inpatients, ***the point of futility***, which provides a clear rationale for a plasma level choice [12].

1 Upper Limits Based on Maximum Approved Dosages for Schizophrenia

The recommendations from BAP and AGNP acknowledge that in certain countries, or in certain practice locations, there are strict limits placed on the highest dose that can be used for a particular antipsychotic derived from what is listed in the approved package insert for schizophrenia treatment [14, 15]. Such decisions represent the compelling interest that national or local health agencies have in limiting unsafe practices, and the choice to enact these policies in a method that applies equally to all antipsychotics, and uses information readily available to every clinician. While the AGNP/ASCP consensus papers describe upper limits estimated from the clinical literature, clinicians must be mindful that certain reviews and laboratory ranges may be based solely on the licensed dosage range for that country, despite abundant subsequent data demonstrating the safety and utility of higher dosages (and higher corresponding plasma levels). This may explain why the upper limits expressed in national or hospital policy documents differ greatly from those espoused in this handbook or the AGNP/ASCP review.

2 Upper Limits Based on PET Imaging of D_2 Occupancy

For antipsychotics whose primary mechanism relies on D_2 antagonism, exceeding 78%–80% D_2 occupancy incurs greater risk for neurological adverse effects, although there are clearly patients who can tolerate > 90% D_2 occupancy [66, 67]. In addition to the more overt neurological manifestations, > 80% D_2 blockade is also associated with decreased subjective well-being for D_2 antagonist antipsychotics [68, 37, 69, 70]. As noted above, the partial agonists aripiprazole and cariprazine operate between 80% and 100% D_2 occupancy, so this relationship with subjective well-being and D_2 occupancy is not found [45]. As the risk for parkinsonism, akathisia, and dystonia emerges at 80% D_2 blockade, this does not imply that the majority of patients at that threshold are experiencing those adverse effects. An early PET imaging study noted that a daily risperidone dose between 6 and 8 mg crossed the 80% occupancy threshold (Figure 2.4) [38], and a subsequent study by that same group found that 80% D_2 blockade corresponded to an active moiety level (risperidone + 9-OH risperidone) of 45 ng/ml, equivalent to 6.43 mg/d of oral risperidone [71]. However, in the pivotal risperidone trial, only 20% required antiparkinsonian medication at

6 mg/d and 31% at 10 mg/d [42]. A decision to use a plasma level that generates 80% D_2 blockade as the upper limit would seem overly conservative, but the choice of higher occupancy levels involves the same judgment decision alluded to above: how much D_2 antagonism is it acceptable to recommend so that a small subgroup of patients are given access to high levels that might be intolerable for most. There is no universal agreement on this point, but the understanding of D_2 occupancy–plasma level relationships for many antipsychotics helps inform the discussion about upper limits. This information does not apply to medications whose antipsychotic response is not dependent on > 60% D_2 antagonism (e.g. aripiprazole, cariprazine, clozapine, lumateperone, quetiapine).

3 95% Effective Dose

The BAP recommendations to consider doses effective in 90% of patients for select cases involves both the decision to use the 90% threshold (as opposed to 80%, 85%, etc.), and acknowledgment of the reality that some patients both respond to and tolerate high plasma antipsychotic levels [14]. The classic graphic on fluphenazine response and adverse effects (Figure 2.7) indicates that, at the level where 90% respond, a nearly equal proportion will experience intolerable adverse effects [16]; however, this is grouped data that may not apply to specific individuals, a finding described in the literature for over 50 years [72]. Using the logic that clinical trials data might provide insight into dosage ranges effective in the majority of chronic schizophrenia patients with acute exacerbation, Stefan Leucht published a meta-analysis in 2020 of 68 placebo-controlled dose-finding studies for oral and long-acting injectable second-generation antipsychotics and for haloperidol [65]. Based on changes in BPRS or PANSS total scores, doses that produced 95% of the maximum symptom reduction were identified, some examples of which are: haloperidol 6.3 mg/d, olanzapine 15.2 mg/d, and risperidone 6.3 mg/d. The limits of using dose to define drug exposure have been discussed previously, but this type of analysis is quite useful for examining trials data in a clinically relatable manner. The risperidone result of 6.3 mg maps very closely to the plasma level associated with 80% D_2 occupancy, but the olanzapine dose of 15.2 mg falls under that threshold, and the expected plasma olanzapine level from 15 mg/d (30 ng/ml) is well below the upper limit of 80 ng/ml suggested by the AGNP/ASCP review [38, 18, 15].

That the conclusions from this analysis vary from other sources does not represent a methodological flaw, but differences between this type of analysis and a responder analysis. This method does not identify the dose at which 95% of patients might respond (with response defined as 30%–50% symptom reduction), but the dose that, on average, is expected to achieve 95% of the possible symptom reduction seen for that antipsychotic. Providing another source of upper limits is important to the evolving literature in this area, but may be confusing to clinicians whose basic question revolves around the maximum plasma level one can pursue in search of adequate response. This meta-analysis also relies heavily on registrational trial data. Industry-sponsored studies typically screen out individuals with certain medical disorders, substance use, and other psychiatric comorbidities, and thus utilize a subgroup of schizophrenia patients who may not be representative of a more general schizophrenia population. For example, the oral olanzapine calculations are based on two studies [65].

The Point of Futility

The multiple definitions of upper limits can be confusing to clinicians who are not intimately familiar with the information each source used. This can lead to situations where providers conflate maximal levels based on responder analyses with imminent safety issues, leading to erroneous conclusions that a level beyond the upper limit must be dangerous and should be reduced immediately [18]. This distinction between an upper limit for response and issues of possible safety is embodied in the AGNP history of separating therapeutic reference ranges from laboratory levels. In discussing this issue, AGNP clearly states that for most psychotropics such as antipsychotics "concentrations in blood with an increased risk of toxicity are normally much higher than the upper threshold levels of the therapeutic reference ranges" [13]. In doing so, they conceptualized a level that would mandate laboratory notification of the prescriber – the **laboratory alert level**. For some psychotropic medications with narrow therapeutic indices (e.g. lithium), these laboratory alert levels are derived from case reports of drug intoxication, but in most instances the alert level was arbitrarily defined as a drug concentration in blood that is two-fold higher than the upper limit of the therapeutic reference range [13]. The underlying method is thus clearly spelt out, and this information is included in the AGNP/ASCP consensus paper [15].

There are some practical issues for implementation of this dual system of reference ranges and laboratory alert levels:

a Laboratory reports generally only contain one range (see Chapter 3), and there has not been acceptance in many countries of this dual limit system, or from laboratories themselves to incorporate the recommended alert levels.

b While laboratories may never adopt the AGNP system, large hospital systems could potentially make this information available internally. As noted previously, having two different limits (an upper limit for the therapeutic range and a laboratory alert level) has the potential to engender confusion, as noted above; moreover, the concept that reported laboratory plasma level ranges for antipsychotics may not represent an imminent safety issue is difficult for most clinicians to accept, often leading to inappropriate sizable dosage decreases in asymptomatic patients [18]. The concern is that, when presented with two systems, clinicians will practice based on one set of values (typically the lower value reported as the upper limit of the therapeutic range) since this is most consistent with what current laboratory reports include.

As a means of simplifying clinical decision making around these upper limits, the term ***point of futility*** was created within the California Department of State Hospitals (Cal-DSH) system as a term of art [12]. Cal-DSH has five campuses with over 6500 patients, 90% of whom have schizophrenia spectrum disorders, with care provided by approximately 200 psychiatrists. Given the varying levels of expertise among the psychiatrists, the term ***point of futility*** was developed to educate clinicians about two important concepts with regards to an upper limit for antipsychotic plasma levels [12]:

a While intolerability is a hard endpoint signaling the end of an antipsychotic trial, a small proportion of patients may never exhibit dose-limiting adverse effects and will tolerate further antipsychotic titration, even with high potency first-generation antipsychotics [72]. Although a plasma fluphenazine level of 4.0 ng/ml is intolerable to > 90% of the population [16], levels ranging from 6.13 to 16.19 ng/ml were documented in early PET studies, and one trial reported a subject with a level of 27.9 ng/ml who was not taking medication for parkinsonism or for akathisia [73, 74].

b Although intolerability may not limit the drug trial in some instances, ongoing titration beyond a certain plasma level (the point of futility) is fruitless as a minuscule fraction of patients will respond to these higher plasma levels [16, 12]. For example, the compelling reason why a fluphenazine level of 4.0 ng/ml is viewed as a point of futility is that the probability of response in those patients who can tolerate a plasma level of 4.0 ng/ml is < 5%, as illustrated elegantly in Figure 2.8 [16, 18].

The latter point is crucial, as clinicians are sometimes wary of starting clozapine and will instead continue to hope that 'more is better' by pursuing seemingly heroic plasma levels of other antipsychotics to achieve schizophrenia response [75, 76]. **The concept of a point of futility also permits the clinician to have a single reference for an upper limit which suffices as both the top of the therapeutic range and**

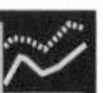

Figure 2.8 Estimated probability of improvement in the absence of disabling adverse effects based on plasma fluphenazine level [16]

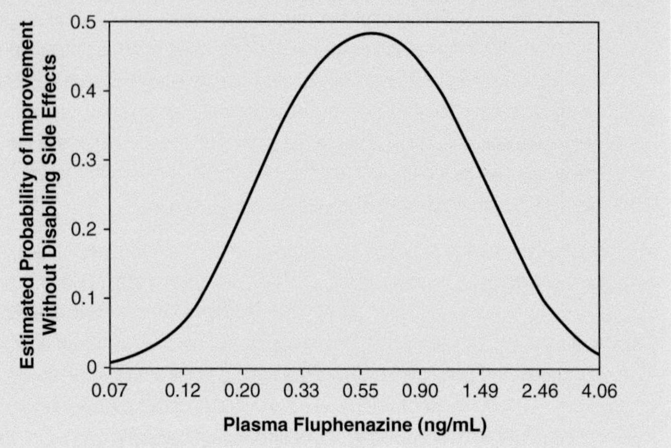

(Adapted from: K. K. Midha, J. W. Hubbard, S. R. Marder, *et al.* [1994]. Impact of clinical pharmacokinetics on neuroleptic therapy in patients with schizophrenia. *J Psychiatry Neurosci*, 19, 254–264.)

an informal alert level demanding that the clinician assess the situation and examine the patient for adverse effects [18]. While the proportion of responders in the interval between the upper limit of the AGNP/ASCP therapeutic range and the alert level is expected to be small, for the management of more severely ill inpatients, that additional yield may be important. If it is deemed reasonable to have a clozapine laboratory alert level of 1000 ng/ml, placing the top of the therapeutic range at 600 ng/ml might dissuade some psychiatrists from pursuing levels of 601–999 ng/ml that could benefit inadequate responders to lower plasma levels [19].

The point of futility largely overlaps with the laboratory alert level, but not in every instance. For example, there appears to be no safety concern to mandate a laboratory alert until fluphenazine levels reach 15 ng/ml [13], yet in clinical trials there are vanishingly few responders at levels above 4.0 ng/ml, as noted in Figures 2.7 and 2.8 and documented elsewhere, so the value of 4.0 ng/ml has been used as the Cal-DSH point of futility for fluphenazine [16, 12]. Throughout this handbook, a justification will be provided for each therapeutic threshold and point of futility estimate, along with the AGNP/ASCP laboratory alert level for comparison. These terminologies represent thoughtful approaches by various groups on how to best educate clinicians about plasma antipsychotic levels, and provide the information in an accessible form to optimize schizophrenia treatment. By outlining the basic evidence supporting a choice of threshold level or point of futility, it is hoped that clinicians will be better able to make sense of conflicting ranges from laboratory reports and other sources, to decide the best course of action for their patient.

Summary Points

a The best sources of information to estimate a therapeutic threshold are ROC curves from multiple fixed-dose schizophrenia studies with plasma level data on responders and nonresponders at various levels. Other types of information (e.g. PET imaging of D_2 occupancy, inference from minimally effective doses) is supportive, but not as robust as the clinically based data.

b What laboratories report as the upper limit of the therapeutic range varies dramatically between sources. The AGNP/ASCP laboratory alert level is a useful construct, although in most instances the alert level was arbitrarily defined as a plasma level two-fold higher than the upper limit of the therapeutic reference range. Nonetheless, it represents a threshold demanding that the clinician be alerted by the laboratory to assess the situation and examine the patient for adverse effects.

c The point of futility is a term devised to provide clinicians a single upper limit value, and to educate clinicians about two important concepts: (1) a small proportion of patients may never exhibit dose-limiting adverse effects and will tolerate further titration; (2) ongoing titration beyond a certain plasma level (the point of futility) is fruitless as $< 5\%$ of patients may respond to these higher plasma levels.

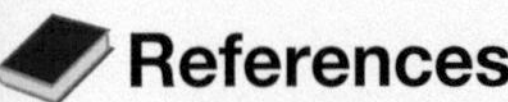

References

1. **Willcox, D. R., Gillan, R., and Hare, E. H. (1965).** Do psychiatric out-patients take their drugs? *BMJ*, 2, 790–792.
2. **Curry, S. H., Davis, J. M., Janowsky, D. S., *et al.* (1970).** Factors affecting chlorpromazine plasma levels in psychiatric patients. *Arch Gen Psychiatry*, 22, 209–215.
3. **Overall, J. E. and Gorham, D. R. (1962).** The Brief Psychiatric Rating Scale. *Psychological Reports*, 10, 799–812.
4. **Curry, S. H. (1968).** The determination and possible significance of plasma levels of chlorpromazine in psychiatric patients. *Agressologie*, 9, 115–121.
5. **Curry, S. H. and Marshall, J. H. (1968).** Plasma levels of chlorpromazine and some of its relatively non-polar metabolites in psychiatric patients. *Life Sci*, 7, 9–17.
6. **Kay, S. R., Fiszbein, A., and Opler, L. A. (1987).** The positive and negative syndrome scale (PANSS) for schizophrenia. *Schizophr Bull*, 13, 261–276.
7. **Sakalis, G., Curry, S. H., Mould, G. P., *et al.* (1972).** Physiologic and clinical effects of chlorpromazine and their relationship to plasma level. *Clin Pharmacol Ther*, 13, 931–946.
8. **Van Putten, T., May, P. R., and Jenden, D. J. (1981).** Does a plasma level of chlorpromazine help? *Psychol Med*, 11, 729–734.
9. **Van Putten, T., Marder, S. R., Wirshing, W. C., *et al.* (1991).** Neuroleptic plasma levels. *Schizophr Bull*, 17, 197–216.
10. **Nielsen, J., Graff, C., Kanters, J. K., *et al.* (2011).** Assessing QT prolongation of antipsychotic drugs. *CNS Drugs*, 25, 473–490.
11. **Van Putten, T., Aravagiri, M., Marder, S. R., *et al.* (1991).** Plasma fluphenazine levels and clinical response in newly admitted schizophrenic patients. *Psychopharmacol Bull*, 27, 91–96.
12. **Meyer, J. M. (2014).** A rational approach to employing high plasma levels of antipsychotics for violence associated with schizophrenia: case vignettes. *CNS Spectr*, 19, 432–438.
13. **Hiemke, C., Bergemann, N., Clement, H. W., *et al.* (2018).** Consensus guidelines for therapeutic drug monitoring in neuropsychopharmacology: update 2017. *Pharmacopsychiatry*, 51, 9–62.
14. **Barnes, T. R., Drake, R., Paton, C., *et al.* (2020).** Evidence-based guidelines for the pharmacological treatment of schizophrenia: Updated recommendations from the British Association for Psychopharmacology. *J Psychopharmacol*, 34, 3–78.
15. **Schoretsanitis, G., Kane, J. M., Correll, C. U., *et al.* (2020).** Blood levels to optimize antipsychotic treatment in clinical practice; a joint consensus statement of the American Society of Clinical Psychopharmacology (ASCP) and the Therapeutic Drug Monitoring (TDM) Task Force of the Arbeitsgemeinschaft für Neuropsychopharmakologie und Pharmakopsychiatrie (AGNP). *J Clin Psychiatry*, 81, https://doi.org/10.4088/JCP.4019cs13169.
16. **Midha, K. K., Hubbard, J. W., Marder, S. R., *et al.* (1994).** Impact of clinical pharmacokinetics on neuroleptic therapy in patients with schizophrenia. *J Psychiatry Neurosci*, 19, 254–264.
17. **Marder, S. R., Davis, J. M., and Janicak, P. G., eds. (1993).** *Clinical Use of Neuroleptic Plasma Levels.* Washington, DC: American Psychiatric Press Inc.
18. **Meyer, J. M. (2020).** Monitoring and improving antipsychotic adherence in outpatient forensic diversion programs. *CNS Spectr*, 25, 136–144.
19. **Remington, G., Agid, O., Foussias, G., *et al.* (2013).** Clozapine and therapeutic drug monitoring: Is there sufficient evidence for an upper threshold? *Psychopharmacology (Berl)*, 225, 505–518.
20. **Lopez, L. V. and Kane, J. M. (2013).** Plasma levels of second-generation antipsychotics and clinical response in acute psychosis: A review of the literature. *Schizophr Res*, 147, 368–374.
21. **Grandjean, E. M. and Aubry, J.-M. (2009).** Lithium: Updated human knowledge using an evidence-based approach. Part II: Clinical pharmacology and therapeutic monitoring. *CNS Drugs*, 23, 331–349.

22. **Machado-Vieira, R., Otaduy, M. C., Zanetti, M. V., *et al.* (2016).** A selective association between central and peripheral lithium levels in remitters in bipolar depression: A 3T-(7) Li magnetic resonance spectroscopy study. *Acta Psychiatr Scand*, 133, 214–220.
23. **Uchida, H., Takeuchi, H., Graff-Guerrero, A., *et al.* (2011).** Predicting dopamine D2 receptor occupancy from plasma levels of antipsychotic drugs: A systematic review and pooled analysis. *J Clin Psychopharmacol*, 31, 318–325.
24. **Takeuchi, H., MacKenzie, N. E., Samaroo, D., *et al.* (2020).** Antipsychotic dose in acute schizophrenia: A meta-analysis. *Schizophr Bull*, 46, 1439–1458.
25. **Melkote, R., Singh, A., Vermeulen, A., *et al.* (2018).** Relationship between antipsychotic blood levels and treatment failure during the Clinical Antipsychotic Trials of Intervention Effectiveness (CATIE) study. *Schizophr Res*, 201, 324–328.
26. **Correll, C. U., Jain, R., Meyer, J. M., *et al.* (2019).** Relationship between the timing of relapse and plasma drug levels following discontinuation of cariprazine treatment in patients with schizophrenia: Indirect comparison with other second-generation antipsychotics after treatment discontinuation. *Neuropsychiatr Dis Treat*, 15, 2537–2550.
27. **Samara, M. T., Leucht, C., Leeflang, M. M., *et al.* (2015).** Early improvement as a predictor of later response to antipsychotics in schizophrenia: A diagnostic test review. *Am J Psychiatry*, 172, 617–629.
28. **Meyer, J. M. and Stahl, S. M. (2019).** *The Clozapine Handbook*. Cambridge: Cambridge University Press.
29. **Van Putten, T., Marder, S. R., and Mintz, J. (1985).** Plasma haloperidol levels: Clinical response and fancy mathematics. *Arch Gen Psychiatry*, 42, 835–838.
30. **Perry, P. J., Miller, D. D., Arndt, S. V., *et al.* (1991).** Clozapine and norclozapine plasma concentrations and clinical response of treatment-refractory schizophrenic patients. *Am J Psychiatry*, 148, 231–235.
31. **Kronig, M. H., Munne, R. A., Szymanski, S., *et al.* (1995).** Plasma clozapine levels and clinical response for treatment-refractory schizophrenic patients. *Am J Psychiatry*, 152, 179–182.
32. **Lu, M. L., Wu, Y. X., Chen, C. H., *et al.* (2016).** Application of plasma levels of olanzapine and N-desmethyl-olanzapine to monitor clinical efficacy in patients with schizophrenia. *PLoS One*, 11, e0148539.
33. **Meyer, J. M. (2018).** Pharmacotherapy of psychosis and mania. In L. L. Brunton, R. Hilal-Dandan, and B. C. Knollmann, eds., *Goodman & Gilman's The Pharmacological Basis of Therapeutics*, 13th edn. Chicago, IL: McGraw-Hill, pp. 279–302.
34. **Farde, L., Hall, H., Ehrin, E., *et al.* (1986).** Quantitative analysis of D2 dopamine receptor binding in the living human brain by PET. *Science*, 231, 258–261.
35. **Kirino, S., Suzuki, T., Takeuchi, H., *et al.* (2017).** Representativeness of clinical PET study participants with schizophrenia: A systematic review. *J Psychiatr Res*, 88, 72–79.
36. **Arakawa, R., Takano, A., and Halldin, C. (2020).** PET technology for drug development in psychiatry. *Neuropsychopharmacol Rep*, 40, 114–121.
37. **de Haan, L., van Bruggen, M., Lavalaye, J., *et al.* (2003).** Subjective experience and D2 receptor occupancy in patients with recent-onset schizophrenia treated with low-dose olanzapine or haloperidol: a randomized, double-blind study. *Am J Psychiatry*, 160, 303–309.
38. **Kapur, S. and Seeman, P. (2001).** Does fast dissociation from the dopamine d(2) receptor explain the action of atypical antipsychotics? A new hypothesis. *Am J Psychiatry*, 158, 360–369.
39. **Perry, P. J., Lund, B. C., Sanger, T., *et al.* (2001).** Olanzapine plasma concentrations and clinical response: Acute phase results of the North American Olanzapine Trial. *J Clin Psychopharmacol*, 21, 14–20.
40. **Preskorn, S. H. (2010).** Outliers on the dose–response curve: How to minimize this problem using therapeutic drug monitoring, an underutilized tool in psychiatry. *J Psychiatr Pract*, 16, 177–182.

41. **Kapur, S., Zipursky, R., Jones, C., *et al.* (2000).** Relationship between dopamine D(2) occupancy, clinical response, and side effects: A double-blind PET study of first-episode schizophrenia. *Am J Psychiatry*, 157, 514–520.
42. **Marder, S. R. and Meibach, R. C. (1994).** Risperidone in the treatment of schizophrenia. *Am J Psychiatry*, 151, 825–835.
43. **Tadori, Y., Forbes, R. A., McQuade, R. D., *et al.* (2011).** In vitro pharmacology of aripiprazole, its metabolite and experimental dopamine partial agonists at human dopamine D2 and D3 receptors. *Eur J Pharmacol*, 668, 355–365.
44. **Maeda, K., Sugino, H., Akazawa, H., *et al.* (2014).** Brexpiprazole I: In vitro and in vivo characterization of a novel serotonin-dopamine activity modulator. *J Pharmacol Exp Ther*, 350, 589–604.
45. **Mizrahi, R., Mamo, D., Rusjan, P., *et al.* (2009).** The relationship between subjective well-being and dopamine D2 receptors in patients treated with a dopamine partial agonist and full antagonist antipsychotics. *Int J Neuropsychopharmacol*, 12, 715–721.
46. **Sparshatt, A., Taylor, D., Patel, M. X., *et al.* (2010).** A systematic review of aripiprazole – dose, plasma concentration, receptor occupancy, and response: Implications for therapeutic drug monitoring. *J Clin Psychiatry*, 71, 1447–1556.
47. **Girgis, R. R., Slifstein, M., D'Souza, D., *et al.* (2016).** Preferential binding to dopamine D3 over D2 receptors by cariprazine in patients with schizophrenia using PET with the D3/D2 receptor ligand [(11)C]-(+)-PHNO. *Psychopharmacology (Berl)*, 233, 3503–3512.
48. **Girgis, R. R., Forbes, A., Abi-Dargham, A., *et al.* (2020).** A positron emission tomography occupancy study of brexpiprazole at dopamine D2 and D3 and serotonin 5-HT1A and 5-HT2A receptors, and serotonin reuptake transporters in subjects with schizophrenia. *Neuropsychopharmacology*, 45, 786–792.
49. **Mamo, D., Graff, A., Mizrahi, R., *et al.* (2007).** Differential effects of aripiprazole on D(2), 5-HT(2), and 5-HT(1A) receptor occupancy in patients with schizophrenia: A triple tracer PET study. *Am J Psychiatry*, 164, 1411–1417.
50. **Wiesel, F. A., Farde, L., Nordstrom, A. L., *et al.* (1990).** Central D1- and D2-receptor occupancy during antipsychotic drug treatment. *Prog Neuro-Psychopharmacol Biol Psychiatry*, 14, 759–767.
51. **Gefvert, O., Bergstrom, M., Langstrom, B., *et al.* (1998).** Time course of central nervous dopamine-D2 and 5-HT2 receptor blockade and plasma drug concentrations after discontinuation of quetiapine (Seroquel) in patients with schizophrenia. *Psychopharmacology*, 135, 119–126.
52. **Vanover, K. E., Davis, R. E., Zhou, Y., *et al.* (2019).** Dopamine D2 receptor occupancy of lumateperone (ITI-007): A Positron Emission Tomography Study in patients with schizophrenia. *Neuropsychopharmacology*, 44, 598–605.
53. **Meltzer, H. Y. and Roth, B. L. (2013).** Lorcaserin and pimavanserin: Emerging selectivity of serotonin receptor subtype-targeted drugs. *J Clin Invest*, 123, 4986–4991.
54. **Stahl, S. M. (2016).** Mechanism of action of pimavanserin in Parkinson's disease psychosis: Targeting serotonin 5HT2A and 5HT2C receptors. *CNS Spectr*, 21, 271–275.
55. **Shekhar, A., Potter, W. Z., Lightfoot, J., *et al.* (2008).** Selective muscarinic receptor agonist xanomeline as a novel treatment approach for schizophrenia. *Am J Psychiatry*, 165, 1033–1039.
56. **Barak, S. and Weiner, I. (2011).** The M_1/M_4 preferring agonist xanomeline reverses amphetamine-, MK801- and scopolamine-induced abnormalities of latent inhibition: Putative efficacy against positive, negative and cognitive symptoms in schizophrenia. *Int J Neuropsychopharmacol*, 14, 1233–1246.
57. **Simmler, L. D., Buchy, D., Chaboz, S., *et al.* (2016).** In vitro characterization of psychoactive substances at rat, mouse, and human trace amine-associated receptor 1. *J Pharmacol Exp Ther*, 357, 134–144.

58. **Dedic, N., Jones, P. G., Hopkins, S. C., *et al.* (2019).** SEP-363856, a novel psychotropic agent with a unique, non-D2 receptor mechanism of action. *J Pharmacol Exp Ther*, 371, 1–14.
59. **Cohen, W. J. and Cohen, N. H. (1974).** Lithium carbonate, haloperidol, and irreversible brain damage. *JAMA*, 230, 1283–1287.
60. **Lieberman, J. A., Stroup, T. S., McEvoy, J. P., *et al.* (2005).** Effectiveness of antipsychotic drugs in patients with chronic schizophrenia. *N Engl J Med*, 353, 1209–1223.
61. **Leucht, S., Samara, M., Heres, S., *et al.* (2014).** Dose equivalents for second-generation antipsychotics: The minimum effective dose method. *Schizophr Bull*, 40, 314–326.
62. **Leucht, S., Samara, M., Heres, S., *et al.* (2016).** Dose equivalents for antipsychotic drugs: The DDD method. *Schizophr Bull*, 42 Suppl 1, S90–94.
63. **Rothe, P. H., Heres, S., and Leucht, S. (2018).** Dose equivalents for second generation long-acting injectable antipsychotics: The minimum effective dose method. *Schizophr Res*, 193, 23–28.
64. **Gardner, D. M., Murphy, A. L., O'Donnell, H., *et al.* (2010).** International consensus study of antipsychotic dosing. *Am J Psychiatry*, 167, 686–693.
65. **Leucht, S., Crippa, A., Siafis, S., *et al.* (2020).** Dose-response meta-analysis of antipsychotic drugs for acute schizophrenia. *Am J Psychiatry*, 177, 342–353.
66. **Kapur, S., Remington, G., Zipursky, R. B., *et al.* (1995).** The D2 dopamine receptor occupancy of risperidone and its relationship to extrapyramidal symptoms: A PET study. *Life Sci*, 57, PL103–107.
67. **Nord, M. and Farde, L. (2011).** Antipsychotic occupancy of dopamine receptors in schizophrenia. *CNS Neurosci Ther*, 17, 97–103.
68. **de Haan, L., Lavalaye, J., Linszen, D., *et al.* (2000).** Subjective experience and striatal dopamine D(2) receptor occupancy in patients with schizophrenia stabilized by olanzapine or risperidone. *Am J Psychiatry*, 157, 1019–1020.
69. **Lataster, J., van Os, J., de Haan, L., *et al.* (2011).** Emotional experience and estimates of D2 receptor occupancy in psychotic patients treated with haloperidol, risperidone, or olanzapine: An experience sampling study. *J Clin Psychiatry*, 72, 1397–1404.
70. **Veselinović, T., Scharpenberg, M., Heinze, M., *et al.* (2019).** Dopamine D2 receptor occupancy estimated from plasma concentrations of four different antipsychotics and the subjective experience of physical and mental well-being in schizophrenia: Results from the randomized NeSSy Trial. *J Clin Psychopharmacol*, 39, 550–560.
71. **Remington, G., Mamo, D., Labelle, A., *et al.* (2006).** A PET study evaluating dopamine D2 receptor occupancy for long-acting injectable risperidone. *Am J Psychiatry*, 163, 396–401.
72. **Simpson, G. M. and Kunz-Bartholini, E. (1968).** Relationship of individual tolerance, behavior and phenothiazine produced extrapyramidal system disturbance. *Dis Nerv System*, 29, 269–274.
73. **Miller, R. S., Peterson, G. M., McLean, S., *et al.* (1995).** Monitoring plasma levels of fluphenazine during chronic therapy with fluphenazine decanoate. *J Clin Pharm Ther*, 20, 55–62.
74. **Nyberg, S., Dencker, S. J., Malm, U., *et al.* (1998).** D(2)- and 5-HT(2) receptor occupancy in high-dose neuroleptic-treated patients. *Int J Neuropsychopharmacol*, 1, 95–101.
75. **Cohen, D. (2014).** Prescribers fear as a major side-effect of clozapine. *Acta Psychiatr Scand*, 130, 154–155.
76. **Gee, S., Vergunst, F., Howes, O., *et al.* (2014).** Practitioner attitudes to clozapine initiation. *Acta Psychiatr Scand*, 130, 16–24.

3 Level Interpretation Including Laboratory Reporting Issues, Responding to High Plasma Levels, Special Situations (Hepatic Dysfunction, Renal Dysfunction and Hemodialysis, Bariatric Surgery)

QUICK CHECK

PRINCIPLES

- Laboratory plasma level reports are often devoid of the underlying rationale, with significant variation between laboratories in their choice of the upper limit of the therapeutic range. Adding to the confusion, some laboratories report a therapeutic range, but others report a reference range based on levels for certain dosages. A response to high plasma levels requires a knowledge of the literature for that particular antipsychotic in order to document a reasonable plan of action. In many instances, no dosing change is needed as the laboratory upper limit may be inconsistent with recommendations from other sources.
- Unexpectedly high plasma levels can occur due to improper timing of specimen collection, dosing errors, and occasionally laboratory error. Clozapine appears more susceptible to laboratory error than other antipsychotics, with false positive and erratic results reported even when using state-of-the-art liquid chromatography–mass spectroscopy.

- **Hepatic dysfunction can alter antipsychotic levels when there is advanced cirrhosis, but there is variation between antipsychotics in the necessary dose adjustments. The best method for staging hepatic dysfunction for drug dosing modification is the Child–Pugh classification, which relies on serum albumin, total bilirubin, and INR. Transaminase values (e.g. AST, ALT) play no role in the staging.**
- **Renal dysfunction also alters antipsychotic clearance, especially at values that are very low (creatinine clearance < 30 ml/min), but with variation between antipsychotics in the necessary dose adjustments. Hemodialysis appears to have limited impact on antipsychotic clearance, possibly due to the high protein binding of antipsychotics.**
- **Stable schizophrenia patients scheduled for bariatric surgery must have preoperative plasma antipsychotic levels checked at steady state to permit postoperative adjustments. This is critical for those on oral antipsychotics, but is also useful for patients on long-acting injectable antipsychotics as dosing adjustments may be necessary due to significant decreases in body mass and adipose tissue mass.**

INTRODUCTION

It is rare that clinicians ordering psychotropic levels must concern themselves with the details of laboratory assay methods, or how the results are reported. For example, knowledge of lithium kinetics has existed for nearly 50 years, and lithium is preferentially administered as a single bedtime dose to minimize the renal dysfunction associated with multiple daily doses, to improve adherence, and to facilitate obtaining levels as 12h troughs in the morning [1–4]. Nearly all commercial laboratories use a standard assay method (ion-selective electrode), and there is limited variation in the laboratory reported therapeutic range: the lower limit is typically 0.5 or 0.6 mEq/l, and the upper limit 1.2 mEq/l, with alerts for levels > 1.2, 1.5 or 1.6 mEq/l [3, 5, 6]. Unlike antipsychotics, the therapeutic index for lithium is quite narrow, the literature on levels more mature, and the ranges reported are based on 12h troughs, with papers specifically devoted to the influence of deviations from the 12h mark on serum levels [7].

Variations in laboratory assay methods do play a certain role in interpretation of antipsychotic levels, and are of particular relevance to clozapine [8]; however, the greatest issue confronting clinicians is the lack of consistent reporting for upper limits, with two-fold to five-fold differences in what laboratory reports recommend [9]. Adding to the confusion, some laboratories report a therapeutic range, but others report a 'reference range' based on levels for certain dosages. As the methods for arriving at these upper limit values are poorly defined and the results not obviously evidence-based, clinicians must be armed with sufficient knowledge about commonly used antipsychotics to permit an intelligent response when a plasma level is beyond the laboratory therapeutic or reference range [9]. Unnecessarily drastic dosage decreases or even discontinuation can result in disastrous outcomes, all of which are avoidable by a systematic approach to the high plasma level, based on patient assessment, ruling out changes in kinetic interactions, and accounting for dosing or phlebotomy timing errors [5, 9, 10].

Schizophrenia patients have higher rates of multiple nonpsychiatric comorbidities compared to the general population [11], including obesity, persistent hepatitis C virus (HCV) infection, nonalcoholic steatohepatitis (NASH), and chronic kidney disease [12–18]. All of these disorders might lead to situations that demand adjustment of antipsychotic exposure in newly treated patients, or in those with declining drug clearance, and plasma level assessment is important in those decisions. The literature in this area has evolved significantly in the last two decades, consistent with more sophisticated language in antipsychotic labeling that provides a precise definition for hepatic dysfunction based on Child–Pugh criteria, wording that was absent prior to 2000 [19–21]. The correlation of Child–Pugh stage with drug metabolism is crucial to the understanding of when and how to adjust antipsychotic dosages, and how to best implement plasma level monitoring. As more cases are published on schizophrenia patients undergoing bariatric surgery and renal dialysis, it is apparent that changes in antipsychotic exposure are expected, placing a premium on timely assessment of plasma levels to prevent relapse from subtherapeutic levels [22–27]. While these are not common events for any one provider, the clinician who develops a comfort level with these situations can serve an important role for peers and the community of schizophrenia patients at large in helping to manage individuals through these lifesaving medical interventions.

Laboratory Assay Methods

As discussed extensively in Chapter 1, plasma antipsychotic levels are best interpreted when obtained at steady state, using 12h troughs for oral agents, or levels drawn 1h–72h prior to the next long-acting injectable dose. The need to avoid morning dosing for oral antipsychotics relates not only to improved tolerability of evening dosing [28], but to the ease of interpreting a plasma level obtained the next morning.

Some sources suggest 12h or 24h troughs depending on when the oral dose is administered (evening versus morning), but provide only one set of therapeutic ranges or laboratory alert levels, most of which appear to be derived from 12h trough levels due to the paucity of 24h trough data [10]. A basic assumption when ordering plasma levels for oral antipsychotics is that the blood was actually drawn at the right time (i.e. a 12h trough ± 2 hours), and that the patient and relevant caregivers were properly informed of the time interval since the evening dose to have the specimen drawn. In the uncommon circumstance of split daily dosing, the morning dose must be held until the level is obtained. If specimens are shipped or delivered to the reference laboratory from a clinic or hospital, those involved should understand the necessary handling procedures (i.e. need for refrigeration, time limits on specimen validity even if refrigerated, etc.) [5].

While the clinician has some control over the timing of dosing and the blood draw, specimen handling procedures and the assay method are at the laboratory's discretion [5]. In most instances, the analytic method is liquid or gas chromatography–tandem mass spectrometry (LC/MS or GC/MS), which has replaced older immunoassay techniques. However, newer immunoassays have been developed that compare favorably to LC/MS or GC/MS, and at times have superior performance [8]. Clozapine is one antipsychotic in particular where a new immunoassay method is superior, and for which LC/MS or GC/MS generates irregular values not seen in other antipsychotic assays. Professor Deanna Kelly at University of Maryland examined results of 117 samples (48 from patients with schizophrenia on clozapine, 24 from patients with schizophrenia not on clozapine, and 45 from healthy controls) sent to a national reference laboratory for clozapine levels by LC/MS, and sent matching samples for levels determined by a novel immunoassay developed by Saladax Biomedical, Inc. (Bethlehem, Pennsylvania) [8]. The reference laboratory sample was split into two tubes, with a frozen aliquot from the same specimen sent to the reference laboratory for repeat testing, while the immunoassay specimens were subjected to three runs. There was good correlation between both methods ($r = 0.84$, $p < 0.0001$), and 16% higher clozapine levels with immunoassay. However, when examining internal consistency of the two assays, the concordance correlation coefficient (CCC) for the three runs of immunoassay was nearly 100% (CCC = 0.99; 95% CI = 0.979–0.997) while that for the two aliquots using LC/MS yielded only 87% (CCC = 0.869; 95% CI = 0.690–0.970). A more disturbing finding is that the reference laboratory generated 18 false positive clozapine results from LC/MS: 3 from schizophrenia patients not on clozapine, and 15 from healthy controls [8]. The plasma clozapine level for these individuals not taking clozapine ranged from 21 to 159 ng/ml. The Saladax assay was just approved in the US in 2020, but the findings from Professor Kelly's study are consistent with the erratic results seen with clozapine assays, with many of the cases involving inexplicably high plasma levels (discussed below) frequently encountered in clozapine-treated patients.

B Laboratory Reporting Issues

As clinical use of plasma antipsychotic levels becomes more widespread, clinicians will be confronted with the fact that reference laboratory ranges differ significantly from each other, with the greatest differences seen in the upper limits. This issue was given little notice in the literature until documented in a 2020 paper examining laboratory levels for four antipsychotics (fluphenazine, haloperidol, clozapine, olanzapine), agents with the highest level of recommendation for plasma level monitoring from the Therapeutic Drug Monitoring (TDM) task force of the German Arbeitsgemeinschaft für Neuropsychopharmakologie und Pharmakopsychiatrie (AGNP) [10]. Based on information from four large US commercial laboratories (Table 3.1), there was a narrow range for recommended threshold plasma levels (when a level was provided); however, for the upper limit there was a two-fold range for haloperidol, five-fold range for fluphenazine, and no upper limits for clozapine provided by two laboratories [9]. Only for olanzapine was there general agreement about the upper limit (75–80 ng/ml), but no laboratory was willing to provide the basis for determining this or any range endpoint when directly queried. As noted previously, another source of confusion relates to the fact that some laboratories report a therapeutic range as understood by clinicians, but others report a 'reference range' based on expected levels for certain dosages, a population kinetic parameter that bears no relationship to therapeutic response.

This lack of transparency presents an obvious problem for clinicians who have come to rely on laboratory therapeutic ranges as evidence-based, and who may incorrectly conclude that any level beyond the upper limit is either unsafe or evidence of substandard practice, and the only appropriate response is dose reduction. As noted in the AGNP and American Society of Clinical Psychopharmacology (ASCP) consensus paper, the appropriate response may involve noting that the laboratory upper limit is not evidence-based (e.g. an upper limit of 600 ng/ml for clozapine despite extensive literature justifying levels up to 1000 ng/ml if tolerated), and an assessment that details the dose taken, prior levels, patient adverse effects, and timing of the specimen [9, 10]. It is hoped that documents such as the AGNP/ASCP consensus paper and this handbook will push laboratories toward greater transparency in defining the reasoning

Table 3.1 Variations in laboratory plasma antipsychotic ranges [9]

	Therapeutic range (ng/ml)*							
	ARUP		LabCorp		Mayo Clinic		Quest	
	Lower	Upper	Lower	Upper	Lower	Upper	Lower	Upper
Fluphenazine	0.5	2.0	1.0	10.0	1.0	10.0	Not provided	
Haloperidol**	5.0	20.0	1.0	10.0	5.0	16.0	5.0	15.0
Olanzapine	20.0	80.0	10.0	80.0	10.0	80.0	5.0	75.0
Clozapine***	Not well established		Not provided		Therapeutic range > 350 ng/ml		See below	

Note: Laboratories may use therapeutic range and reference range interchangeably, but these represent different concepts. The therapeutic range is based on response and tolerability analyses, while reference ranges are derived from expected plasma levels for certain dosages, typically with allowance for outliers (e.g. on the basis of standard deviations or confidence intervals around an expected mean level). Even more confusing, laboratories may report therapeutic ranges for some agents (e.g. clozapine) and reference ranges for others.

* Sites accessed July 15, 2020:

ARUP Laboratories: www.aruplab.com

LabCorp: www.labcorp.com/test-menu/search

Mayo Clinic Laboratories: www.mayomedicallaboratories.com

Quest: www.questdiagnostics.com/testcenter/TestDetail.action

** ARUP reports that the toxic haloperidol level is > 42.0 mg/ml; LabCorp reports a potentially toxic haloperidol level is > 50.0 mg/ml; Mayo provides the following text: "A therapeutic window exists for haloperidol; patients who respond at serum concentrations between 5 to 16 ng/mL show no additional improvement at concentrations > 16 to 20 ng/mL. Some patients may respond at concentrations < 5 ng/mL, and others may require concentrations significantly > 20 ng/mL before an adequate response is attained."

*** ARUP reports that the toxic clozapine level is ≥ 1500 mg/ml; Quest reports a level range only for norclozapine: 25–400 ng/ml. Patient reports contain the following referring to the plasma clozapine level: "The therapeutic response begins to appear at 100 mcg/L. Refractory schizophrenia appears to require a therapeutic concentration of at least 350 mcg/L (trough, at steady state). Toxic range: > 1000 mcg/L." **(NB: mcg/L = ng/mL)**

behind, and greater uniformity in reporting, antipsychotic plasma levels as therapeutic ranges, and clearly indicating when the range is a 'reference range' based on kinetic data for certain dosages. Until such time, clinicians must develop the sophistication to understand that variations exist between laboratories for antipsychotic ranges in a manner not seen with other psychotropics, and how to respond appropriately to levels beyond the upper limit [9].

Responding to High Levels

Whenever any drug level result is out of range, the appropriate clinical response involves a patient safety assessment, investigation into possible causes, and **documentation of the reasoning** behind the clinical decision based on the findings from the investigation [9]. Reflexively reducing medication dosages for high antipsychotic levels without documentation of a patient assessment and medical reasoning is a grossly inappropriate and unprofessional response, especially given the limitations on laboratory reporting methods noted above. Box 3.1 describes a systematic approach to the evaluation of high plasma levels for oral and long-acting injectable (LAI) dosing, and how to document the response.

Box 3.1 How to Respond to High Plasma Antipsychotic Levels [29]

The first rule of thumb is patient safety as assessed by clinical evaluation. Many clinicians become alarmed when high levels are reported and reflexively reduce doses without first determining whether the level fits the clinical picture. Most patients with high plasma levels typically exhibit adverse effects consistent with the level. Moreover, as noted in Chapter 2, there is wide variation in what laboratories refer to as a 'high' antipsychotic level. Before any action is taken, a few steps need to be performed.

Assessment

- **a** The patient should be evaluated in person if inpatient, or outpatients can be contacted and queried by phone if unable to come to the clinic. The goal is to assess changes in response, including the presence of any new adverse effects, or change in severity of adverse effects.
- **b** Determine whether the oral intended dose was indeed ingested, or whether there was an accidental or intentional overdose. For LAI medications, assess whether the intended doses were administered and the recent schedule of injections.
- **c** For oral antipsychotics, determine whether the level was a 12h ± 2h trough; for LAIs, whether the level was obtained at peak concentrations based on the kinetics of that preparation, or if it was drawn at trough levels 1h–72h prior to the next scheduled dose.
- **d** For those on divided daily oral doses, determine whether the morning dose was inadvertently given prior to the blood draw.
- **e** Determine whether a metabolic inhibitor was recently added, or whether an inducer was recently discontinued.

Responses

- **a** New or worsening adverse effects present:
  - **i** **Oral medications:** As plasma level results may not return for 1–14 days, the fact that the patient continues to have adverse effects implies that

this is unlikely to be a one-time dosing error. A hypothesis should be recorded in the chart for the high level (e.g. dose increase, dosing error, metabolic inhibitor added, or inducer removed). In these circumstances, the next oral dose should be held, and modest dose reduction for subsequent doses is preferable to discontinuation. If the incorrect dose was ingested, then this should be corrected. If no error exists, a cause must be sought and documented. The amount of dose reduction should be based on the prior tolerated level or dose. If that information is not available, consider reductions of 25%–33%, ideally based on the reduction needed to reach the **point of futility**, not the upper end of the laboratory range, or to the prior tolerated dose.

ii **LAI medications:** The time to next injection should be delayed until adverse effects have abated, and the subsequent dose reduced to the prior tolerated dose. For some LAIs, the dosing interval can be increased on an ongoing basis in lieu of dose reduction. Prolonged treatment of certain adverse effects (e.g. akathisia, parkinsonism) may be needed until plasma levels drop sufficiently.

b New or worsening adverse effects absent:

i When there is a complete absence of adverse effects or exacerbation of prior adverse effects, and no obvious safety issue present (e.g. QT prolongation from a first-generation antipsychotic), this must be noted in the record as the reason for not changing the dose immediately and for ordering a repeat level. Clinicians should review prior doses and levels to determine whether the level is comparable to other levels for that dose. A hypothesis should be recorded in the chart for the high level (e.g. consistent with other prior levels and the dose, probable laboratory error). Occasional patients will be encountered who both tolerate and respond to high antipsychotic plasma levels beyond what the local laboratory recommends. An assessment of whether there has been marked benefit from plasma antipsychotic levels above the point of futility can be helpful in planning a dose reduction.

ii If the repeat level remains above the point of futility, and there is no marked benefit from levels beyond that point (even if tolerated), dose reduction ought to be pursued. For patients on strong D_2 antagonists (e.g. first-generation antipsychotics), decreases must be very slow (e.g. 10% per month) to prevent rebound or dopamine supersensitivity psychosis [30, 31, 32]. For the second-generation antipsychotics, dopamine supersensitivity psychosis is less of a concern, but slow decreases (10%–20%/month) are best to prevent other rebound effects (e.g. insomnia) due to decreased muscarinic or histamine H_1 antagonism. This is particularly true for clozapine, quetiapine, and olanzapine.

Case 3.1 Response to High Haloperidol Level – Kinetic Interaction

A 35-year-old female with schizophrenia on a stable haloperidol dose of 15 mg PO QHS has a trough plasma level of 11.7 ng/ml obtained after one month on that dose. When the patient complained about depression, a covering psychiatrist starts bupropion extended release 300 mg qam. Two weeks later, the patient has new onset of moderate restlessness and parkinsonism. The plasma level is 23.4 ng/ml, and the laboratory upper limit is 15 ng/ml.

Documentation

a **Assessment:** Haloperidol is metabolized partly via cytochrome P450 (CYP) 2D6, and bupropion is a strong CYP 2D6 inhibitor, resulting in doubling of the plasma level and new adverse effects. The level and the adverse effects are thus consistent with the scenario.

b **Response:** As the patient has new adverse effects, reduction back to the prior tolerated plasma level is necessary. An appropriate response is to discontinue bupropion without taper (it lacks the withdrawal syndrome seen with many antidepressants), hold haloperidol for one night, and resume in 24 hours at bedtime. The 48-hour hiatus between doses will allow the haloperidol level to drop by about 75%, and also decrease the levels of bupropion and their effects on 2D6 activity. A different antidepressant without kinetic interactions should be considered (e.g. sertraline).

Case 3.2 Response to High Clozapine Level – No Suspected Laboratory Error

A 47-year-old male nonsmoker with treatment-resistant schizophrenia treated as an outpatient transfers to a new clinic where a 12h trough plasma clozapine level of 1107 ng/ml and norclozapine level of 455 ng/ml are obtained on 450 mg QHS. This patient has been on the same dose for 5 months. The laboratory upper limit is 600 ng/ml. The patient complains of mild sialorrhea and constipation, but these adverse effects are unchanged for the past 3 months. The last available level, 3.5 months prior was: clozapine 982 ng/ml, norclozapine 401 ng/ml on 450 mg QHS for 3 weeks.

Documentation

a **Assessment:** Queries revealed no dosing error and the patient denied hoarding and ingesting excessive doses of clozapine. The dose is unchanged, and the increase in clozapine level is consistent with expected modest fluctuations between determinations (± 30%) seen with oral antipsychotics (see Chapter 4) [33]. The absence of any change in the severity of adverse effects, and the increase of < 13% are all consistent with good adherence. Having multiple trough levels showing consistent dose–plasma level relationships will strengthen the case for good adherence [34]. Of note, the clozapine–norclozapine ratio of 2.4 is higher than expected and reflects that this patient is both a nonsmoker and a poor metabolizer of clozapine, a variant common in some populations [29, 35]. The level and the lack of worsening adverse effects are thus consistent with the scenario.

b Response: The documentation will note that laboratory error is not suspected, and normal variation in plasma trough levels is the leading hypothesis. The appropriate response is no change in the clozapine dose and consideration of a repeat level with next routine blood draw.

Case 3.3 Response to High Clozapine Level – Suspected Laboratory Error

A 58-year-old male with treatment-resistant schizophrenia treated as an inpatient in a nonsmoking facility had a plasma clozapine level of 287 ng/ml on 250 mg QHS. The dosage was increased to 300 mg QHS, and after 4 days a trough plasma level was drawn. The level returned from the laboratory 3 days later was 1200 ng/ml, and the laboratory upper limit is 600 ng/ml. The patient complained of no adverse effects.

Documentation

a Assessment: Queries revealed no dosing error and the patient denied hoarding and ingesting excessive doses of clozapine. The dose was increased only 20%, but the level jumped almost five-fold. No new medications were added, and no inducers were stopped. Patients with clozapine levels > 1000 ng/ml often have complaints of sedation, orthostasis, or sialorrhea, or may experience a seizure, but none of these were present. The level and the lack of adverse effects are thus inconsistent with the scenario.

b Response: The documentation will note laboratory error as the leading hypothesis. The appropriate response is to repeat the level with no change in the clozapine dose.

1 Considerations for Dose Reduction in Patients with High Plasma Levels

In some patients, the plasma level will be consistently above the point of futility and without documented benefit for levels above that cutoff. In these patients, dose reduction ought to be considered as the patient is being subjected to excessive systemic exposure without the obvious tradeoff of enhanced psychiatric response. The concern for any dose reduction is relapse, and a recent publication outlined certain variables that pose greater risk. This 2020 review found 40 papers describing dose reduction or discontinuation using a variety of strategies (n = 1677 patients), and noted the risk for psychotic relapse (the event rate) was 55% per patient-year [36]. The event rate was significantly higher in the following situations: inpatients, patients with a shorter duration of illness, patients in whom antipsychotics were discontinued or in whom the dose was reduced to less than 5 mg/d of haloperidol equivalent doses, studies with a short follow-up or published before 1990, and studies in which relapse was based on clinical judgment (i.e. rating scales were not used). Another consideration when pursuing dose reduction is based on antipsychotic-related changes in dopamine D_2 receptors, and the potential for unmasking supersensitivity psychosis [37–38, 32]. Most are familiar with the proposed mechanism of tardive dyskinesia (TD): excessive postsynaptic D_2 blockade in the nigrostriatal pathway (dorsal striatum) leads to upregulation of supersensitive D_2 receptors [39, 40]. When antipsychotics are decreased or discontinued, these upregulated supersensitive receptors have greater access to dopamine, resulting in an exacerbation of TD symptoms. When the problem of TD was not clinically obvious, this is termed withdrawal dyskinesia, and reflects an unmasking of these upregulated supersensitive receptors.

This same process is also hypothesized to occur in the mesolimbic pathway (associative striatum) in certain patients. While D_2 antagonism decreases the positive symptoms of psychosis in this pathway, decreased antipsychotic exposure results in a degree of psychotic rebound greater than expected ***for some patients*** as the upregulated and supersensitive receptors overreact to dopamine binding [37–38, 32]. In a manner akin to TD, the greatest risk factor for supersensitivity psychosis is chronic exposure to potent D_2 antagonists, particularly first-generation antipsychotics, and there is also a strong association with comorbid TD. To avoid marked exacerbation of positive psychosis symptoms from dose reduction, those with plasma levels above the point of futility who are receiving potent D_2 antagonists should have doses lowered by no more than 10% per month [9, 32]. The hope is that gradual reduction will permit these upregulated supersensitive D_2 receptors to normalize without the spike in postsynaptic D_2 activity that markedly increases positive symptoms. The slowness of this downward titration must be adjusted based on patient symptoms, but the eventual goal is the lowest level consistent with stability. For second-generation agents, avoidance of rebound effects (e.g. insomnia) due to withdrawal of muscarinic cholinergic or histamine H_1 antagonism is a concern, especially for extremely sedating medications such as clozapine, quetiapine or olanzapine.

Hepatic Dysfunction and Impact on Drug Metabolism and Plasma Antipsychotic Levels

Many clinicians have been trained using vague concepts of drug metabolism in patients with hepatic disease, as seen in this statement from a 2000 review of psychotropic use in the medically ill: “In general, for any patient with liver disease, the initial dose of neuroleptic drugs should be reduced to one third or half of the usual dose for healthy patients" [41]. Absent from this review is any language on severity, or the necessary laboratory parameters to define severity, of hepatic disease. The confusion provided by such papers was considerable, leading prescribers to labor under the incorrect notion that any abnormality of liver function tests (LFTs) necessitates some type of antipsychotic dosage adjustment, or demands preferential use of certain antipsychotics that are less dependent on hepatic metabolism. Starting in the early 2000s, regulatory agencies such as the US Food and Drug Administration (FDA) provided more explicit guidance to industry on how to perform pharmacokinetic studies in patients with impaired hepatic function, and how to report the data for labeling purposes [42]. These initiatives have resulted in modern drug labeling, with precise definitions of hepatic impairment and dosage adjustments corresponding to various stages of hepatic disease. The basis for FDA choices about liver disease staging relates to research into those aspects of hepatic dysfunction that best correlate with decreased ability to metabolize medications.

The liver plays a central role in biotransformation of most drugs, and with advanced hepatic disease changes in multiple parameters impact drug clearance: hepatic blood flow, biliary excretion of metabolites, and plasma protein concentrations. Orally administered drugs must pass through the enzyme-containing intestinal epithelium as well as the liver, and extensive metabolism in these tissues greatly reduces the amount of drug entering the systemic circulation [43]. The initial metabolism process involves phase I reactions such as oxidation, reduction, hydrolysis, addition of oxygen, or removal of hydrogen. These processes are carried out by mixed-function oxidases, of which the cytochrome P450 (CYP) system is widely known to clinicians [21]. The resulting metabolites are often conjugated in phase II reactions (e.g. sulfation, glucuronidation) to produce molecules that are less active, and more easily transported and excreted. The extent of this first pass effect varies between medications, and is expressed as the hepatic extraction (EH) ratio. An EH < 0.3 is low, EH 0.3–0.7 intermediate, and EH > 0.7 high [21].

Complicating the assessment of drug metabolism in the liver is the absence of a single test for hepatic function analogous to the creatinine clearance (CrCl) or estimated glomerular filtration rate (eGFR) used to quantify renal function [42]. Hepatic disease can alter drug kinetics by multiple mechanisms, including changes of intrahepatic blood flow associated with cirrhosis, changes in enzyme expression or function, and the impact of advanced hepatic disease on kidney function, all of which can lead to accumulation of a drug and its metabolites. As a way around this complexity, investigators have performed dynamic tests with drugs having low or high EH values, and whose hepatic elimination is minimally affected by altered hepatic drug flow (e.g. the intravenous injection of caffeine or lidocaine to examine the rate of metabolite formation) [42]. While the results of these tests correlate with other measures of hepatic impairment, they cannot be used in routine clinical practice. To arrive at a clinically feasible measure of hepatic impairment, the FDA analyzed 57 pharmacokinetic studies in patients with hepatic impairment from new drug applications submitted in 1995–1998. Of the 57 studies, 31 used the Child–Pugh scale to assess hepatic impairment, and 19/57 estimated oral drug clearance in normal controls and for patients in more than one Child–Pugh category (i.e., mild, moderate, or severe). Of those 19 studies, 17 demonstrated a negative correlation (r^2 between 0.5 to 1.0) between oral drug clearance and hepatic impairment, and 16 showed impaired hepatic metabolism for the moderate Child–Pugh category [42]. From this analysis, the FDA concluded in their 2003 guidance document: "Other approaches to assess varying degrees of hepatic impairment may be appropriate, but a Child–Pugh categorization should still be included for each patient." The FDA also noted that results of dynamic tests for hepatic function had not proven superior to the Child–Pugh classification, and that dynamic probes using medications with high and low EH highly correlated with Child–Pugh scores [42].

What is the Child–Pugh scoring system? This classification scheme was developed in 1964 to predict surgical mortality for patients with advanced liver disease, and was subsequently modified in 1972 to derive prognostic information on necessity of liver transplantation based on predicted survival [44]. Child–Pugh staging correlates with the extent of cirrhosis, and the FDA's analysis indicates that it is cirrhosis which decreases the ability to metabolize medications. Cirrhosis is a diffuse process characterized by fibrosis and conversion of normal liver architecture into abnormal modules, leading to the abnormalities noted above associated with advanced hepatic disease [21]. As hepatic tissue is lost, all enzymatic activity decreases proportionally, although certain enzymes (e.g. 2C19) may be more greatly affected in earlier stages [43]. Cirrhosis also alters hepatic blood flow, and in advanced stages will impact renal blood flow. The sum of these components is complex, but the net result is that Child–Pugh classification correlates with directly measured changes in drug kinetics. The FDA states that a full pharmacokinetic study must be carried out in patients in the three Child–Pugh categories (mild, moderate, and severe), as well as in controls. At least six subjects in each arm should be evaluated; the control group should be derived from the intended patient population and not from young, healthy volunteers; and, to the extent possible, the control group should be similar to patients with respect to age, weight, and gender [42]. These studies are required in the following circumstances: when hepatic metabolism and/or excretion accounts for a substantial portion of the elimination of a parent drug or active metabolite (> 20% of the absorbed drug); if the literature suggests the drug has a narrow therapeutic range even if hepatic metabolism is < 20%; or when the drug's metabolism is unknown and other information is lacking to suggest that hepatic elimination routes are minor [42].

Mathematically complex models are sometimes used for transplant considerations but do not perform better than Child–Pugh when determining the need for dosing adjustments [34, 45]. The value of the Child–Pugh classification also lies in its ease of use. The three laboratory parameters are total bilirubin, serum albumin, and the International Normalized Ratio (INR), a calculation that reflects the ratio of a patient's prothrombin time to a control sample, normalized for that manufacturer's equipment and assay [44]. The latter two, albumin and INR, reflect the loss of hepatic tissue and the ability to synthesize proteins. There are also two clinical criteria: hepatic encephalopathy and ascites. Absent are measures of inflammation such as alanine aminotransferase (ALT) and aspartate transaminase (AST), as those values do not correlate with loss of hepatic architecture. Classification by severity (A – mild; B – moderate; C – severe) is calculated with a point system (Table 3.2), and manufacturer recommendations for dosing adjustments are based on the impact of different Child–Pugh stages. Outside of industry studies, there tends to be limited systematic information regarding the effects of Child–Pugh stages on the kinetics of individual antipsychotics, so package inserts are often the best source of this information [46].

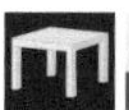

Table 3.2 Child–Pugh criteria scoring and interpretation [44]

Measure	1 point	2 points	3 points
Total bilirubin (mg/dl)	< 2.0	2.0–3.0	> 3.0
Serum albumin (g/dl)	> 3.5	2.8–3.5	< 2.8
INR*	< 1.70	1.71–2.30	> 2.30
Ascites	None	Mild	Moderate/Severe
Hepatic encephalopathy	None	Grade I–II (suppressed with meds)	Grade III–IV (or refractory)

Points	Class	1-year survival	2-year survival
5–6	A	100%	85%
7–9	B	81%	57%
10–15	C	45%	35%

* International normalized ratio (INR): this calculation reflects the ratio of a patient's prothrombin time to a control sample, normalized for that manufacturer's equipment and assay

That inflammation without cirrhosis is not a significant factor in drug metabolism was seen in the FDA analysis, and is corroborated by other literature. Persistent HCV infection and NASH (i.e. fatty liver disease) are conditions seen with higher prevalence in schizophrenia patients, and are model illnesses for studying changes in hepatic function due to inflammation that has not progressed to cirrhosis [12, 13, 15, 18]. By 1995, it was recognized that inflammation by itself without the presence of cirrhosis is not associated with changes in the expression, or activity, of the two major cytochrome P450 (CYP) enzymes CYP 3A4 and CYP 2D6 [47]. Only CYP 1A2 exhibited some evidence of decreased activity without cirrhosis in animal and human studies of NASH [47]. The conclusion from an extensive 1995 review on the pharmacokinetic effects of liver diseases including chronic active hepatitis, primary or secondary liver cancer, and hepatosplenic schistosomiasis, is that **hepatic disease without cirrhosis does not result in significant alterations in drug pharmacokinetics** [47]. **Significantly impaired hepatic elimination only occurs when cirrhosis is present, and this is captured by Child–Pugh classification.** Clinicians unfamiliar with these concepts may inappropriately fixate on elevated AST and ALT, since these are commonly encountered and may demand discontinuation of offending medications, but those liver function tests play no role in dosing decisions.

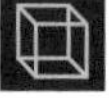

Box 3.2 Approach to Antipsychotic Dosing in Patients with Abnormal Liver Function Tests

Except in rare cases of fulminant hepatic failure due to toxins or severe drug reaction with eosinophilia and systemic symptoms (DRESS syndrome), hepatic ability to metabolize medications correlates with Child–Pugh staging [42]. The laboratory elements of Child–Pugh classification include: serum albumin, total bilirubin, and INR (see Table 3.2). Transaminases (AST, ALT, GGT) and alkaline phosphatase are not part of the staging as models have found that they do not correlate with hepatic ability to metabolize medications. For those classified as Child–Pugh A, no adjustment to antipsychotic dosing is necessary. For patients who meet Child–Pugh B (moderate) or C (severe) criteria, dosing considerations include whether this is a new start, or if this is a patient on established antipsychotic treatment.

a **New antipsychotic starts:** Antipsychotics approved in the last 10–15 years contain language on dosage adjustments for those with mild (Child–Pugh A), moderate (Child–Pugh B), or severe (Child–Pugh C) hepatic dysfunction from kinetic studies performed by the manufacturer. The recommended adjustments differ considerably between medications, so blanket statements should be ignored in lieu of the specific labeling guidance. For example, no dosage adjustment for cariprazine is required in patients with mild to moderate hepatic impairment (Child–Pugh A/B, score 5–9), but use is not recommended in patients with severe hepatic impairment (Child–Pugh

C, score 10–15). Oral aripiprazole notes no dosage adjustment is needed for Child–Pugh A–C (score 5–15). By way of contrast, lurasidone labeling notes that the recommended starting dose in moderate (Child–Pugh B, score 5–9) and severe hepatic impairment (Child–Pugh C, score 10–15) is 20 mg/d. The maximum daily dose is 80 mg/d in moderate hepatic impairment, and 40 mg/d in severe hepatic impairment, corresponding to 50% and 25% of the approved maximum daily dosage. Both labels also provide the exact scoring corresponding to moderate and severe hepatic impairment.

When one wants to prescribe a first-generation antipsychotic whose label lacks such guidance, one should preferentially use a medication for which plasma level testing is readily available in the local area, and with quick turnaround on the results. Based on the labels for multiple medications, an estimated dose reduction of 50% is reasonable for Child–Pugh B and C; however, subsequent dosing must be based on the results of the 12h trough plasma level obtained at steady state. **Example:** A Child–Pugh B patient is to be started on haloperidol due to prior history of response, and the clinician's desire to eventually use the long-acting injectable form. When younger, with normal hepatic function, 10 mg/d was sufficient with plasma levels in the 7–9 ng/ml range. As an initial estimate, an oral dose of 5 mg QHS is used and a plasma level of 7.4 ng/ml obtained six days later at steady state. For that dose, the expected level is 3.9 ng/ml, indicating that doses in this patient will need to be decreased by 50%.

b **Patients on existing antipsychotic therapy:** As with renal dysfunction, the two questions to address are: (a) Has there been a recent categorical decline in hepatic function (Child–Pugh A->B, or B->C)? (b) Are there any new or worsening adverse effects? If the Child–Pugh stage has remained stable or declined, but the patient is not experiencing any new or worsening adverse effects, no urgent action need be taken. If there is concern that the level might be beyond the point of futility, a trough level should be drawn and the appropriate actions taken (see Box 3.1). When there are new or worsening adverse effects, a trough plasma level should be drawn prior to dosing changes to use as a benchmark. For patients on long-acting injectable formulations, the adverse effect will need to be managed until the trough level can be drawn 1h–72h before the next scheduled injection date. However, this next injection will need to be held, sometimes for 1–3 weeks or more, until the adverse effects wane. At this point, one can use the plasma level obtained recently to help with deciding on dosage adjustments.

Case 3.4 Which Antipsychotic Can One Choose with these Abnormal Liver Function Tests?

A 31-year-old female with schizophrenia is admitted with her second relapse since initial diagnosis 2 years earlier. She has shown prior response to risperidone, but discontinued due to weight gain and prolactin-related adverse effects (dysmenorrhea, gynecomastia). This patient has a history of asymptomatic HCV infection, genotype 1b, which was diagnosed during her first psychiatric hospitalization. She has yet to follow through with plans for treatment. Given her history of oral medication nonadherence and adverse effects, the plan is a trial of oral aripiprazole and a switch to a long-acting injectable (aripiprazole monohydrate or lauroxil) prior to discharge if she responds adequately. Her admission laboratory results are as follows:

CBC: Normal WBC, normal platelets, normal hemoglobin and hematocrit, MCV normal

Chemistry panel: Normal electrolytes and calcium, renal function

Liver function tests: ALT 66 U/L (high), AST 54 U/L (high), total bilirubin 1.0 mg/dl (normal), albumin 4.0 g/dl (normal), INR 1.0 (normal), alkaline phosphatase 74 U/L (normal)

HCV viral load: 4 x 10^6

Urine pregnancy testing: negative

Consultation: Due to the abnormal transaminase values (AST, ALT), a consultation is requested from a colleague, who suggests that the antipsychotics paliperidone and ziprasidone are least dependent on hepatic metabolism and should be considered. However, the treating clinician has concerns that the adverse effect profile of paliperidone is exactly the same as for risperidone, and that ziprasidone is not available as a long-acting injectable.

Assessment and plan: A review of the laboratory results indicates that this patient is Child–Pugh A, **and therefore can be treated with any antipsychotic at any dose that is clinically appropriate.** Neither AST nor ALT are part of the Child–Pugh scoring system, and the patient's serum albumin, total bilirubin, and INR are normal. There is no reason to avoid use of aripiprazole.

Severe Chronic Kidney Disease and Hemodialysis

Schizophrenia also increases risk for chronic kidney disease, so clinicians must be familiar with decisions about dosing in these circumstances, and how to use plasma antipsychotic levels when faced with declining and abnormal renal function [14]. Fortunately, there are two basic ways to measure renal function that are easily understood and widely accepted: creatinine clearance (CrCl) and estimated glomerular filtration rate (eGFR) [48, 49]. The former measures the amount of creatinine that is removed from the blood over a given time interval (expressed as ml/min), while the latter is the volume of fluid filtered from the renal glomerular capillaries into the proximal part of the filtering system (Bowman's capsule) per unit of time, also expressed as ml/min. To directly measure GFR requires infusing a protein such as inulin that is neither reabsorbed nor secreted after glomerular filtration: the rate of excretion is therefore directly proportional to the rate of filtration. Creatinine is very close in these regards, since it is present in steady state amounts in the blood and is freely filtered, but tiny amounts are secreted, and calculations of CrCl tend to overestimate GFR [50]. There are extensive debates on the appropriate weighting of variables such as muscle mass (which generates higher serum creatinine values), age, gender, body mass or surface area, and race to generate formulas for CrCl and eGFR, but in routine clinical care eGFR is often provided with laboratory reports when the patient age and gender are known to the laboratory, and is the parameter mostly used for decisions about staging of chronic kidney disease (Table 3.3) (CKD), using values normalized for an average body surface area of 1.73 m^2 [48, 51].

While it is often difficult to find schizophrenia patients with more severe forms of hepatic disease (especially Child–Pugh C), renal dysfunction is common, so the impact of low CrCl or eGFR on individual antipsychotics can sometimes be found in the literature [52, 46]. For newer antipsychotics, the product label might have the only available data, the sources of which are single-dose kinetic studies of volunteers with normal or impaired renal function. These studies are required for drug approval, and correlate with naturalistic data derived from larger patient samples [52, 46].

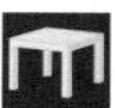

Table 3.3 Staging of kidney disease [51]

Stage	eGFR (ml/min*)
1. Normal	≥ 90
2. Mild	60–89
3a. Moderate	45–59
3b. Moderate	30–44
4. Severe	15–29
5. Failure	< 15

* This is based on the average body surface area of 1.73 m^2. Individuals with eGFR < 60 ml/min/1.73 m^2 for 3 months are classified as having chronic kidney disease.

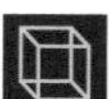

Box 3.3 Approach to Antipsychotic Dosing in Patients with Abnormal Renal Function

Estimated glomerular filtration rate (eGFR) is used in clinical practice to stage chronic kidney disease (CKD) and is reported by most laboratories, but antipsychotic labeling more commonly uses creatinine clearance (CrCl). There are multiple smartphone and web-based calculators to generate CrCl from the Cockroft–Gault formula using age, gender, weight, and serum creatinine, but for the purposes of adjusting antipsychotic dosing eGFR is an acceptable substitute, with values 10%–20% higher than CrCl [46]. Dosing considerations include whether this is a new start, if this is a patient on established antipsychotic treatment, whether the eGFR is stable or declining, and whether the patient is on hemodialysis.

a **New antipsychotic starts (not on dialysis):** Antipsychotic labels contain language on dose adjustments for renal dysfunction from kinetic studies performed by the manufacturer and expressed in CrCl. For older antipsychotics, the published literature is another source of information. The manufacturer-recommended adjustments differ considerably between medications, so one should refer to the specific labeling. For example, no dosage adjustment for cariprazine is required when CrCl is ≥ 30 ml/min, but use is not recommended when CrCl is < 30 ml/min as cariprazine was not evaluated in that patient population. For risperidone, a 60% dose decrease is recommended when CrCl is < 30 ml/min [52].

  In any patient with low CrCl (< 30 ml/min), initial dosing should be oral, decreased by the recommended amount, and then followed up with a 12h trough plasma level at steady state. The antipsychotic should be among those with data in patients with CrCl < 30 ml/min, and for which plasma levels are readily obtainable to compare the expected level with the dose, and thus make timely adjustments (see example in Box 3.2). Due to the inflexibility in dose adjustments, long-acting injectable antipsychotics are best avoided out of concern that there may be further decreases in renal function, but could be continued in certain cases with regular plasma level monitoring.

b **New antipsychotic starts (on dialysis):** The available data on hemodialysis suggests that it has minimal impact on drug kinetics for oral or long-acting injectable antipsychotics, likely due to the fact that these medications are highly protein bound [53–55]. Assuming the patient will continue with routine hemodialysis, there is no concern about further decreases in renal function, so dosing should be based on the usual clinical variables (e.g. comedication, age, etc.). Initiation with oral medication should be followed with a 12h trough plasma level at steady state. Based on these levels, one can choose the appropriate dose of a long-acting injectable if desired, and follow the patient with plasma levels at steady state.

c **Patients on existing antipsychotic therapy (not on dialysis):** The two questions to address are: (a) Has there been a recent marked decline in renal function? (b) Are there any new or worsening adverse effects? If the eGFR has remained stable or declined but the patient is not experiencing any new or worsening adverse effects, no urgent action need be taken. If there is concern that the level might be beyond the point of futility, a trough level should be drawn and the appropriate actions taken (see Box 3.1). When there are new or worsening adverse effects, a trough plasma level should be drawn prior to dosing changes to use as a benchmark. For patients on long-acting injectable formulations, the adverse effect will need to be managed until the trough level can be drawn 1h–72h before the next scheduled injection date. However, this next injection will need to be held, sometimes for 1–3 weeks or more, until the adverse effects wane. At this point, one should consider switching to an oral formulation as there may be further decreases in renal function, and long-acting injectable antipsychotics do not permit rapid dosing adjustments should significant adverse effects appear. In select cases, the LAI could be continued with regular plasma level monitoring.

d **Patients on existing antipsychotic therapy (on dialysis):** Given the limited impact on plasma antipsychotic levels, these patients should be evaluated and managed in a manner akin to those not on dialysis, bearing in mind the medical comorbidities and other factors (e.g. concurrent medications, age) that might influence drug kinetics. As with all medically complex patients, plasma antipsychotic levels can be very useful in making treatment decisions.

The bulk of the antipsychotic literature focuses on plasma level increases from moderate or severe renal dysfunction, but with surprisingly little published on plasma levels during hemodialysis [22–25]. The theoretical concern is that active removal of drug and metabolites by dialysis results in a kinetic profile different from that seen in patients with very low eGFR not receiving dialysis. Most antipsychotic labels are silent on the issue, but some comment on the fact that antipsychotics tend to be highly protein bound and unlikely to be influenced by dialysis (brexpiprazole), or that the agent is not removed by hemodialysis (ziprasidone) [56, 57]. The limited case literature substantiates this position and indicates that hemodialysis appears to have limited impact on the half-lives or plasma levels of oral or long-acting injectable antipsychotics [53–55]. Ritanserin is an agent studied for schizophrenia with very high affinity for serotonin $5HT_{2A}$ receptors and low dopamine D_2 affinity. Its ability to lessen the negative symptoms and neurological adverse effects of haloperidol led to the development of risperidone, an agent that combines the high $5HT_{2A}$ affinity and less D_2 antagonism than first-generation antipsychotics [58]. A 1991 paper examined ritanserin kinetics in five study subjects on regular hemodialysis every 2–3 days who were given single 10 mg oral doses on nondialysis days. The authors noted that dialysis did not affect ritanserin's elimination rate, with the half-life in these patients (39 ± 23 hours) nearly identical to that in healthy volunteers (41 ± 14 hours), although they did not specifically comment on the impact of dialysis the following day [53]. A Japanese case series of four hemodialysis patients with delirium managed with oral or intravenous haloperidol found that blood levels after dialysis were not lower than expected, but overall seemed to be higher for the dosage [54]. More recently, detailed records on plasma aripiprazole levels were obtained in a 64-year-old male schizophrenia patient with a long history of medication nonadherence whose eGFR was 4 ml/min/1.73 m^2 when admitted for a psychotic relapse. Hemodialysis was immediately commenced, and the decision was made to choose a long-acting injectable (LAI) antipsychotic due to his poor insight and repeated episodes of nonadherence [55]. LAI aripiprazole was chosen, and serum aripiprazole levels were checked before and after each hemodialysis session for the first 14 weeks from the beginning of the dialysis treatment. As seen in Figure 3.1, there was minimal effect of hemodialysis on aripiprazole levels. Dialysis patients have multiple comorbidities, so other factors may influence drug disposition in this population (e.g. concurrent medications); however, the available data suggest that hemodialysis has a limited influence on plasma antipsychotic levels.

Figure 3.1 Limited impact of hemodialysis on antipsychotic levels: example of a patient on monthly 400 mg injections of long-acting aripiprazole [55]

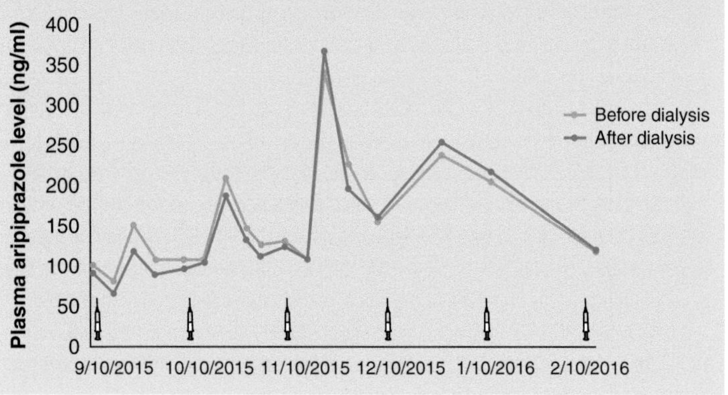

- Syringes at the bottom of the graph represent injections

(Adapted from: D. De Donatis, S. Porcelli, A. Serretti, *et al.* [2020]. Serum aripiprazole concentrations prehemodialysis and posthemodialysis in a schizophrenic patient with chronic renal failure: a case report. *J Clin Psychopharmacol*, 40, 200–202.)

Bariatric Surgery

Schizophrenia patients have higher rates of overweight and obesity than the general population due to numerous factors, including illness-related lifestyle behaviors and medications [16]. Given the tremendous health benefits that can result from bariatric surgery, there has been increasing acceptance that stable, higher-functioning schizophrenia patients are appropriate candidates for these procedures. The weight loss outcomes for those with mental illness are comparable to those for other patients, but one large study noted that patients with preoperative severe depression or anxiety, bipolar disorder, psychotic or schizophrenia spectrum disorders had higher follow-up levels of emergency department visits and hospital days compared to those with no mental illness [59]. The types of bariatric surgery procedures now utilized include gastric bypass to limit absorption (e.g. duodenal switch, Roux-en-Y bypass), or restrictive procedures that create a sense of fullness by physically shrinking the stomach size (gastric banding, sleeve gastrectomy) or by inserting objects that occupy space in the stomach (intragastric balloons) [16]. It is a reasonable assumption that any procedure which alters gastrointestinal absorptive capacity can influence the kinetics of orally administered antipsychotics, but the effects are not always predictable depending on the delivery mechanism and the need for food to enhance absorption. One of the earliest published cases from 1986 documented that a patient was eventually stabilized postoperatively on the same haloperidol dose (20 mg/d) she took preoperatively, but preoperative levels were not checked to compare changes in absorption [60]. Decreased oral antipsychotic absorption has been demonstrated in cases involving clozapine, lurasidone, and paliperidone, highlighting the need to draw preoperative plasma levels and adjust doses postoperatively using preoperative levels as the target [26, 61, 27]. Preoperative levels are also useful for patients on long-acting injectable antipsychotics, as the significant decreases in body mass and adipose tissue mass can influence levels and require dosing adjustments [62]. With forethought and advanced planning, tracking plasma antipsychotic levels can help to alleviate uncertainties surrounding the impact of bariatric surgery, and allow patients to have the best chance at a stable postoperative course.

Box 3.4 Approach to Antipsychotic Dosing in Patients Undergoing Bariatric Surgery

Patients who are candidates for these procedures must be psychiatrically stable, and thus should be on stable doses of an antipsychotic. For those on a long-acting injectable antipsychotic there is no immediate impact on drug kinetics from gastrointestinal surgery, but longer-term monitoring is recommended (see (d) below). Below are some considerations in the management of antipsychotic-treated individuals:

a Check pre-surgery trough antipsychotic plasma levels: Obtain a steady state 12h trough plasma level for all patients on oral agents, or 1h–72h prior to the next LAI injection. For patients on an oral antipsychotic for which plasma levels cannot be obtained, serious consideration should be given to finding an alternative (if possible) that will permit plasma level monitoring. If not possible, postoperative dosing will be based on clinical response. Clinicians should also bear in mind that postoperative doses might be significantly higher than preoperative doses and may exceed approved limits. The use of plasma levels will provide sufficient justification to exceed approved label dosages, but whether this is permissible for a specific antipsychotic in that country or hospital must be investigated to avoid the need to change therapy postoperatively.

b **Patients on oral antipsychotics – Option 1:** Many patients are adherent with oral antipsychotics, or respond best to a medication for which there is no LAI option (e.g. clozapine). A postoperative plasma level should be obtained as soon as possible once oral intake is resumed and at steady state for that antipsychotic. Until the level is returned, adjust doses based on clinical response. The postoperative level will provide exact information on the degree to which the dose will need to be increased to reach the preoperative stable plasma level. As long as there are ongoing declines in body mass, levels should be checked monthly and doses adjusted accordingly [62].

c **Patients on oral antipsychotics – Option 2: Switching to a long-acting injectable antipsychotic:** As noted above, transitioning a patient to an LAI avoids all of the immediate concerns surrounding postoperative changes in gastric absorption. Enough time should elapse prior to surgery for the patient to be at steady state on the LAI and psychiatrically stable. This is a decision best made when surgery is contemplated to permit sufficient time (up to 6 months) for LAI dosing adjustments if needed. As long as there are ongoing declines in body mass, levels should be checked monthly and doses adjusted accordingly [62].

d **Patients on long-acting injectable antipsychotics:** Surgery will have no immediate effect on plasma levels, but decreases in body mass can alter plasma levels over time. As long as there are ongoing declines in body mass, levels should be checked monthly and doses adjusted accordingly [62].

Summary Points

a What laboratories report as the upper limit of the therapeutic range varies dramatically between sources and is not always evidence-based. Clinicians must know how to respond to high levels based on an assessment of response, adverse effects, prior levels, and hypothesized factors that may have contributed to the high level, including the possibility of laboratory error. Documentation of the rationale is crucial, and in many instances dose reduction is not necessary.

b The extent of cirrhosis is associated with decreased ability to metabolize medications. The staging tool for hepatic dysfunction which correlates with the degree of cirrhosis is the Child–Pugh classification, and this is the basis for decisions regarding dose adjustments. The laboratory criteria include total bilirubin, serum albumin, and INR, not AST or ALT. Package labeling is often the best source of dosing adjustments for various Child–Pugh stages (A, B, C).

c For patients not on hemodialysis, dosing decisions are made based on estimated glomerular filtration rate, which is derived from creatinine clearance. Package labeling is often the best source of dosing adjustments based on renal dysfunction, typically reported by creatinine clearance. Hemodialysis does not have a marked effect on antipsychotic kinetics.

d Trough antipsychotic levels at steady state should be drawn prior to bariatric surgery. For those on oral antipsychotics, this will permit rapid dose adjustment from postoperative levels. For all patients, including those on long-acting injectable antipsychotics, monthly plasma level monitoring during ongoing weight loss will permit dosing adjustments related to the decrease in body mass and adipose tissue mass.

References

1. **Amdisen, A. (1977).** Serum level monitoring and clinical pharmacokinetics of lithium. *Clin Pharmacokinet*, 2, 73–92.
2. **Swartz, C. M. (1987).** Correction of lithium levels for dose and blood sampling times. *J Clin Psychiatry*, 48, 60–64.
3. **Grandjean, E. M. and Aubry, J.-M. (2009).** Lithium: Updated human knowledge using an evidence-based approach. Part II: Clinical pharmacology and therapeutic monitoring. *CNS Drugs*, 23, 331–349.
4. **Castro, V. M., Roberson, A. M., McCoy, T. H., *et al.* (2016).** Stratifying risk for renal insufficiency among lithium-treated patients: An electronic health record study. *Neuropsychopharmacology*, 41, 1138–1143.
5. **Hiemke, C., Bergemann, N., Clement, H. W., *et al.* (2018).** Consensus guidelines for therapeutic drug monitoring in neuropsychopharmacology: Update 2017. *Pharmacopsychiatry*, 51, 9–62.
6. **Schoot, T. S., Molmans, T. H. J., Grootens, K. P., *et al.* (2020).** Systematic review and practical guideline for the prevention and management of the renal side effects of lithium therapy. *Eur Neuropsychopharmacol*, 31, 16–32.
7. **Malhi, G. S. and Tanious, M. (2011).** Optimal frequency of lithium administration in the treatment of bipolar disorder: Clinical and dosing considerations. *CNS Drugs*, 25, 289–298.
8. **Buckley, T., Kitchen, C., Vyas, G., *et al.* (2020).** Comparison of novel immunoassay with liquid chromatography / tandem mass spectrometry (LC–MS/MS) for therapeutic drug monitoring of clozapine. *Ther Drug Monit*, 42, 771–777.
9. **Meyer, J. M. (2020).** Monitoring and improving antipsychotic adherence in outpatient forensic diversion programs. *CNS Spectr*, 25, 136–144.
10. **Schoretsanitis, G., Kane, J. M., Correll, C. U., *et al.* (2020).** Blood levels to optimize antipsychotic treatment in clinical practice: A joint consensus statement of the American Society of Clinical Psychopharmacology (ASCP) and the Therapeutic Drug Monitoring (TDM) Task Force of the Arbeitsgemeinschaft für Neuropsychopharmakologie und Pharmakopsychiatrie (AGNP). *J Clin Psychiatry*, 81, https://doi.org/10.4088/JCP.4019cs13169.
11. **Meyer, J. M. and Nasrallah, H. A., eds. (2009).** *Medical Illness and Schizophrenia*, 2nd edn. Washington, DC: American Psychiatric Press, Inc.
12. **Meyer, J. M. (2003).** Prevalence of hepatitis A, hepatitis B, and HIV among hepatitis C-seropositive state hospital patients: Results from Oregon State Hospital. *J Clin Psychiatry*, 64, 540–545.
13. **Hsu, J. H., Chien, I. C., Lin, C. H., *et al.* (2014).** Increased risk of chronic liver disease in patients with schizophrenia: A population-based cohort study. *Psychosomatics*, 55, 163–171.
14. **Tzeng, N. S., Hsu, Y. H., Ho, S. Y., *et al.* (2015).** Is schizophrenia associated with an increased risk of chronic kidney disease? A nationwide matched-cohort study. *BMJ Open*, 5, e006777.
15. **Morlán-Coarasa, M. J., Arias-Loste, M. T., Ortiz-García de la Foz, V., *et al.* (2016).** Incidence of non-alcoholic fatty liver disease and metabolic dysfunction in first episode schizophrenia and related psychotic disorders: A 3-year prospective randomized interventional study. *Psychopharmacology (Berl)*, 233, 3947–3952.
16. **Kouidrat, Y., Amad, A., Stubbs, B., *et al.* (2017).** Surgical management of obesity among people with schizophrenia and bipolar disorder: A systematic review of outcomes and recommendations for future research. *Obes Surg*, 27, 1889–1895.
17. **Yan, J., Hou, C., and Liang, Y. (2017).** The prevalence and risk factors of young male schizophrenics with non-alcoholic fatty liver disease. *Neuropsychiatr Dis Treat*, 13, 1493–1498.
18. **Xu, H. and Zhuang, X. (2019).** Atypical antipsychotics-induced metabolic syndrome and nonalcoholic fatty liver disease: A critical review. *Neuropsychiatr Dis Treat*, 15, 2087–2099.

19. **Everson, G., Lasseter, K. C., Anderson, K. E., *et al.* (2000).** The pharmacokinetics of ziprasidone in subjects with normal and impaired hepatic function. *Br J Clin Pharmacol*, 49 Suppl 1, 21s–26s.
20. **Roerig Division of Pfizer Inc. (2001).** Geodon package insert. New York.
21. **Verbeeck, R. K. (2008).** Pharmacokinetics and dosage adjustment in patients with hepatic dysfunction. *Eur J Clin Pharmacol*, 64, 1147–1161.
22. **Levy, N. B. (1985).** Use of psychotropics in patients with kidney failure. *Psychosomatics*, 26, 699–701, 705, 709.
23. **Levy, N. B. (1990).** Psychopharmacology in patients with renal failure. *Int J Psychiatry Med*, 20, 325–334.
24. **Levy, N. B., Blumenfield, M., Beasley, C. M., Jr., *et al.* (1996).** Fluoxetine in depressed patients with renal failure and in depressed patients with normal kidney function. *Gen Hosp Psychiatry*, 18, 8–13.
25. **Cohen, L. M., Tessier, E. G., Germain, M. J., *et al.* (2004).** Update on psychotropic medication use in renal disease. *Psychosomatics*, 45, 34–48.
26. **Mahgoub, Y. and Jacob, T. (2019).** Schizoaffective exacerbation in a Roux-en-Y gastric bypass patient maintained on clozapine. *Prim Care Companion CNS Disord*, 21, 19l02462–19l02463.
27. **McGrane, I. R., Salyers, L. A., Molinaro, J. R., *et al.* (2020).** Roux-en-Y gastric bypass and antipsychotic therapeutic drug monitoring: Two cases. *J Pharm Pract*, 897190020905467.
28. **Hagi, K., Tadashi, N., and Pikalov, A. (2020).** S5. Does the time of drug administration alter the adverse event risk of lurasidone? *Schizophr Bull*, 46, S31–32.
29. **Meyer, J. M. and Stahl, S. M. (2019).** *The Clozapine Handbook.* Cambridge: Cambridge University Press.
30. **Iyo, M., Tadokoro, S., Kanahara, N., *et al.* (2013).** Optimal extent of dopamine D2 receptor occupancy by antipsychotics for treatment of dopamine supersensitivity psychosis and late-onset psychosis. *J Clin Psychopharmacol*, 33, 398–404.
31. **Servonnet, A. and Samaha, A. N. (2020).** Antipsychotic-evoked dopamine supersensitivity. *Neuropharmacology*, 163, 107630.
32. **Horowitz, M. A., Jauhar, S., Natesan, S., *et al.* (2021).** A method for tapering antipsychotic treatment that may minimize the risk of relapse. *Schizophr Bull*, doi:10.1093/schbul/sbab017, 1–14.
33. **Velligan, D. I., Wang, M., Diamond, P., *et al.* (2007).** Relationships among subjective and objective measures of adherence to oral antipsychotic medications. *Psychiatr Serv*, 58, 1187–1192.
34. **Pérez-Ruixo, C., Remmerie, B., Peréz-Ruixo, J. J., *et al.* (2019).** A receiver operating characteristic framework for non-adherence detection using drug concentration thresholds – application to simulated risperidone data in schizophrenic patients. *AAPS J*, 21, 40.
35. **Ruan, C. J., Zang, Y. N., Wang, C. Y., *et al.* (2019).** Clozapine metabolism in East Asians and Caucasians: A pilot exploration of the prevalence of poor metabolizers and a systematic review. *J Clin Psychopharmacol*, 39, 135–144.
36. **Bogers, J. P. A. M., Hambarian, G., Michiels, M., *et al.* (2020).** Risk factors for psychotic relapse after dose reduction or discontinuation of antipsychotics in patients with chronic schizophrenia: A systematic review and meta-analysis. *Schizophr Bull Open*, 10.1093/schizbullopen/sgaa1002/5771215.
37. **Nakata, Y., Kanahara, N., and Iyo, M. (2017).** Dopamine supersensitivity psychosis in schizophrenia: Concepts and implications in clinical practice. *J Psychopharmacol*, 31, 1511–1518.
38. **Emsley, R., Nuamah, I., Gopal, S., *et al.* (2018).** Relapse after antipsychotic discontinuation in schizophrenia as a withdrawal phenomenon vs illness recurrence: A post hoc analysis of a randomized placebo-controlled study. *J Clin Psychiatry*, 79, e1–e9.
39. **Meyer, J. M. (2016).** Forgotten but not gone: New developments in the understanding and treatment of tardive dyskinesia. *CNS Spectr*, 21, 13–24.
40. **Meyer, J. M. (2018).** Future directions in tardive dyskinesia research. *J Neurol Sci*, 389, 76–80.

41. **Robinson, M. J. and Levenson, J. L. (2000).** The use of psychotropics in the medically ill. *Curr Psychiatry Rep*, 2, 247–255.
42. **Food and Drug Administration Center for Drug Evaluation and Research (2003).** Guidance for industry – pharmacokinetics in patients with impaired hepatic function: Study design, data analysis, and impact on dosing and labeling, www.fda.gov/cder/guidance/index.htm.
43. **Frye, R. F., Zgheib, N. K., Matzke, G. R., *et al.* (2006).** Liver disease selectively modulates cytochrome P450-mediated metabolism. *Clin Pharmacol Ther*, 80, 235–245.
44. **Cholongitas, E., Papatheodoridis, G. V., Vangeli, M., *et al.* (2005).** Systematic review: The model for end-stage liver disease – should it replace Child–Pugh's classification for assessing prognosis in cirrhosis? *Aliment Pharmacol Ther*, 22, 1079–1089.
45. **Kamath, P. S. and Kim, W. R. (2007).** The model for end-stage liver disease (MELD). *Hepatology*, 45, 797–805.
46. **Preskorn, S. (2019).** Three clinically important but underutilized and misunderstood tools: Formulas to estimate creatinine clearance, the package insert, and therapeutic drug monitoring. *J Clin Psychiatry*, 80, e1–e2.
47. **Morgan, D. J. and McLean, A. J. (1995).** Clinical pharmacokinetic and pharmacodynamic considerations in patients with liver disease: An update. *Clin Pharmacokinet*, 29, 370–391.
48. **Rule, A. D., Gussak, H. M., Pond, G. R., *et al.* (2004).** Measured and estimated GFR in healthy potential kidney donors. *Am J Kidney Dis*, 43, 112–119.
49. **Chiu, C.-C., Shen, W. W., Chen, K.-P., *et al.* (2007).** Application of the Cockcroft–Gault method to estimate lithium dosage requirement. *Psychiatry Clin Neurosci*, 61, 269–274.
50. **Pottel, H., Hoste, L., Dubourg, L., *et al.* (2016).** An estimated glomerular filtration rate equation for the full age spectrum. *Nephrol Dial Transplant*, 31, 798–806.
51. **Hill, N. R., Fatoba, S. T., Oke, J. L., *et al.* (2016).** Global prevalence of chronic kidney disease – a systematic review and meta-analysis. *PLoS One*, 11, e0158765.
52. **Grunder, P., Augustin, M., Paulzen, M., *et al.* (2019).** Influence of kidney function on serum risperidone concentrations in patients treated with risperidone. *J Clin Psychiatry*, 80.
53. **Zazgornik, J., Kuska, J., Kokot, F., *et al.* (1991).** Pharmacokinetics of ritanserin in patients undergoing hemodialysis. *J Clin Pharmacol*, 31, 657–661.
54. **Sanga, M. and Shigemura, J. (1998).** [Pharmacokinetics of haloperidol in patients on hemodialysis]. *Nihon Shinkei Seishin Yakurigaku Zasshi*, 18, 45–47.
55. **De Donatis, D., Porcelli, S., Serretti, A., *et al.* (2020).** Serum aripiprazole concentrations prehemodialysis and posthemodialysis in a schizophrenic patient with chronic renal failure: A case report. *J Clin Psychopharmacol*, 40, 200–202.
56. **Otsuka America Pharmaceutical Inc. (2020).** Rexulti package insert. Rockville, MD.
57. **Roerig Division of Pfizer Inc. (2020).** Geodon package insert. New York.
58. **Grant, S. and Fitton, A. (1994).** Risperidone: A review of its pharmacology and therapeutic potential in the treatment of schizophrenia. *Drugs*, 48, 253–273.
59. **Fisher, D., Coleman, K. J., Arterburn, D. E., *et al.* (2017).** Mental illness in bariatric surgery: A cohort study from the PORTAL network. *Obesity (Silver Spring)*, 25, 850–856.
60. **Fuller, A. K., Tingle, D., DeVane, C. L., *et al.* (1986).** Haloperidol pharmacokinetics following gastric bypass surgery. *J Clin Psychopharmacol*, 6, 376–378.
61. **Ward, H. B., Yudkoff, B. L., and Fromson, J. A. (2019).** Lurasidone malabsorption following bariatric surgery: A case report. *J Psychiatr Pract*, 25, 313–317.
62. **Schoretsanitis, G., Kirner-Veselinovic, A., Gründer, G., *et al.* (2017).** Clinically relevant changes in clozapine serum concentrations after breast reduction surgery. *Aust N Z J Psychiatry*, 51, 1059–1060.

4 Tracking Oral Antipsychotic Adherence

QUICK CHECK

PRINCIPLES

- There are multiple ways in which oral medication adherence is defined and measured. Electronic pill caps are the gold standard but usually reserved for research. Pill counts, plasma levels, and third-party information are the most easily used evidence-based sources. Patient self-report and clinician estimates correlate poorly with oral antipsychotic adherence.
- The expected variation in plasma levels for individual patients is approximately ± 30% from their baseline. Variations > 50% are likely due to nonadherence, assuming timing and dosing errors have been minimized.
- Causes for low levels must be sought, including improper timing of the blood draw, dosing errors, or exposure to metabolic inducers. One level may not be enough to indicate nonadherence when no baseline levels exist.
- Clinicians must develop a nonjudgmental language for discussing adherence and lower than expected plasma levels with patients.
- Kinetic failures can happen due to genetic variations that result in an ultrarapid metabolizer phenotype. This should be suspected when levels are low but are very consistent, and lack the variation seen with poor adherence.

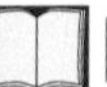

INTRODUCTION

That people with chronic illness do not take all of their oral medications is well established, and schizophrenia is not unique in this regard. A World Health Organization study estimated that medication adherence among patients with chronic diseases averages only 50% in developed countries, with recent data indicating a rate of 45% for hypertension specifically [1, 2]. Unlike hypertension, where the impact of nonadherence might not be felt for years, poor adherence with oral antipsychotic therapy can result in psychotic relapse within days or weeks, leading to hospitalization, social disruption, and legal sequelae (e.g. increased risk for violence) [3, 4]. Another concern is that schizophrenia relapse is also a disease-modifying event, based on the association between relapse among nonadherent individuals and decreased likelihood of subsequent antipsychotic response. The strongest evidence for this conclusion comes from a 2019 paper that analyzed clinical outcomes for 130 schizophrenia spectrum patients treated in a specialized first-episode psychosis program in Toronto from 2003 to 2013, and who met the following criteria: (a) treated with an oral second-generation antipsychotic (SGA) with remission of positive symptoms; (b) subsequent relapse due to nonadherence; and (c) reintroduction of the same SGA used in the first episode. Although all patients took the same SGA in both episodes, the proportion who achieved 50% symptom reduction was significantly greater after the first episode versus the second episode, despite the need for significantly higher doses in the second episode – week 7 responders: 48.7% (first episode) versus 10.4% (second episode); week 27 responders: 88.2% (first episode) versus 27.8% (second episode) [5].

The development of long-acting injectable (LAI) antipsychotics is an ideal solution for many patients, and LAI antipsychotics are associated with improved adherence, which translates into improved psychiatric outcomes in most studies, depending somewhat on the population chosen and study methodology (e.g. mirror-image, naturalistic, etc.) [6–8]. Nonadherence is present in schizophrenia patients at all stages of illness, and there is increased enthusiasm in recent years for LAI use in first-episode (FE) schizophrenia patients to forestall the social, legal, and psychiatric consequences of relapse. Multiple studies have demonstrated that FE patients will not only accept LAI treatment, but have improved adherence, lower relapse and hospitalization rates compared to those on oral antipsychotic therapy [9–13]. The first large-scale, randomized trial of LAI use versus clinician's choice of care (n = 289) was published in 2020, and enrolled patients in the early phase of their schizophrenia illness (mean age 25.2, mean duration of illness 3.59 years) [14]. In this population, use of an LAI (aripiprazole monohydrate once monthly) produced a significant 44%

reduction in the incidence rate of first hospitalization compared to clinician's choice of care, with a number needed to treat (NNT) of 7 for prevention of hospitalization [14].

Clinicians who work in FE programs readily use LAI treatment in those patients identified as having poor prognostic factors (male gender, lower premorbid functioning, homelessness, substance use disorder, and schizophrenia spectrum diagnoses) [15]. However, clinicians incorrectly assume that certain functional aspects (e.g. current employment or school attendance, living with family, lower rates of legal problems prior to program enrollment) are indicative of future adherence. Unfortunately, research in this area indicates that these assumptions might not be true. Naturalistic data acquired from a Montreal FE program from 2005–2015 demonstrated that the group offered oral antipsychotics first were more likely to relapse and be rehospitalized **although they manifested better functioning at baseline than those started on LAIs** [13]. At the end of 1 year, over 50% initially given oral antipsychotics had relapsed, a rate twice as fast as those started on LAI treatment. By year 3, 82.3% of those started initially on oral antipsychotics had been hospitalized, compared to 52% for patients started on LAIs, despite lower baseline functioning in the latter group [13]. By virtue of their involvement in school, work, and the presence of family connections, more functional FE patients have the most to lose due to relapse, including antipsychotic responsiveness. Depriving FE schizophrenia patients of LAI treatment is no longer considered medically acceptable or justifiable.

Unfortunately, even in 2021, there is a limited range of pharmacological options for LAI antipsychotics, all of which can be broken down into one of four categories, based on similar mechanism of action and adverse effect profile: (a) first-generation antipsychotics (FGAs); (b) risperidone or its active metabolite 9-OH risperidone (paliperidone); (c) aripiprazole; (d) olanzapine. This limited array of LAI choices is but one of many reasons some patients are on oral antipsychotics, including: (a) an ideal antipsychotic option cannot be found in an LAI preparation (e.g. clozapine); (b) the patient refuses LAI treatment; (c) the patient has a history of good adherence to and response to an oral medication; (d) clinician behavior. Clinician behavior is one of the more significant barriers to LAI use, often related to the common practice of restricting clinical discussions about LAIs to those patients with nonadherence or repeated hospitalizations, thereby excluding FE patients or those who might simply prefer the convenience of an LAI option over daily pill taking [16]. Other clinician-related issues include concerns about LAIs being perceived as coercive, lack of familiarity with dosing adjustments, and less dosing flexibility compared to oral antipsychotics [17]. While improved communication from prescribing clinicians and support from other treatment team members can decrease patient barriers to LAI antipsychotic utilization

[16], it must be acknowledged that the majority of schizophrenia patients are on oral medication, so measures to track adherence need to be implemented in their care. The targeted use of plasma level monitoring is thus part of an integrated approach to oral antipsychotic adherence whose goal is to enhance the odds of maximal functional benefit from antipsychotic treatment.

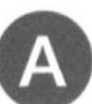

Measuring and Discussing Adherence

What is adherence? Although this is a basic question, a 2020 review notes the lack of a standardized definition, and the numerous methods employed in adherence studies (Figure 4.1) [4]. While our understanding of schizophrenia pathophysiology has evolved rapidly in the past 15 years, in the decade from 2006 through 2017 much of the adherence literature continued to report outcomes based on the least evidence-based method, patient self-report, with < 15% using any of the three most rigorous methods: plasma levels, pill counts, or electronic pill containers (Figure 4.2) [4].

The gold standard for measuring oral medication adherence is electronic monitoring of pill bottle opening, typically using devices such as the Medication Event Monitoring System (MEMS), a cap with a microprocessor that records each bottle opening [18]. It is considered the standard for prospective research, and MEMS cap results correlate extremely highly with pill counts in controlled and naturalistic studies [19, 18]. As discussed extensively in this handbook, ingesting the antipsychotic is no guarantee of efficacy, as variations in drug metabolism create a range of values even for patients who are 100% adherent. Moreover, there are also marked interindividual differences in response to any given plasma antipsychotic level. Nonetheless, plasma levels correlate significantly with electronic data and are crucial to making clinical inferences about adherence; however, as a measure of adherence, levels are less exact than pill counts or MEMS cap data unless repeated on a regular basis [18].

Reviews of electronic device studies (almost exclusively using the MEMS cap) have defined three types of adherence parameters for oral medications, from least stringent to most stringent: taking adherence, regimen adherence, and timing adherence [20]. In an ideal world, clinicians would want high levels of timing adherence wherein patients take the appropriate doses within the prescribed time frame each day. Generally speaking, those who manage any patients with chronic illness are satisfied with high levels of regimen adherence, meaning that the percentage of days with the appropriate number of doses taken is as close to 100% as possible. By recording the time and occurrence of each bottle opening, MEMS studies have the potential to report all three parameters, but the most common outcome measure is taking adherence: the

Figure 4.1 Types of adherence methods in 300 papers (2007–2017) [4]

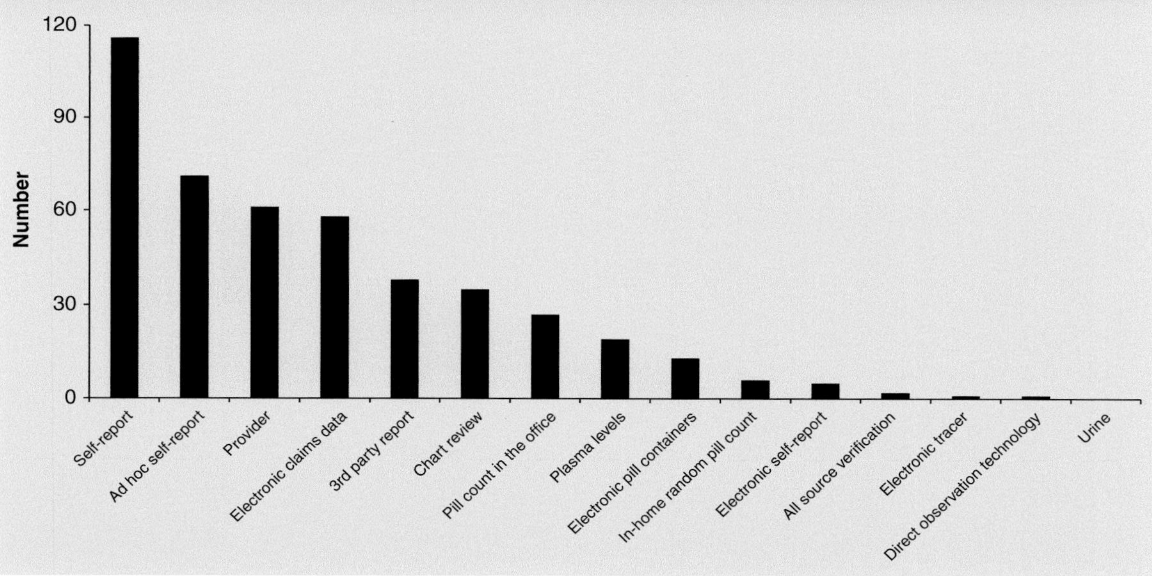

(Adapted from: D. I. Velligan, N. J. Maples, J. J. Pokorny, *et al*. [2020]. Assessment of adherence to oral antipsychotic medications: What has changed over the past decade? *Schizophr Res*, 215, 17–24.)

Figure 4.2 Trends in methods used in adherence studies (prior to 2006, and 2007–2017) [4]

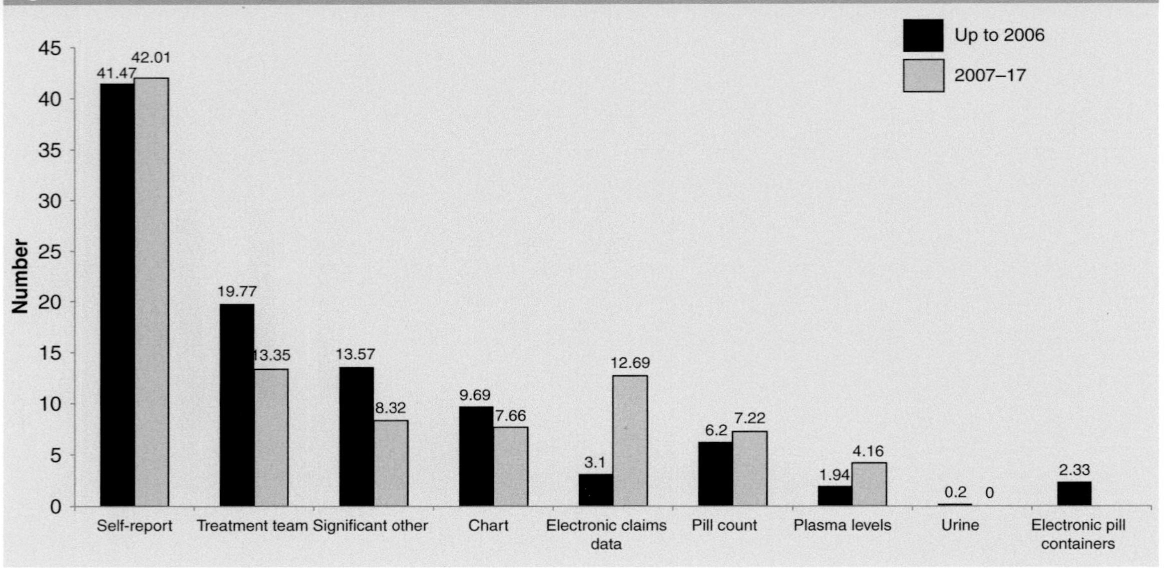

(Adapted from: D. I. Velligan, N. J. Maples, J. J., Pokorny, *et al.* [2020]. Assessment of adherence to oral antipsychotic medications: What has changed over the past decade? *Schizophr Res*, 215, 17–24.)

Figure 4.3 The three forms of oral antipsychotic adherence documented by electronic methods [20]

	Mean	Standard error	Variance	Lower limit	Upper limit	Z-value	p-value
Taking adherence	0.711	0.067	0.004	0.580	0.841	10.680	0.000
Regimen adherence	0.700	0.033	0.001	0.636	0.764	21.409	0.000
Timing adherence	0.649	0.060	0.004	0.532	0.766	10.884	0.000

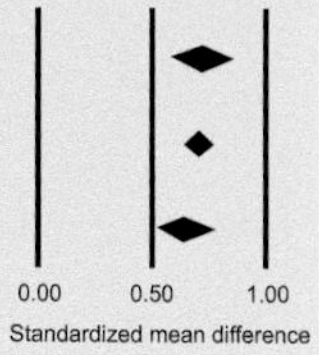

Three levels of adherence in order of increasing stringency:

1. **Taking adherence:** the number of bottle cap openings divided by the number of prescribed doses during the monitoring period.
2. **Regimen adherence:** the percentage of days that the correct number of doses was taken.
3. **Timing adherence:** the percentage of doses taken within an assigned time window.

(Adapted from: H. Yaegashi, S. Kirino, G. Remington, *et al.* [2020]. Adherence to oral antipsychotics measured by electronic adherence monitoring in schizophrenia: A systematic review and meta-analysis. *CNS Drugs*, 34, 579–598.)

number of bottle cap openings divided by the number of prescribed doses during the monitoring period [20]. The overlap between these three measures is considerable, with taking adherence and regimen adherence having the highest concordance (Figure 4.3). For the sake of simplicity, the term **adherence** throughout this volume should be considered synonymous with taking adherence.

From electronic data, various thresholds for adherence have been utilized, ranging from 70%–80% of prescribed oral antipsychotic dosages [21, 22, 18]. In a one-month MEMS cap study of stable outpatients with schizophrenia (n = 52) at the Centre for Addiction and Mental Health (CAMH) in Toronto, the range of nonadherence can readily be seen (Figure 4.4) [22]. The 80% mark seemed to best discriminate adherent from nonadherent in this study, but there was considerable variation in the extent of nonadherence. While the CAMH study found that ≤ 80% adherence in doses taken was an appropriate cutoff for defining nonadherence, a 2020 meta-analysis of 19 electronic monitoring studies involving 2184 patients found that the proportion of patients with oral antipsychotic adherence ranged from 50%–78.3% for the 70% threshold to 47.8%–75.7% for the 80% threshold, suggesting that either threshold value is appropriate [20]. When defined as a continuous variable, 71.1% of doses were taken, based on electronic data records of pill bottle openings (7 studies, n = 256). If

Figure 4.4 Rates of adherence in stable schizophrenia patients monitored over four weeks [22].

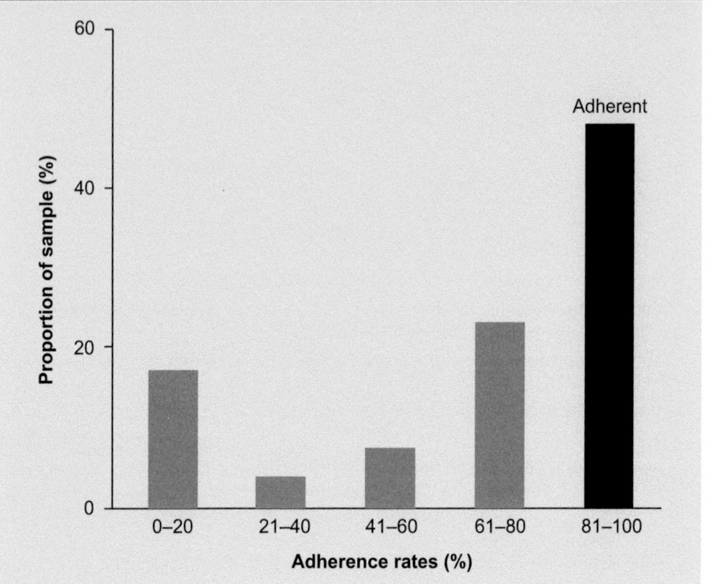

(Adapted from: G. Remington, C. Teo, S. Mann, *et al.* [2013]. Examining levels of antipsychotic adherence to better understand nonadherence. *J Clin Psychopharmacol*, 33, 261–263.)

each patient took 71% of their doses, there would be 100% adherence using the 70% threshold [20]. That the range of adherence for the 70% threshold was 50%–78.3% reinforces the findings from the CAMH trial: some patients take nearly all of their daily doses, while others struggle with a range of nonadherence.

Adherence is not static, so efforts to monitor adherence must be part of an ongoing treatment plan for patients on oral antipsychotics and mood stabilizers. The best illustration of temporal patterns in nonadherence can be seen in a large retrospective analysis of three US insurance databases (2007–2013), using claims data on adult schizophrenia patients followed for 1 year after a new prescription for an oral second-generation antipsychotic [23]. Adherence was defined by the proportion of days covered (PDC) by the antipsychotic prescription, based on the 80% threshold. PDC was calculated as the number of days of antipsychotic supply in the 12 months following antipsychotic initiation divided by 365, with a maximum value of 100% [23]. Among

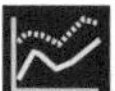

Figure 4.5 Temporal adherence patterns in adult schizophrenia patients newly started on an oral second-generation antipsychotic (SGA) with no SGA prescriptions during the prior 6 months [23]

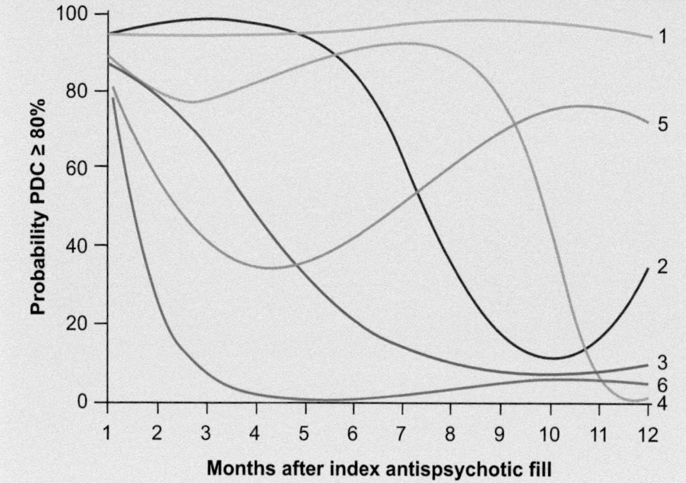

Adherence was defined as having ≥ 80% of the proportion of days covered (PDC).

PDC was calculated as the number of days of antipsychotic supply in the 12 months following therapy initiation, divided by 365 days, with a maximum value of 100%.

Group descriptions:

Group 1 = adherent; group 2 = discontinuation at 6 months; group 3 = discontinuation at 3 months; group 4 = discontinuation at 9 months; group 5 = stop/start at 6 months; group 6 = immediate discontinuation.

(Adapted from: J. P. MacEwan, F. M. Forma, J. Shafrin, *et al*. [2016]. Patterns of adherence to oral atypical antipsychotics among patients diagnosed with schizophrenia. *J Manag Care Spec Pharm*, 22, 1349–1361.)

the 29,607 patients who met inclusion criteria, six distinct adherence-trajectory groups emerged from the data (Figure 4.5): adherent (33%); gradual discontinuation after 3 months (15%), 6 months (7%), and 9 months (5%); stop-start after 6 months (15%); and immediate discontinuation (25%). Compared to patients 18–24 years of age in the adherent group, patients displaying a stop-start pattern after 6 months had greater odds of a substance use history and concurrent major depressive disorder, and were under 35 years old [23]. While these results are dispiriting, the large, naturalistic nature of this study should underscore the dynamic nature of nonadherence, and the need for regular monitoring of oral antipsychotic therapy.

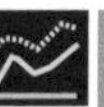

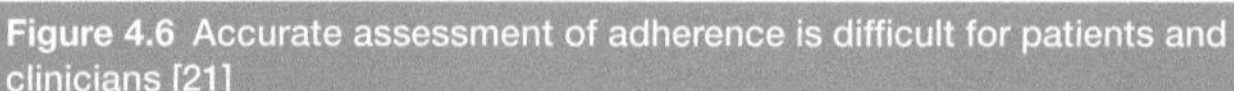

Figure 4.6 Accurate assessment of adherence is difficult for patients and clinicians [21]

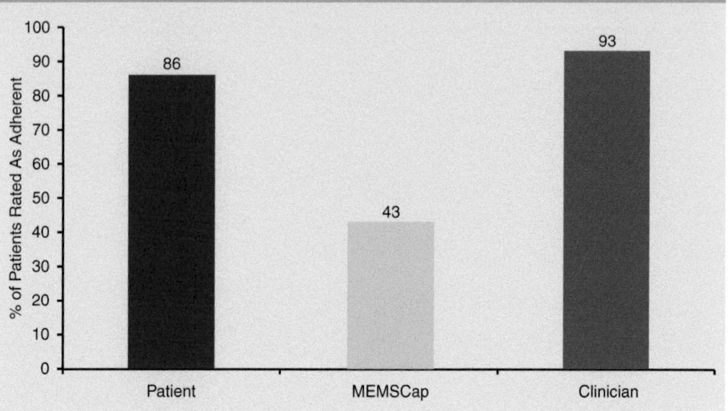

(Adapted from: M. J. Byerly, A. Thompson, T. Carmody, *et al.* [2007]. Validity of electronically monitored medication adherence and conventional adherence measures in schizophrenia. *Psychiatr Serv*, 58, 844–847.)

The retrospective 1-year data and the numerous prospective MEMS cap studies provide compelling evidence that nonadherence is a common and enduring issue with oral antipsychotic treatment, but patients and clinicians are poor estimators of oral nonadherence [21, 19, 18]. Figure 4.6 presents 6-month data from a group of 61 schizophrenia spectrum adult outpatients followed in Dallas mental health clinics [21]. As part of this study, patients and clinicians were questioned about their perceptions of medication adherence, and objective information on taking adherence was collected by MEMS cap [21]. Using the 70% threshold to define adherence from the MEMS cap data, 57% of patients were nonadherent; however, clinicians opined that only 7% of their patients could not take their medications 5 days out of 7 (i.e. 70% of the time), and only 5% of patients thought they were nonadherent [21]. The issue of clinician overestimation of adherence has been replicated in other settings, including an emergency room study that showed a significant disconnect between plasma antipsychotic levels and staff opinions about adherence [24]. When patients appear stable, prescribers may use clinical state as a proxy for adherence despite objective data indicating a poor correlation between these two variables [19].

To examine factors that might influence clinician perception of adherence, an international survey was performed across 11 countries (Australia, Brazil, Canada, China, Denmark, Greece, New Zealand, Portugal, Taiwan, United States, United Kingdom), which asked psychiatrists to estimate the percentage of patients they see who are adherent (> 75% of doses taken), partially adherent (taking 50%–75%), or poor/non-adherent (< 50% of doses taken) [25]. The survey received 1316 responses: 65.2% of the respondents were attending psychiatrists (qualified specialists) and 27.4% in residency, with a mean psychiatric experience of 12.9 ± 11.0 years. Overall, 45.4% ± 23.4% of the patients were estimated to be adherent using the 75% threshold, but practice setting and experience played important roles in clinician perception. Years of experience were positively correlated with good adherence estimation ($r = 0.205$, $p < 0.001$), to the extent that attending physicians were significantly more likely to consider patients adherent than did residents ($p = 0.011$). Psychiatrists who mainly see outpatients were also more likely to consider patients adherent than those seeing mostly inpatients or those seeing both inpatients and outpatients ($p < 0.001$, $p < 0.001$, respectively) [25]. Unfortunately, the most optimistic quartile of psychiatrists regarding patient adherence were less likely to confirm adherence by asking caregivers ($p < 0.001$), and were more likely to confirm adherence by utilizing the least reliable methods such as "asking the patient" and "self-report" ($p < 0.001$, $p < 0.001$, respectively) [25]. It appears counterintuitive that seasoned clinicians are more optimistic regarding patient adherence, but the authors hypothesized that more experienced psychiatrists may be better at building rapport, and therefore (incorrectly) assume their patients are adherent, while lacking good-quality data to test this hypothesis. This optimistic bias was noted in the 6-month Dallas study and is a cognitive error that can only be corrected through diligent monitoring to capture the extent of adherence issues. Oral antipsychotic nonadherence is not a problem that only happens to other people's patients.

In addition to the use of plasma antipsychotic levels, other steps should be taken to improve adherence (Table 4.1). As MEMS caps are not typically used outside of research studies, pill counts and third-party information are evidence-based strategies that are easily employed [26, 19, 18, 1]. Given the negative effects of nonadherence and relapse, clinicians should use every tool at their disposal to promote adherence, even though the literature is not very encouraging regarding any one method [27]. While the impact of patient rapport on adherence may be overestimated by experienced outpatient clinicians [25], there is a known correlation between the use of declarative questions [28], or the use of shared decision-making principles, and adherence [29]. When working with FE schizophrenia patients in particular, the lack of prior medication experience elevates the importance of the clinician relationship, and this relationship stands out as a significant factor promoting adherence among the FE population [30]. Instruments have been developed to assess adherence – including the 30-item Drug Attitude Inventory (DAI-30), and the Brief Adherence Rating Scale (BARS) – but may overestimate ongoing adherence compared with unannounced pill

Table 4.1 Tips to maximize adherence

Intervention	Comments
1. Dosing	• Once daily dosing and fewer changes improve adherence [36]
2. Gather objective data	• Prescription refills, third-party information, home visits with unannounced pill counts, and plasma antipsychotic levels are all evidence-based strategies [19, 4] • Do not assume or infer any level of adherence based on patient stability or patient self-report
3. Remind patients	• Utilize every tool possible (e.g. reminders via text, phone, or email; timed pill boxes with alerts) despite literature suggesting modest benefits [27, 37–39]
4. Communicate effectively	• Normalize nonadherence to draw out the extent of the problem [29] o **Appropriate question:** Most people who take medicines every day miss some doses. How many do you think you missed in the past four weeks? o **Inappropriate question:** Did you take your pills? • Drug attitude predicts adherence, so solicit reasons and concerns that relate to adherence and respond to them in a nonjudgmental manner [40, 41] • Employ shared decision-making principles as much as possible [29] • Declarative questions during patient encounters improve therapeutic alliance and adherence [28]. These questions are of the form "so, you were (feeling, experiencing, etc.) x," in which the clinician is trying to show an understanding of what the patient is conveying, and which the patient might then clarify. • **Example:** o Patient: "My mom is getting older and it's harder for her to do things for me." o Clinician: "So, what you're saying is that sometimes you are worried or anxious about the future – is that right?" o Patient: "Yeah. I don't know if I can manage everything myself."
5. Recognize that nonadherence is a persistent and pervasive issue	• Do not become complacent, regardless of your level of expertise [25] • Adherence is dynamic and changes over time [23]

counts [31–33]. The DAI-30 is also intended for research purposes, but the BARS only takes 5 minutes (Figure 4.7), with good sensitivity (73%) and specificity (74%) [32]. A recent analysis of baseline BARS data from a prospective long-term randomized trial (up to 24 months) of paliperidone palmitate and haloperidol decanoate also showed that those with lower baseline BARS scores had better response to LAI therapy [34]. An ROC analysis of the **summary visual analog scale** on the BARS determined that a clinician summary rating of 66% adherence or less best discriminated patients likely to respond to LAI treatment ($p = 0.025$). The study patients whose clinician-rated

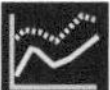

Figure 4.7 The Brief Adherence Rating Scale (BARS) [32]

|·········|·········|·········|·········|·········|·········|·········|·········|·········|·········|

0% 10% 20% 30% 40% 50% 60% 70% 80% 90% 100%

Response struck on above line (%) = ___________

(Adapted from: M. J. Byerly, P. A. Nakonezny, and A. J. Rush [2008]. The Brief Adherence Rating Scale (BARS) validated against electronic monitoring in assessing the antipsychotic medication adherence of outpatients with schizophrenia and schizoaffective disorder. *Schizophr Res*, 100, 60–69.)

adherence was ≤ 66% on the BARS summary visual analog scale had 3.46 times the predicted odds (95% CI = 1.604 to 7.480, p = 0.001) of responding to LAI treatment than subjects initially rated above 66% [35]. As noted from the Montreal FE study, initial clinician impression of adherence may not prove true, so even a high baseline rating on the BARS summary visual analog scale should not dissuade a clinician from routine oral antipsychotic adherence monitoring of all schizophrenia patients.

B Expected Variation in Plasma Antipsychotic Levels

To effectively use plasma levels as an adherence tracking tool requires an understanding of the expected variation in drug levels so adherent patients are not unfairly labeled as nonadherent due to other factors impacting levels (Box 4.1). The approach to higher-than-expected plasma levels is discussed in Chapter 3, and the assessment of lower than expected antipsychotic levels deserves a similar careful examination. This is especially true in instances where there is no prior level to use as a reference, and gives rise to the dictum: **a single level not enough**. If the level is zero, or close to zero, one can conclude that nonadherence is the likely culprit even without prior levels, but patients who are ultrarapid metabolizers (UM) may have antipsychotic levels more than 70% below that predicted for the prescribed dose [42]. With only one data point and no baseline, one can only rule out certain reasons for low levels (e.g. timing errors), but with a second data point the nature of the problem becomes much clearer. If there is marked variation, as noted by an increase in the next plasma level by 50% or more, the prior low level was the product of nonadherence; however, if the level is low with limited variation from the last determination, this suggests an etiology other than poor adherence. Additional information can be gleaned when the levels of active metabolites are reported, as is generally true for risperidone or clozapine. When plasma levels for oral risperidone or clozapine remain low but with high consistency (i.e. with limited variability), the ratio of the parent compound to its metabolite (**the metabolic ratio, MR**) will indicate whether the patient is a

UM. For patients who are metabolizing these medications 'normally', the MR will be comparable to population mean MR values, but for UM the MR will be significantly lower than the population average (see Case 4.1) [43].

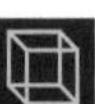

Box 4.1 Factors Resulting in Lower than Expected Plasma Levels among Adherent Patients [44]

- **a** Ultrarapid metabolism due to genetic factors
- **b** Increased drug metabolism related to cytochrome P450 inducers (e.g. other medications, smoking)
- **c** Timing of the plasma level collection significantly beyond 14h post-dose
- **d** Poor drug absorption

Case 4.1 Is This Nonsmoking Male Patient Taking His Clozapine?

Concurrent CYP or Drug Transporter (BCRP, PGP, OATP*) Inducers: None
Levels are in ng/ml

Date	Clozapine	Norclozapine	MR**	Dose
11 Sept. 2017	336	237	1.42	800 mg QHS
20 Oct. 2017	436	339	1.29	900 mg QHS
13 Apr. 2018	502	366	1.37	900 mg QHS

* CYP = cytochrome P450; BCRP = breast cancer resistance protein; OATP1A2 = organic anion transporting polypeptide)

** MR = metabolic ratio. This patient's mean MR = 1.33

Considerations

- **a** For a nonsmoking male who is an extensive metabolizer at CYP 1A2, the plasma clozapine level is 1.08 times the oral dose [44]. The mean of the last two plasma levels on 900 mg/d is 469 ng/ml, approximately half of the expected value of 972 ng/ml.
- **b** The expected metabolic ratio (MR) of clozapine to its metabolite norclozapine in large studies is 1.32 [43]. (Note: In Asia this ratio may be higher.) Although the plasma level is low, this patient's MR is exactly as expected, 1.33, so his low clozapine level is not due to ultrarapid metabolism.
- **c** While we have only three data points on 900 mg QHS, the level fluctuates only ± 7% from the mean value of 469 ng/ml indicating excellent adherence over the 6-month interval.
- **d** **Conclusion: This patient appears adherent and he is not an ultrarapid metabolizer, so some other explanation is responsible for his consistent and unvarying low plasma levels, with poor absorption being the only viable candidate. The reason is unclear, but may relate to overexpression of a drug transporter in the intestinal epithelium [45].**

As with all laboratory assays, a certain degree of variation in the result is expected, some of which is related to the assay itself, but mostly related to patient factors (e.g. adherence, timing of the blood draw). This variability is represented by the coefficient of variation (CV), a number that reflects the distribution of data compared to the average (i.e. mean) (Box 4.2). Laboratory variance is minimized by the use of quality-control samples provided by the assay manufacturer to guarantee precision, and thereby limit variation from one run to the next (i.e. to minimize the interassay variation). In the largest published data set on antipsychotic plasma level monitoring, more than 100,000 samples were examined from the therapeutic drug monitoring service at St. Olav University Hospital, Trondheim, Norway, covering October 1999 – December 2015. Plasma level data on 12 antipsychotics were reported, and for these 12 antipsychotics the interassay CV was generally less than 10% [46]. Patient-related factors present the greatest source of variability in plasma levels due to nonadherence and the additional items listed in Box 4.1. Investigators examining the St. Olav data were able to use antipsychotic dose information from the laboratory requisition form, and could usually infer whether the plasma level was obtained at steady state conditions. Information on concomitant medications, however, was not available. Despite these limitations, the enormous volume of data analyzed, combined with the multiple results present for many patients, permitted calculation of within-patient CVs for each of the 12 antipsychotics [46]. For most of the antipsychotics, the within-individual CVs were in the range of 30%–50%, with the very short half-life antipsychotic quetiapine being a notable outlier (76%).

How does this naturalistic data on within-subject CV, where the exact time since last dose and use of concomitant medications are unknown, compare to results in well-characterized patient groups? Psychiatrists associated with CAMH in Toronto assessed 723 clozapine and norclozapine levels obtained at steady state from 61 individuals with schizophrenia receiving outpatient treatment at their facility from January 2009 to December 2010 [47]. A median value of five plasma clozapine levels per patient was available (range 2–56), and within-subject (intraindividual) CVs were calculated based on the predicted clozapine level for each patient, using a well-validated model that accounted for variables known to influence clozapine kinetics (e.g. gender, smoking status, age, dose, concurrent medications) [48]. The observed within-subject CV was 29.8% ± 17.2% for clozapine, and 27.4% ± 16.4% for the metabolite norclozapine, providing further evidence that suspicion of nonadherence with oral antipsychotic therapy should only begin when levels are more than 30% from that expected [47]. Not surprisingly, CVs are closer to 25% on inpatient psychiatric units, since the administered dose and the time since dose are tightly controlled, and trough plasma levels are obtained consistently around 12h after the evening dose [49]. This assertion comes

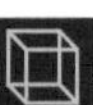

Box 4.2 Understanding Coefficient of Variation (CV)

a In its most basic interpretation, the CV is calculated as the standard deviation (SD) divided by the mean:

CV = SD/μ (where μ = mean)

(More sophisticated estimates of CV from the within-subject error component of an analysis of variance are often employed for large, complex data sets [46].)

Using some algebra, we can take a known CV and mean to figure out the SD:

SD = CV x μ

b Since the intraindividual CV is typically 30% for plasma antipsychotic levels, we can now translate this into something that can be clinically applied:

Example: Clozapine mean plasma level for a patient = 400 ng/ml, and the expected CV (from the literature) = 30%.

SD = 0.30 x 400 ng/ml = 120 ng/ml

c **Interpretation:** Since the SD is 120 ng/ml, we would expect 68.2% of the plasma levels to fall within the range of ± 120 ng/ml from the mean value of 400 ng/ml (i.e. 280–520 ng/ml). To put this numerically, 68.2% of the plasma levels will fall within the range of ± 30% from the mean value.

d **How much variation seems reasonable:** For an individual patient, the CV might be greater than 30%, but the literature indicates that, for most antipsychotics, CV values > 50% are uncommon. **It is for this reason that fluctuations up to 30% from the patient's average level do not necessarily indicate an adherence issue, but that repeated decreases (or rarely increases) > 30% from the average value without explanation (see** Box 4.1**) raise questions about adherence that need to be investigated.** Fluctuations > 50% almost certainly are due to nonadherence.

e **Clinical use:** Establish a baseline average (mean) plasma level on the current oral antipsychotic dose, ideally during a period where adherence is high (based on one's best judgment), such as in an inpatient facility, or during a period of frequent pill counts. Levels more than 30% below that mean value without explanation (see Box 4.1) require a follow-up level after a nonjudgmental discussion with the patient (see Box 4.3). Levels more than 50% below the mean (without explanation), or the presence of symptomatic worsening, require more urgency in the communication with the patient and in repeating the plasma level (Figure 4.8). In some instances, the dose may have to be adjusted before the next level; if so, the level should be obtained at steady state and the expected plasma level for this higher dose estimated from the mean value on the lower dose. A subsequent level close to the mean (if unchanged), or to the expected value (if increased), establishes that nonadherence was the issue and should prompt a discussion about causes (e.g. avoidance of adverse effects, uncertainty about the need, etc.) and ways to address this using principles of shared decision making as much as possible [29]. Unless the patient is a candidate for an LAI, ongoing random 12h trough plasma level monitoring will be helpful.

Figure 4.8 Case example: use of plasma levels to identify nonadherence

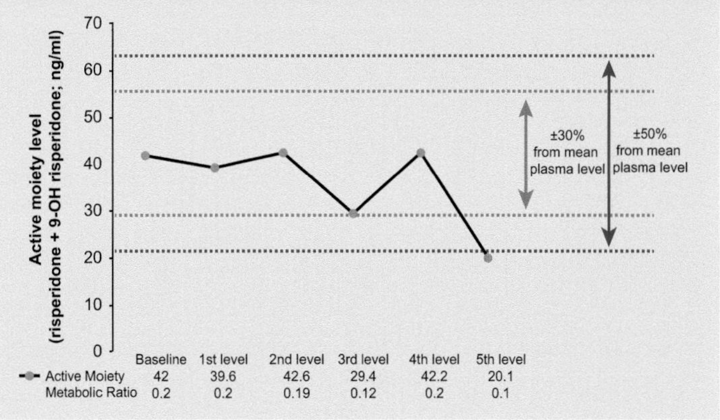

from studies that compare CV data on plasma antipsychotic levels for both inpatients and outpatients. One of the better-documented papers examined plasma levels from inpatients and outpatients with schizophrenia, in which patients were randomized to fixed doses of one of three antipsychotics (haloperidol, thioridazine, mesoridazine). Repeated sampling took place, and during the 3-week inpatient study 4–6 trough levels were drawn between days 6 and 24, while the outpatients had weekly levels during month 1, every 2 weeks during month 2, and monthly thereafter. The outpatient data was analyzed only for the fixed-dose portion of the study (months 1–3), with a range of 4–10 plasma levels available for each subject. To improve adherence, outpatients were given pill boxes with the doses distributed for each day until the next visit, and also asked to keep medication diaries and note any deviation from the dosing schedule [49]. While the mean CV for inpatients was nearly identical across all three antipsychotics (range 24.4%–24.9%), the range of mean CVs for outpatients was much broader (34.7%–49.4%), and the values markedly higher than for the inpatients (39%–99%) (Table 4.2) [49]. LAI antipsychotics offer a number of advantages to schizophrenia patients, and, based on the absence of adherence and timing issues, one might expect the variation in trough plasma levels to be low, yet data from a 1-year study of 43 adult schizophrenia patients on stables dose of fluphenazine decanoate found the median within-subject CV was 31%, almost identical to that with oral therapy and good adherence [50]. The data from this LAI study and that from the inpatient fixed-dose study provide the best evidence that, even under ideal circumstances with limited nonadherence, variations of 25%–30% are seen with oral antipsychotic treatment.

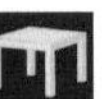

Table 4.2 Outpatients with schizophrenia have larger within-subject (intraindividual) coefficients of variation for plasma antipsychotic levels than do inpatients [49]

	Inpatient intraindividual CV	Outpatient intraindividual CV	*P*
Haloperidol	24.9% ± 15.3% (n = 38)	34.7% ± 17.1% (n = 15)	< .05
Thioridazine	24.4% ± 13.4% (n = 40)	45.3% ± 28.1% (n = 17)	< .001
Mesoridazine	24.8% ± 13.4% (n = 40)	49.4% ± 34.8% (n = 17)	< .01

Appreciating that trough antipsychotic values ± 30% from an established baseline are expected in adherent patients should shape the conversation when levels drop. The goal is to avoid accusing patients of nonadherence due to level fluctuations within the expected range, and to have relevant discussions when levels fluctuate 30% or more, ideally when the patient remains stable (Box 4.3). **While information on threshold plasma levels and the point of futility apply specifically to schizophrenia, one can use variation in plasma levels to track oral antipsychotic adherence regardless of indication (e.g. bipolar I disorder).** Whether an individual patient will relapse when the trough antipsychotic level is still within ± 30% of the baseline (or average) plasma level depends on the clinical indication; only sampling over an extended time frame can provide that answer for a specific patient and their diagnosis. Given the slow turnaround in some locales for plasma level results, these should be obtained with enough time before a planned visit for the result to be available so it can be reviewed with the patient. Due to the extended lag time between drawing the level and the clinic visit, it also might be difficult to correlate the antipsychotic level obtained 1–2 weeks ago with the current patient presentation; however, the information is useful nonetheless. If the patient is more symptomatic and the prior level very close to baseline, one can look for recent changes in adherence or other issues (e.g. substance use, psychosocial stressors). If the prior level was low and the patient is stable, then an adherence conversation ensues. When the prior level is low and the patient is more symptomatic, urgent discussions with all parties involved (including case managers and caregivers) must occur, focusing on immediate steps that can be taken to improve adherence, and whether an increased level of care is needed to manage the situation. In the near future, point-of-care devices will be available that provide plasma antipsychotic levels in real time, thereby allowing clinicians to schedule visits at 12h trough times, obtain the results, and then engage the patient in a meaningful interchange about adherence based on those (and prior) results.

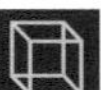

Box 4.3 How to Talk with a Patient about Low Plasma Antipsychotic Levels and Create a Follow-Up Plan

- Rule out other factors (see Box 4.1 and Case 4.1)
- After normalizing that people miss doses, explain that the level is lower than expected, inquire regarding how many doses might have been missed in the past two weeks and explore reasons why.
- Remain nonjudgmental. Patients with chronic illnesses have low rates of oral medication adherence. Schizophrenia patients also wrestle with cognitive dysfunction, and may have limited insight into the need for daily adherence despite psychoeducational efforts.
- Create a plan for improving adherence and rechecking the 12h trough level. (If the level has decreased > 50%, or the patient is symptomatic, see Box 4.2).
- Remain vigilant and repeat levels randomly as often as is deemed reasonable, based on distance to the laboratory, cost, patient fragility, risk factors (homelessness, substance use), and prior patterns on nonadherence. Clinical stability is not a good proxy for adherence.

C Identifying Kinetic Failure due to Genetic Variations – Role of Pharmacogenomics

The value in ongoing level sampling lies in the ability to rapidly identify subtherapeutic plasma levels, and differentiate treatment failure due to nonadherence from that related to other factors [51]. Without ongoing examination of plasma antipsychotic levels, one may erroneously assume, based on dose alone, that a patient is a nonresponder [52]. A 2018 analysis of 99 outpatients with schizophrenia, all of whom were deemed treatment-resistant and candidates for clozapine, found that 35% had plasma antipsychotic levels that were subtherapeutic [53]. Moreover, of the 35% with subtherapeutic antipsychotic levels, 34% of that group had undetectable levels [53]. A similar result was seen from a Norwegian database covering 2005–2017: 10.8% of patients had undetectable or subtherapeutic plasma antipsychotic levels in the year prior to starting clozapine [54]. By examining variation in plasma levels, one will often find patterns consistent with nonadherence, but what about the patient with persistently low levels without marked variation (i.e. variations less than ± 30%)? Assuming that trough levels are obtained approximately 12h ± 2h post-dose, there is a small list of possibilities to consider: the presence of inducers, genetic variants in drug-metabolizing enzymes, or poor drug absorption. Clinicians should know the major cytochrome P450 (CYP) metabolizing enzymes for each medication, and whether that CYP enzyme plays a significant role in the disposition of the medication. Ziprasidone is a notable example where CYP 3A4 is cited as the CYP enzyme that is responsible for drug metabolism

[51]. Technically, this is correct, but CYP-mediated metabolism is a minor pathway, and strong 3A4 inhibitors increase ziprasidone drug exposure only 35% [55]. Two-thirds of ziprasidone metabolism is via the aldehyde oxidase pathway, a highly expressed system not implicated in drug–drug interactions [56, 57]. (The major CYP enzymes and other metabolic pathways will be noted in the chapters for each antipsychotic.)

As part of the initial investigation into unexplained and unvaryingly low antipsychotic levels, clinicians must review a patient's medications to look for potential inducers of various CYP enzymes (Table 4.3). Smoking is a strong inducer of CYP 1A2 and must be noted, especially since there are genetic variants that increase the impact of smoking-mediated CYP 1A2 induction beyond its usual effect

Table 4.3 Prevalence of ultrarapid phenotypes for cytochrome P450 (CYP) enzymes primarily responsible for antipsychotic metabolism [58, 59]

Cytochrome P450 enzyme, and extent of activity in the human GI tract	Basic facts	Moderate/strong inducers	Ultrarapid phenotypes
CYP 3A4: 30% of all hepatic cytochrome activity, 70% of all gut cytochrome activity	Chromosome 7 Relatively few functional polymorphisms Low affinity / high capacity enzyme	Carbamazepine Efavirenz Nevirapine Oxcarbazepine Phenobarbital Phenytoin Rifampin	Yes, rare
CYP 2D6: 20% of all hepatic cytochrome activity, but only 1%–2% by weight	Chromosome 15 Multiple polymorphisms High affinity / low capacity enzyme	Not inducible	Ethiopian 29% Saudi 19% Spain 10% Italy 8.3% US Whites 3.5%
CYP 2C9: 20% of liver cytochrome activity (in combination with 2C19)	Chromosome 10 Multiple polymorphisms	Carbamazepine Efavirenz Lopinavir Nelfinavir Nevirapine Phenobarbital Phenytoin Rifampin Ritonavir	Unclear if this phenotype exists

Cytochrome P450 enzyme, and extent of activity in the human GI tract	Basic facts	Moderate/strong inducers	Ultrarapid phenotypes
CYP 1A2: 10%–15% of all CYP P450 activity	Chromosome 15 Multiple polymorphisms Low affinity / high capacity enzyme Located only in the liver	Cigarette smoke (but not by vaping) Omeprazole	No However, a variant (CYP 1A2*1F) exists that increases the inducing effects of smoking
CYP 2C19: 10% all CYP P450 activity	Chromosome 10 Multiple polymorphisms	Carbamazepine Efavirenz Rifampin Ritonavir	Yes, 2–7%

on CYP 1A2 expression [58]. When the presence of inducers is not found, the other possibility is increased drug metabolism via genetic variants. These UM phenotypes are due to gene duplications or gain-of-function mutations, the prevalence of which varies for each CYP enzyme and for various populations [59]. Figure 4.9 illustrates the range of activities of CYP 2D6 for a northern European cohort. While prevalence of the UM phenotype is low in northern Europeans, UM prevalence is extremely high in northern Africa and is also elevated (but not to the same degree) in surrounding Mediterranean regions such as Italy and Spain [58]. Laboratory reports for risperidone and clozapine plasma levels include the principal metabolites, so one can easily see whether the MR is significantly below the population mean, implying an UM phenotype. For other antipsychotics, relevant genetic testing should be ordered to avoid having the same issue with other medications which share that CYP isoenzyme. Although psychiatric genetic panels promoted by for-profit corporations do include CYP 450 polymorphisms, the field has expanded so rapidly that there is a significant chance these panels are out of date and only include variants identified 10 or more years ago. For this reason, it is strongly urged that samples be sent to a well-known reference laboratory, but even they miss newly reported variants, so patients can be PM or UM despite the lab not reporting this result [60]. Most antipsychotics have only one or two CYP pathways, so the genetic testing is ordered only for those CYPs predominantly responsible for drug metabolism. If the patient is found to have an UM phenotype, this must be flagged in the chart, and an antipsychotic chosen that might avoid such issues. For instances when no inducers or UM variants are found and the CV is $< 30\%$, the unsatisfying conclusion is that, for unclear reasons, the medication

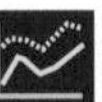

Figure 4.9 Frequency of various 2D6 phenotypes in a northern European cohort [58]

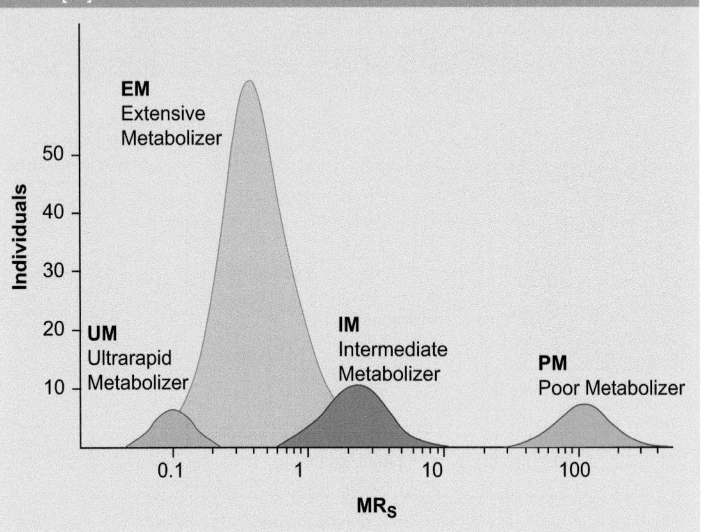

(Adapted from: U. M. Zanger and M. Schwab [2013]. Cytochrome P450 enzymes in drug metabolism: regulation of gene expression, enzyme activities, and impact of genetic variation. *Pharmacol Ther*, 138, 103–141.)

is not being absorbed (see Case 4.1). It is certainly possible that polymorphisms in drug transporters play a role in poor absorption, but investigating this may be costly and fruitless. An LAI avoids these issues entirely, but if an oral antipsychotic is to be used more frequent plasma level monitoring is necessary. If antipsychotic switching is not an option (e.g. a patient with treatment-resistant schizophrenia on clozapine), expert consultation should be sought to determine the safest way to increase plasma levels [61].

Summary Points

a Pill counts, regular plasma antipsychotic levels and third-party information are the most evidence-based methods for tracking oral antipsychotic adherence. Clinicians routinely overestimate oral antipsychotic adherence, and often use stability inappropriately as a proxy for adherence.

b Plasma levels in adherent patients may still vary ± 30% between determinations, with slightly smaller values on inpatient units (± 25%), and higher values for outpatients. Variations > 50% are likely due to nonadherence, assuming timing and dosing errors have been minimized.

c Causes for low levels must be sought before concluding that nonadherence is the culprit. One level may not be enough to conclude that nonadherence is the issue when no baseline levels exist, as the patient could be an UM. Having a second data point is immensely useful.

d Clinicians must learn to normalize problems with oral medication adherence as this is common with all chronic diseases. Develop a nonjudgmental language to converse with patients about lower than expected plasma levels, and use this language to create a plan for improved adherence with as much of the patient's input as is possible.

e Ultrarapid metabolizer phenotypes exist for various CYP enzymes, especially CYP 2D6. This should be suspected when levels are persistently low but also vary little, eliminating the possibility of nonadherence. Laboratories may not assay all CYP known variants, so the UM phenotype is still possible despite the lack of lab confirmation. Low levels with a low CV can also be due to poor absorption.

References

1. **Lam, W. Y. and Fresco, P. (2015).** Medication adherence measures: An overview. *Biomed Res Int*, 2015, 217047.
2. **Abegaz, T. M., Shehab, A., Gebreyohannes, E. A., *et al.* (2017).** Nonadherence to antihypertensive drugs: A systematic review and meta-analysis. *Medicine (Baltimore)*, 96, e5641.
3. **Buchanan, A., Sint, K., Swanson, J., *et al.* (2019).** Correlates of future violence in people being treated for schizophrenia. *Am J Psychiatry*, 176, 694–701.
4. **Velligan, D. I., Maples, N. J., Pokorny, J. J., *et al.* (2020).** Assessment of adherence to oral antipsychotic medications: What has changed over the past decade? *Schizophr Res*, 215, 17–24.
5. **Takeuchi, H., Siu, C., Remington, G., *et al.* (2019).** Does relapse contribute to treatment resistance? Antipsychotic response in first- vs. second-episode schizophrenia. *Neuropsychopharmacology*, 44, 1036–1042.
6. **Kishi, T., Oya, K., and Iwata, N. (2016).** Long-acting injectable antipsychotics for the prevention of relapse in patients with recent-onset psychotic disorders: A systematic review and meta-analysis of randomized controlled trials. *Psychiatry Res*, 246, 750–755.
7. **Kishimoto, T., Hagi, K., Nitta, M., *et al.* (2018).** Effectiveness of long-acting injectable vs oral antipsychotics in patients with schizophrenia: A meta-analysis of prospective and retrospective cohort studies. *Schizophr Bull*, 44, 603–619.
8. **Miura, G., Misawa, F., Kawade, Y., *et al.* (2019).** Long-acting injectables versus oral antipsychotics: A retrospective bidirectional mirror-image study. *J Clin Psychopharmacol*, 39, 441–445.
9. **Weiden, P. J., Schooler, N. R., Weedon, J. C., *et al.* (2009).** A randomized controlled trial of long-acting injectable risperidone vs continuation on oral atypical antipsychotics for first-episode schizophrenia patients: Initial adherence outcome. *J Clin Psychiatry*, 70, 1397–1406.
10. **Weiden, P. J., Schooler, N. R., Weedon, J. C., *et al.* (2012).** Maintenance treatment with long-acting injectable risperidone in first-episode schizophrenia: A randomized effectiveness study. *J Clin Psychiatry*, 73, 1224–1233.
11. **Subotnik, K. L., Casaus, L. R., Ventura, J., *et al.* (2015).** Long-acting injectable risperidone for relapse prevention and control of breakthrough symptoms after a recent first episode of schizophrenia: A randomized clinical trial. *JAMA Psychiatry*, 72, 822–829.
12. **Kane, J. M., Schooler, N. R., Marcy, P., *et al.* (2019).** Patients with early-phase schizophrenia will accept treatment with sustained-release medication (long-acting injectable antipsychotics): Results from the recruitment phase of the PRELAPSE trial. *J Clin Psychiatry*, 80, 18m12546.
13. **Abdel-Baki, A., Medrano, S., Maranda, C., *et al.* (2020).** Impact of early use of long-acting injectable antipsychotics on psychotic relapses and hospitalizations in first-episode psychosis. *Int Clin Psychopharmacol*, 35, 221–228.
14. **Kane, J. M., Schooler, N. R., Marcy, P., *et al.* (2020).** Effect of long-acting injectable antipsychotics vs usual care on time to first hospitalization in early-phase schizophrenia: A randomized clinical trial. *JAMA Psychiatry*, 77, 1–8.
15. **Medrano, S., Abdel-Baki, A., Stip, E., *et al.* (2018).** Three-year naturalistic study on early use of long-acting injectable antipsychotics in first episode psychosis. *Psychopharmacol Bull*, 48, 25–61.
16. **Robinson, D. G., Subramaniam, A., Fearis, P. J., *et al.* (2019).** Focused ethnographic examination of barriers to use of long-acting injectable antipsychotics. *Psychiatr Serv*, appips201900236.
17. **Lindenmayer, J. P., Glick, I. D., Talreja, H., *et al.* (2020).** Persistent barriers to the use of long-acting injectable antipsychotics for the treatment of schizophrenia. *J Clin Psychopharmacol*, 40, 346–349.

18. **Brain, C., Sameby, B., Allerby, K., *et al.* (2014).** Twelve months of electronic monitoring (MEMS) in the Swedish COAST-study: A comparison of methods for the measurement of adherence in schizophrenia. *Eur Neuropsychopharmacol*, 24, 215–222.

19. **Velligan, D. I., Wang, M., Diamond, P., *et al.* (2007).** Relationships among subjective and objective measures of adherence to oral antipsychotic medications. *Psychiatr Serv*, 58, 1187–1192.

20. **Yaegashi, H., Kirino, S., Remington, G., *et al.* (2020).** Adherence to oral antipsychotics measured by electronic adherence monitoring in schizophrenia: A systematic review and meta-analysis. *CNS Drugs*, 34, 579–598.

21. **Byerly, M. J., Thompson, A., Carmody, T., *et al.* (2007).** Validity of electronically monitored medication adherence and conventional adherence measures in schizophrenia. *Psychiatr Serv*, 58, 844–847.

22. **Remington, G., Teo, C., Mann, S., *et al.* (2013).** Examining levels of antipsychotic adherence to better understand nonadherence. *J Clin Psychopharmacol*, 33, 261–263.

23. **MacEwan, J. P., Forma, F. M., Shafrin, J., *et al.* (2016).** Patterns of adherence to oral atypical antipsychotics among patients diagnosed with schizophrenia. *J Manag Care Spec Pharm*, 22, 1349–1361.

24. **Lopez, V. L., Shaikh, A., Merson, J., *et al.* (2017).** Accuracy of clinician assessments of medication status in the emergency setting – a comparison of clinician assessment of antipsychotic usage and plasma level determination. *J Clin Psychopharmacol*, 37, 310–314.

25. **Kurokawa, S., Kishimoto, T., Su, K.-P., *et al.* (2019).** Psychiatrists' perceptions of medication adherence among patients with schizophrenia: An international survey. *Schizophr Res*, 211, 105–107.

26. **Velligan, D. I., Lam, Y. W., Glahn, D. C., *et al.* (2006).** Defining and assessing adherence to oral antipsychotics: A review of the literature. *Schizophr Bull*, 32, 724–742.

27. **Nieuwlaat, R., Wilczynski, N., Navarro, T., *et al.* (2014).** Interventions for enhancing medication adherence. *Cochrane Database Syst Rev*, 2014, CD000011.

28. **Thompson, L., Howes, C., and McCabe, R. (2016).** Effect of questions used by psychiatrists on therapeutic alliance and adherence. *Br J Psychiatry*, 209, 40–47.

29. **McCabe, R., Healey, P. G., Priebe, S., *et al.* (2013).** Shared understanding in psychiatrist–patient communication: Association with treatment adherence in schizophrenia. *Patient Educ Couns*, 93, 73–79.

30. **Sapra, M., Weiden, P. J., Schooler, N. R., *et al.* (2014).** Reasons for adherence and nonadherence: A pilot study comparing first- and multi-episode schizophrenia patients. *Clin Schizophr Relat Psychoses*, 7, 199–206.

31. **Hogan, T. P., Awad, A. G., and Eastwood, R. (1983).** A self-report scale predictive of drug compliance in schizophrenics: Reliability and discriminative validity. *Psychol Med*, 13, 177–183.

32. **Byerly, M. J., Nakonezny, P. A., and Rush, A. J. (2008).** The Brief Adherence Rating Scale (BARS) validated against electronic monitoring in assessing the antipsychotic medication adherence of outpatients with schizophrenia and schizoaffective disorder. *Schizophr Res*, 100, 60–69.

33. **Xu, D. R., Gong, W., Gloyd, S., *et al.* (2018).** Measuring adherence to antipsychotic medications for schizophrenia: Concordance and validity among a community sample in rural China. *Schizophr Res*, 201, 307–314.

34. **McEvoy, J. P., Byerly, M., Hamer, R. M., *et al.* (2014).** Effectiveness of paliperidone palmitate vs haloperidol decanoate for maintenance treatment of schizophrenia: A randomized clinical trial. *JAMA*, 311, 1978–1987.

35. **Nakonezny, P. A., Lindow, J. C., Stroup, T. S., *et al.* (2020).** A single assessment with the Brief Adherence Rating Scale (BARS) discriminates responders to long-acting injectable antipsychotic treatment in patients with schizophrenia. *Schizophr Res*, 220, 92–97.

36. **Pfeiffer, P. N., Ganoczy, D., and Valenstein, M. (2008).** Dosing frequency and adherence to antipsychotic medications. *Psychiatr Serv*, 59, 1207–1210.

37. **Beebe, L. H., Smith, K., and Phillips, C. (2017).** Effect of a telephone intervention on measures of psychiatric and nonpsychiatric medication adherence in outpatients with schizophrenia spectrum disorders. *J Psychosoc Nurs Ment Health Serv*, 55, 29–36.

38. **Xu, D. R., Xiao, S., He, H., *et al.* (2019).** Lay health supporters aided by mobile text messaging to improve adherence, symptoms, and functioning among people with schizophrenia in a resource-poor community in rural China (LEAN): A randomized controlled trial. *PLoS Med*, 16, e1002785.

39. **Uslu, E. and Buldukoglu, K. (2020).** Randomized controlled trial of the effects of nursing care based on a telephone intervention for medication adherence in schizophrenia. *Perspect Psychiatr Care*, 56, 63–71.

40. **Gaebel, W., Riesbeck, M., von Wilmsdorff, M., *et al.* (2010).** Drug attitude as predictor for effectiveness in first-episode schizophrenia: Results of an open randomized trial (EUFEST). *Eur Neuropsychopharmacol*, 20, 310–316.

41. **Quirk, A., Chaplin, R., Hamilton, S., *et al.* (2013).** Communication about adherence to long-term antipsychotic prescribing: An observational study of psychiatric practice. *Soc Psychiatry Psychiatr Epidemiol*, 48, 639–647.

42. **Meyer, J. M. (2014).** A rational approach to employing high plasma levels of antipsychotics for violence associated with schizophrenia: Case vignettes. *CNS Spectr*, 19, 432–438.

43. **Rostami-Hodjegan, A., Amin, A. M., Spencer, E. P., *et al.* (2004).** Influence of dose, cigarette smoking, age, sex, and metabolic activity on plasma clozapine concentrations: A predictive model and nomograms to aid clozapine dose adjustment and to assess compliance in individual patients. *J Clin Psychopharmacol*, 24, 70–78.

44. **Meyer, J. M. (2020).** Monitoring and improving antipsychotic adherence in outpatient forensic diversion programs. *CNS Spectr*, 25, 136–144.

45. **Müller, J., Keiser, M., Drozdzik, M., *et al.* (2017).** Expression, regulation and function of intestinal drug transporters: An update. *Biol Chem*, 398, 175–192.

46. **Jönsson, A. K., Spigset, O., and Reis, M. (2019).** A compilation of serum concentrations of 12 antipsychotic drugs in a therapeutic drug monitoring setting. *Ther Drug Monit*, 41, 348–356.

47. **Lee, J., Bies, R., Takeuchi, H., *et al.* (2016).** Quantifying intraindividual variations in plasma clozapine levels: A population pharmacokinetic approach. *J Clin Psychiatry*, 77, 681–687.

48. **Ng, W., Uchida, H., Ismail, Z., *et al.* (2009).** Clozapine exposure and the impact of smoking and gender: A population pharmacokinetic study. *Ther Drug Monit*, 31, 360–366.

49. **Shvartsburd, A., Sajadi, C., Morton, V., *et al.* (1984).** Blood levels of haloperidol and thioridazine during maintenance neuroleptic treatment of schizophrenic outpatients. *J Clin Psychopharmacol*, 4, 194–198.

50. **Gitlin, M. J., Nuechterlein, K. H., Mintz, J., *et al.* (2000).** Fluphenazine levels during maintenance treatment of recent-onset schizophrenia: Relation to side effects, psychosocial function and depression. *Psychopharmacology*, 148, 350–354.

51. **Schoretsanitis, G., Kane, J. M., Correll, C. U., *et al.* (2020).** Blood levels to optimize antipsychotic treatment in clinical practice: A joint consensus statement of the American Society of Clinical Psychopharmacology (ASCP) and the Therapeutic Drug Monitoring (TDM) Task Force of the Arbeitsgemeinschaft für Neuropsychopharmakologie und Pharmakopsychiatrie (AGNP). *J Clin Psychiatry*, 81, https://doi.org/10.4088/JCP.4019cs13169.

52. **McCutcheon, R., Beck, K., Bloomfield, M. A., *et al.* (2015).** Treatment resistant or resistant to treatment? Antipsychotic plasma levels in patients with poorly controlled psychotic symptoms. *J Psychopharmacol*, 29, 892–897.

53. **McCutcheon, R., Beck, K., D'Ambrosio, E., *et al.* (2018).** Antipsychotic plasma levels in the assessment of poor treatment response in schizophrenia. *Acta Psychiatr Scand*, 137, 39–46.

54. **Kylleso, L., Smith, R. L., Karlstad, O., *et al.* (2020).** Undetectable or subtherapeutic serum levels of antipsychotic drugs preceding switch to clozapine. *NPJ Schizophr*, 6, 17.
55. **Roerig Division of Pfizer Inc. (2020).** Geodon package insert. New York.
56. **Beedham, C., Miceli, J. J., and Obach, R. S. (2003).** Ziprasidone metabolism, aldehyde oxidase, and clinical implications. *J Clin Psychopharmacol*, 23, 229–232.
57. **Dalvie, D. and Di, L. (2019).** Aldehyde oxidase and its role as a drug metabolizing enzyme. *Pharmacol Ther*, 201, 137–180.
58. **Zanger, U. M. and Schwab, M. (2013).** Cytochrome P450 enzymes in drug metabolism: Regulation of gene expression, enzyme activities, and impact of genetic variation. *Pharmacol Ther*, 138, 103–141.
59. **Zanger, U. M., Klein, K., Thomas, M., *et al.* (2014).** Genetics, epigenetics, and regulation of drug-metabolizing cytochrome p450 enzymes. *Clin Pharmacol Ther*, 95, 258–261.
60. **Manikandan, P. and Nagini, S. (2018).** Cytochrome P450 structure, function and clinical significance: A review. *Curr Drug Targets*, 19, 38–54.
61. **Meyer, J. M. and Stahl, S. M. (2019).** *The Clozapine Handbook*. Cambridge: Cambridge University Press.

5 What Is an Adequate Antipsychotic Trial? Using Plasma Levels to Optimize Psychiatric Response and Tolerability

QUICK CHECK

PRINCIPLES

- The concept of delayed antipsychotic response in schizophrenia was disproven over 15 years ago. The 2-week rule for oral antipsychotic treatment notes that lack of early improvement (i.e. < 20% improvement) at week 2 predicts later nonresponse. Lack of early improvement demands assessment of plasma levels to determine if adherence or kinetic issues are an issue, and to guide dose increases.
- The Clinical Global Impressions improvement and severity scales can be clinically useful in deciding if a patient has met the 20% threshold for early improvement.
- For long-acting injectable (LAI) antipsychotics, the time frames for making response decisions are different, and depend on whether the LAI was loaded.

Plasma levels obtained 1h–72h before the LAI dose is due (typically 4–5 weeks after a loading or initiation regimen is administered) can help greatly in assessing response.

- **There are four reasons to terminate an antipsychotic drug for acute schizophrenia: substantial improvement; intolerable adverse effects; a point of futility has been reached for the plasma antipsychotic level; local or national formulary regulations preclude higher dosages. When none of these conditions has been met, ongoing titration guided by response and levels is the best course of action.**
- **Plasma level monitoring of oral antipsychotic therapy is necessary beyond the acute episode to track adherence and minimize relapse risk. For LAI antipsychotics, checking levels during the first year permits dosing adjustments as levels slowly rise to steady state.**

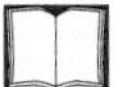

INTRODUCTION

Psychiatry is the youngest medical specialty, with continually evolving methods of disease classification, models of pathogenesis, and concepts about evidence-based management. One of the greatest advances in the treatment of schizophrenia comes from sophisticated analyses of clinical trials data, with a view to identifying patients who appear unlikely to respond to the current treatment condition (i.e. the current dose of the psychotropic) regardless of how much time they are given [1]. These analyses are not a trivial exercise, but a concerted effort to minimize unnecessary patient suffering when clinicians delay changes in dose (or medication), waiting for delayed response. The delayed response concept was reified in the old dictum that an adequate trial of an antipsychotic for an acute exacerbation of schizophrenia was 6 weeks of an "adequate dose," with vague definitions of what constituted an adequate dose [2]. Starting in the early 2000s, the 6-week rule came under attack as a group led by Professor Ofer Agid (the Centre for Addiction and Mental Health [Toronto, Canada], and the Department of Psychiatry, University of Toronto) re-examined results from all randomized, double-blind, placebo, or active controlled antipsychotic studies from 1976 to 2001 for temporal patterns of symptom improvement in schizophrenia spectrum disorder patients [3]. The 42 trials involved 7450 subjects (olanzapine, n = 3750; risperidone, n = 896; haloperidol, n = 2447; chlorpromazine, n = 95; and placebo, n = 262), with 52.4% performed in inpatients, and study duration ranging from 28 to 196 days. Subject age was 16 years and above, but most participants were not experiencing their first episode of psychosis, as noted by a mean age of 37.6 years and mean illness duration of 15.5 years. As illustrated by Figures 5.1a and 5.1b, it was

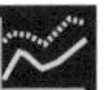

Figure 5.1a Time course of overall symptom improvement over weeks 1–4 in schizophrenia spectrum disorders (age 16 and above) [3]

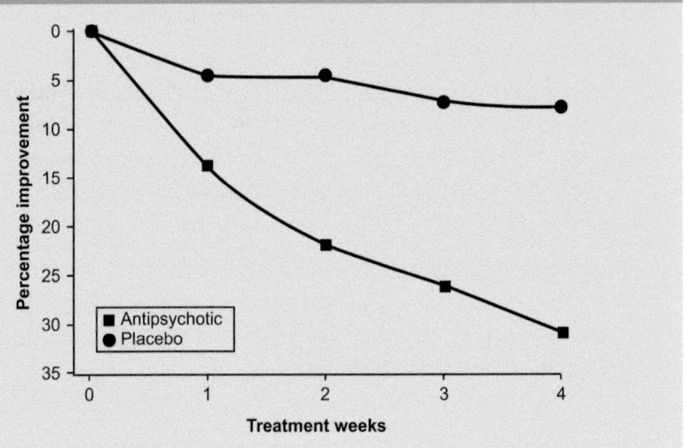

(Adapted from O. Agid, S. Kapur, T. Arenovich, *et al.* [2003]. Delayed-onset hypothesis of antipsychotic action: A hypothesis tested and rejected. *Arch Gen Psychiatry*, 60, 1228–1235.)

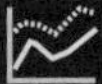

Figure 5.1b Percentage of overall symptom improvement over weeks 1–4 in schizophrenia spectrum disorder patients [3]

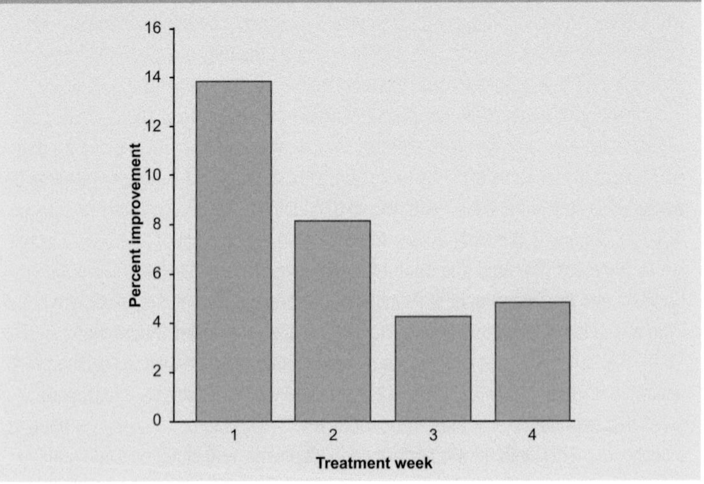

(Adapted from O. Agid, S. Kapur, T. Arenovich, *et al.* [2003]. Delayed-onset hypothesis of antipsychotic action: A hypothesis tested and rejected. *Arch Gen Psychiatry*, 60, 1228–1235.)

clear that the greatest extent of acute response to antipsychotic treatment occurred in the first two weeks, with less incremental change over time [3]. The groundbreaking paper by Agid and colleagues was published in 2003, and subsequently validated in 2005 in a paper by Professor Stefan Leucht (the Department of Psychiatry and Psychotherapy, Klinikum rechts der Isar der Technischen Universität München, Munich). The 2005 Leucht publication analyzed data from 1708 patients in seven randomized, double-blind antipsychotic trials of amisulpride (4–51 weeks duration), all of which had active comparators (e.g. haloperidol, fluphenazine, or risperidone) and no placebo arm [2]. Leucht and colleagues concluded that the early-onset hypothesis of antipsychotic activity was indeed confirmed, "as the reduction of overall and positive symptoms until week 2 was larger than the additional reduction until week four ($p < .0001$)" [2]. This conclusion held even when the analysis was confined to studies of 1-year duration (n = 748) (Figure 5.1c).

The US Food and Drug Administration (FDA) continues to require placebo controlled antipsychotic trials to support an indication for acute treatment of schizophrenia,

Figure 5.1c Percentage of overall symptom improvement over weeks 1–51 in schizophrenia spectrum disorder patients [2]

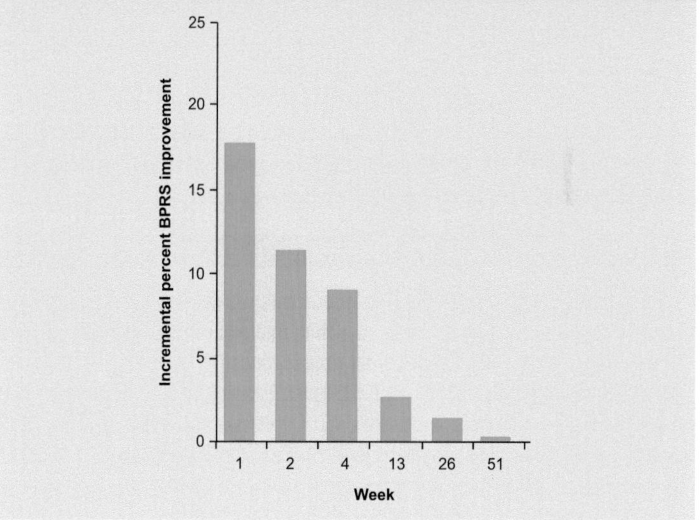

(Adapted from: S. Leucht, R. Busch, J. Hamann, *et al.* [2005]. Early-onset hypothesis of antipsychotic drug action: A hypothesis tested, confirmed and extended. *Biol Psychiatry*, 57, 1543–1549.)

thus subjecting one cohort to the risk of untreated psychosis. One fortuitous result of this conceptual shift in the view of response trajectory was the evidence-based recommendation to shorten placebo controlled acute antipsychotic trials from 6 weeks to 4 weeks. The goal is to minimize risk in the placebo arm, especially when there is no greater yield for response signal detection with trials of longer duration [4]. This strategy was recently employed for the US approval of lumateperone: two of the three pivotal studies were 4 weeks, and only one was 6 weeks; moreover, all three trials were performed on inpatients to enhance subject safety [5, 6]. Another consequence of these insights into early antipsychotic response has been the elaboration of the 2-week rule that provides a strong rationale for taking action when less than minimal clinical improvement is seen after 2 weeks of oral antipsychotic therapy [7]. Researchers in this area applied the same mathematical methods as those used for determining plasma level response thresholds (e.g. receiver operating characteristic [ROC] analysis – see Chapter 1), but in this instance to elucidate what degree of early nonresponse predicts later nonresponse. While the derivations are mathematical, the conclusions provide clinicians easy-to-implement criteria for deciding if a patient is an early nonresponder. How the criteria were elucidated and how they are applied to oral and long-acting injectable (LAI) antipsychotic therapy is the cornerstone of modern schizophrenia treatment. Importantly, antipsychotic plasma level monitoring plays a key role in determining whether nonresponse is related to underdosing, nonadherence, or kinetic failure [8, 9], and also when further titration is an act of futility with minimal odds of achieving substantial patient improvement [10]. By grasping these concepts, clinicians will be more adept at minimizing prolonged periods of undertreatment and curtailing excessive exposure to treatments that may be ineffective for that patient, regardless of how high the plasma level is pushed.

A The 2-Week Rule for Acute Response to Oral Antipsychotic Therapy

In its most basic form, the 2-week rule for oral antipsychotic therapy of an acute exacerbation of schizophrenia states: **less than minimal clinical response at week 2 is significantly associated with later nonresponse** [7]. (How this rule is modified for LAI treatment is covered in Section C below.) Following up the papers documenting early antipsychotic response, Professor Leucht, Professor Myrto Samara, and colleagues published a meta-analysis in 2015 of 34 studies with 9460 participants to test whether antipsychotic nonimprovement at week 2 predicts later nonresponse in patients with schizophrenia spectrum disorders [7]. In addition, the authors sought to calculate the optimal threshold of early nonresponse that predicts endpoint nonresponse, and to translate this into clinically useful language. The conclusions reached from this meta-analysis were considered robust not only due to the enormity of the database, but also to the fact that detailed patient-level data was available for 32 of the 34 studies. Moreover, the authors chose a clinically relevant criterion for response at study endpoint: 50% or greater reduction in symptoms using a standard rating scale (Positive and Negative Syndrome Scale [PANSS] or the Brief Psychiatric Rating Scale [BPRS]).

The first step was to examine various thresholds for ***early nonimprovement*** to determine the best predictor of later nonresponse. Table 5.1 presents the basic arrangement of a 2x2 array in which a test is performed with a binary result (Yes or no – Does this patient have early lack of improvement?), and there are two results (the patient is, or is not, a responder at endpoint). Recall that our test is one of early

Table 5.1 Understanding sensitivity, specificity, and positive predictive value (PPV) of early nonresponse based on the standard presentation of data in a 2x2 table

	Early responder **(our initial test on nonresponse is negative)**	Early nonresponder **(our initial test on nonresponse is positive)**
Patient is a responder at endpoint **(our test was wrong [early nonresponse did not predict later nonresponse] – a negative test result)**	**a**	**b**
Patient is a nonresponder at endpoint **(our test was correct [early nonresponse did predict later nonresponse] – a positive test result)**	**c**	**d**

Basic concepts:

1. **Our test is based on early nonresponse.** A negative (incorrect) result is that the patient turns out to be a responder at endpoint.
2. **Specificity = the true negative rate.** High specificity means low rates of false positives. Calculated from the table as:

   a/(a+b)
3. **Sensitivity = the true positive rate.** High specificity means low rates of false negatives. Calculated from the table as:

   d/(c+d)
4. **PPV** = the probability that a patient with a positive test result (in this case, a positive result is someone identified with early nonresponse), will indeed be a nonresponder at endpoint. Calculated from the table as:

   d/(b+d)

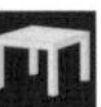

Table 5.2 Initial exploration of various lack of early improvement cutoffs as predictors of later endpoint antipsychotic nonresponse (< 50% symptom reduction at endpoint). The < 20% threshold maximizes specificity and PPV without unduly sacrificing sensitivity [7]

Cutoff for defining lack of early improvement based on % symptom reduction at week 2	Sensitivity (CI)	Specificity (CI)	PPV (CI)
≤ 0%	0.26 (0.23–0.30)	0.98 (0.96–0.98)	0.95 (0.93–0.96)
< 10%	0.43 (0.40–0.47)	0.94 (0.92–0.96)	0.93 (0.91–0.95)
< 15%	0.54 (0.51–0.58)	0.91 (0.88–0.93)	0.92 (0.89–0.94)
< 20%	**0.63 (0.59–0.66)**	**0.86 (0.82–0.89)**	**0.90 (0.86–0.91)**
< 25%	0.73 (0.69–0.76)	0.81 (0.77–0.85)	0.88 (0.85–0.91)
< 30%	0.80 (0.77–0.83)	0.74 (0.68–0.79)	0.86 (0.82–0.89)
< 40%	0.92 (0.89–0.93)	0.57 (0.48–0.66)	0.80 (0.76–0.84)
< 50%	0.97 (0.96–0.98)	0.39 (0.31–0.48)	0.76 (0.72–0.80)

CI = confidence interval; PPV = positive predictive value

lack of improvement – when the test is accurate, most of those identified early on by lack of improvement will have < 50% reduction in their symptoms at study endpoint. When looking at various thresholds for early nonimprovement (Table 5.2), another parameter was examined, namely that of positive predictive value (PPV). PPV reflects the probability that a patient with a positive test result (i.e. someone identified with early lack of improvement), will indeed be a nonresponder at endpoint. When treating patients with schizophrenia, specificity and PPV are important for the diagnostic test (i.e. the threshold for identifying early nonimprovement) for the following reasons:

a High specificity means low false positives. In this case, a false positive (i.e. there is early lack of improvement but the patient would have responded at endpoint) would cause the antipsychotic or the dose to be changed unnecessarily at week 2.

b High PPV means that early lack of improvement predicts endpoint nonresponse satisfactorily.

When analyzing any clinical test, one might value sensitivity or specificity more, depending on a variety of factors. For example, if the test were for a deadly and highly contagious disease (e.g. Ebola virus), one might want a test that has 100% sensitivity (no false negatives), with the tradeoff that you may have to quarantine some false positives. With these values in mind, the ROC analysis was performed and a cutpoint chosen that maximized specificity and PPV without unduly sacrificing sensitivity [7]. **The conclusion from this meta-analysis is that less than 20% improvement by week 2 is a significant predictor of eventual nonresponse. Moreover, the < 20% threshold has 90% PPV, meaning that out of 100 patients showing nonimprovement at week 2 (< 20% symptom reduction on PANSS or BPRS score), 90 will not show significant improvement at endpoint (< 50% PANSS or BPRS score reduction)** (see Box 5.1). These results held regardless of subject characteristics (gender, age, first episode, or chronic schizophrenia), study design (blinded, use of a placebo arm, randomized clinical trial or naturalistic, fixed or flexible dosing), the presence of industry sponsorship, or whether the antipsychotics involved were first or second generation. Further sensitivity analyses were performed, and the results remained unchanged when using observed cases only (as opposed to using

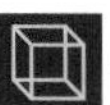

Box 5.1 The 2-Week Early Nonimprovement Rule for Oral Antipsychotics

The basic rule: Less than 20% improvement by week 2 is a significant predictor of eventual nonresponse.

Corollary 1: The < 20% threshold has 90% positive predictive value, meaning that out of 100 patients showing nonimprovement at week 2 (< 20% symptom reduction on PANSS or BPRS score), 90 will not show clinically relevant improvement at endpoint (< 50% PANSS or BPRS score reduction).

Corollary 2: Deciding whether nonresponse is due to nonadherence, subtherapeutic antipsychotic exposure, or treatment resistance will necessitate checking plasma antipsychotic levels, and consideration of further titration unless adverse effects are limiting, or the point of futility has been reached.

Corollary 3: Even among patients who are adherent with a level beyond the therapeutic threshold, < 20% response after two weeks predicts nonresponse. Allowing more time on the same antipsychotic dose with the same level hoping for 'late response' is not the appropriate clinical reaction to this scenario.

Example: The concept of late response with clozapine was often based on the prolonged titration needed to reach the therapeutic plasma level [11]. When studied systematically in a dose titration trial, the mean time to response (± SD) once a patient reached the clozapine dose (and level) at which they finally responded was 17 (± 14) days. In this treatment-resistant group, the range of time to response was broader than for other antipsychotics (2–56 days). Importantly, no late response was found among nonresponders despite a mean follow-up period of 75 weeks [12]. The conclusion from this data is that the 2-week rule might be modified for clozapine once plasma levels are beyond the therapeutic threshold of 350 ng/ml to allow a bit more time for response (e.g. 1 month, which represents one standard deviation from the mean time to response). Under no circumstances should a patient be left on the same dose and plasma level for months with inadequate improvement, hoping for late response.

statistical methods to impute missing data points), when treatment-resistant patients were removed from the analysis, when the few studies employing quicker titration were removed, or when the analysis was confined to specific medications with large sample sizes (e.g. haloperidol, olanzapine, risperidone, amisulpride) [7].

As noted above, early nonimprovement has a 90% PPV, meaning that 90 out of 100 patients showing nonimprovement at week 2 will not have significant clinical improvement at endpoint (i.e. will have < 50% PANSS or BPRS score reduction). Further analysis also indicated that, of the 100 patients exhibiting lack of early improvement, 55 will not even be minimally improved at endpoint (i.e. < 20% PANSS or BPRS score reduction). One should not infer from this that 55% of schizophrenia patients are treatment resistant, as the literature clearly shows that a substantial fraction might have subtherapeutic plasma levels [8, 9]. However, the PPV of early nonimprovement becomes more significant as the population rate of nonresponders increases (Figure 5.2). One of the limitations of this meta-

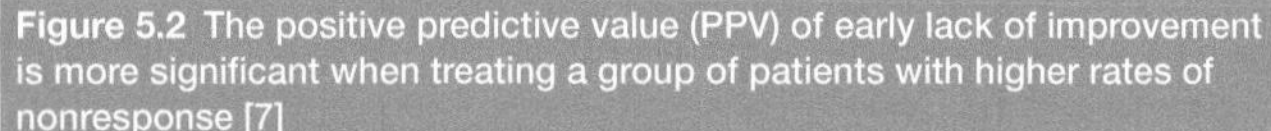

Figure 5.2 The positive predictive value (PPV) of early lack of improvement is more significant when treating a group of patients with higher rates of nonresponse [7]

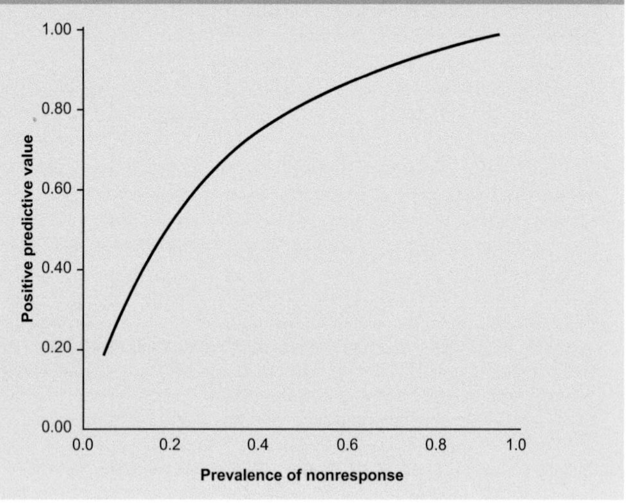

(Adapted from: M. T. Samara, C. Leucht, M. M. Leeflang, *et al.* [2015]. Early improvement as a predictor of later response to antipsychotics in schizophrenia: A diagnostic test review. *Am J Psychiatry*, 172, 617–629.)

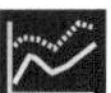

Figure 5.3 Difference in response rates between first-episode schizophrenia patients and those with a history of prior treatment [13]

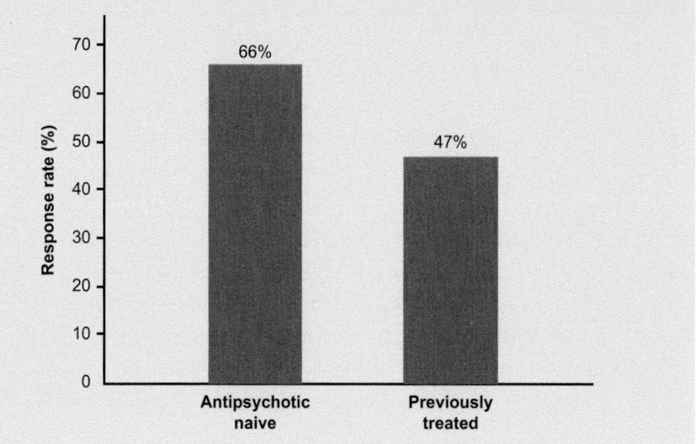

(Adapted from: P. M. Haddad and C. U. Correll [2018]. The acute efficacy of antipsychotics in schizophrenia: A review of recent meta-analyses. *Ther Adv Psychopharmacol*, 8, 303–318.)

analysis is that there were six studies with first-episode schizophrenia patients, and only one with treatment-resistant patients [13]. First-episode schizophrenia patients have higher response rates than previously treated individuals (Figure 5.3), so clinicians should consider extending the 2-week rule, although there is insufficient data to indicate exactly how long to wait before acting. As a matter of prudence, waiting more than 4 weeks may simply not be feasible, but a trial of 2–4 weeks will allow one to obtain a plasma level at steady state for nearly every oral antipsychotic. For clinicians working in facilities with higher rates of resistant schizophrenia (e.g. forensic psychiatric or state hospitals), the 2-week rule may have even greater predictive value, bearing in mind that only one study of resistant patients was analyzed [12, 7]. Despite that limitation, a prospective trial of clozapine treatment indicates that once patients reach a level where they will respond, this response occurs on average after 17 ± 14 days, with a range of 2–56 days (Box 5.1) [12].

For important reasons, particularly subtherapeutic plasma levels, lack of early improvement is not synonymous with treatment-resistant schizophrenia [13]. In the absence of intolerable adverse effects, most patients will warrant further titration, with termination of that specific antipsychotic trial based on the considerations outlined in Section D and Box 5.3. Nonetheless, the pool of schizophrenia patients who exhibit early nonimprovement captures a group whose eventual antipsychotic response is often less robust than early improvers. This claim is substantiated by findings from a recent double-blind, placebo-controlled trial of acutely exacerbated adult schizophrenia patients (mean age 40.8 years) that employed the 2-week rule. As part of the study design, those with lack of early improvement to a known effective lurasidone dose after 2 weeks (i.e. patients with < 20% reduction in the PANSS total score) were then re-randomized on a 1:1 basis to continue the original dose (80 mg taken with an evening meal), or a higher dose of 160 mg (also taken with an evening meal) [14]. Compared to those with early improvement (Figure 5.4a), those who lacked early improvement and whose dose was increased to 160 mg (Figure 5.4b) still had 1/3 less symptom improvement at the 6-week study endpoint; moreover, the patients who remained on 80 mg fared no better than the placebo arm [14]. This prospective study confirms the concept underlying the 2-week rule for managing acute exacerbations of schizophrenia: more time is not the answer. It also points to the fact that lack of improvement identifies a distinct group from early improvers – further dose titration makes sense in the absence of adverse effects, but the extent of response may be limited by inherent biological factors [15, 14].

To what extent early improvement predicts long-term stability is a separate question that was recently addressed in a 1-year follow-up study of 132 first-episode schizophrenia patients. Based on symptom ratings, ROC analyses were performed to identify the predictive validity of improvement from week 1 to week 8 for identifying odds of maintaining response through week 52 [16]. While the 2-week rule clearly defines those who are endpoint nonresponders, the authors found that a 51.6% PANSS total score improvement starting with week 6 correctly identified those who maintained response during follow-up, with a sensitivity of 74.7% [16]. The important clinical point is that early improvement is a strong indicator of endpoint response (i.e. ≥ 50% reduction in symptoms), but it is not a guarantee. Not all early improvers will achieve that ≥ 50% symptom reduction mark – therefore, those early improvers who fail to respond adequately over time might benefit from assessment of plasma levels to check for nonadherence, and ongoing antipsychotic titration if adherence is not the issue (see Section D below.)

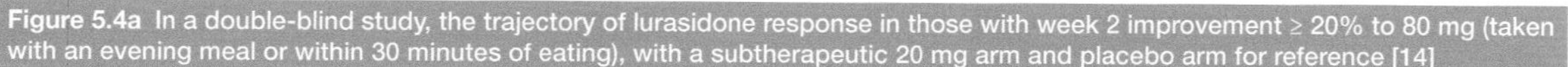

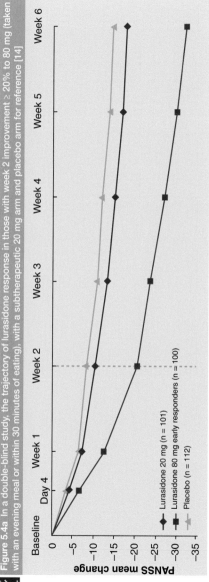

Figure 5.4a In a double-blind study, the trajectory of lurasidone response in those with week 2 improvement ≥ 20% to 80 mg (taken with an evening meal or within 30 minutes of eating), with a subtherapeutic 20 mg arm and placebo arm for reference [14]

(Adapted from: A. Loebel, R. Silva, R. Goldman, *et al*. [2016]. Lurasidone dose escalation in early nonresponding patients with schizophrenia: A randomized, double-blind, placebo-controlled study. *J Clin Psychiatry*, 77, 1672–1680.)

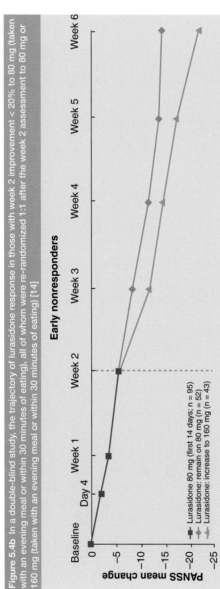

Figure 5.4b In a double-blind study, the trajectory of lurasidone response in those with week 2 improvement < 20% to 80 mg (taken with an evening meal or within 30 minutes of eating), all of whom were re-randomized 1:1 after the week 2 assessment to 80 mg or 160 mg (taken with an evening meal or within 30 minutes of eating) [14]

(Adapted from: A. Loebel, R. Silva, R. Goldman, *et al*. [2016]. Lurasidone dose escalation in early nonresponding patients with schizophrenia: A randomized, double-blind, placebo-controlled study. *J Clin Psychiatry*, 77, 1672–1680.)

Using the Clinical Global Impressions of Severity (CGI-S) and Improvement (CGI-I) Rating Scales to Track Nonresponse

Certain rating scales have gained traction in mental health when they are evidence based and, importantly, easy to use [17]. Standardized, anchored rating scales used in schizophrenia research trials, such as the Positive and Negative Syndrome Scale (PANSS) and the Brief Psychiatric Rating Scale (BPRS), require extensive and ongoing training to minimize rater error, and are not designed for routine clinical work [18, 19]. Those detailed instruments provide a breadth of nuanced information; however, when confronted with a schizophrenia patient experiencing an acute exacerbation, the overriding question is: How can I determine if this patient is 20% better by the end of week 2? In routine practice, clinicians use their best judgment about severity and extent of improvement to decide when to increase antipsychotic dosages or change to a different agent. Prior to 2013, patients would receive a score on the Global Assessment of Functioning (GAF) scale incorporated into the *Diagnostic and Statistical Manual of Mental Disorders* (DSM) multiaxial assessment. With the publication of DSM-5 in May 2013, the GAF was removed, partly because it combined severity and functioning into one scale, elements that should be rated separately [20]. In the DSM-5 section on Emerging Measures and Models, a Dimensional Assessment of Psychosis Symptom Severity scale was described (pages 742–744), with anchored ratings for eight symptom dimensions seen in chronic psychotic disorders: hallucinations, delusions, disorganized speech, abnormal psychomotor behavior, negative symptoms, impaired cognition, depression, mania [20]. The psychometric properties of this scale were unknown in 2013, but two papers emerged in 2013 [21] and 2016 [22]. Limitations of the 2013 study related to their use of a nine-item draft version, although they did find high internal consistency and inter-rater reliability (IRR) among the three raters [21]. The 2016 paper did not examine IRR, but found good correlation with information gleaned from the BPRS. Both studies appeared to use trained raters and did not examine scoring by clinical providers without research backgrounds.

A study was finally published in 2020 based on an analysis of multiple assessments (using the Dimensional Assessment of Psychosis Symptom Severity scale) of 335 consecutive adult schizophrenia outpatients recruited at the Academic Medical Center clinic in Amsterdam [23]. For this group, 179 PANSS ratings were also available. The point of this study was to examine whether daily information exchange between professionals results in reliable assessment of psychopathological dimension severity, and thereby calculate an IRR as this instrument is applied in typical practice settings. The study methodology was quite unique in this regard. A diagnostic patient interview was performed by a psychiatry and a psychology resident, together with an attending psychiatrist present, and the case presented in a formal staff meeting with other psychiatry residents, interns, psychologists, and psychiatrists. Prior to the staff meeting, a dimensional rating score was assigned by the attending psychiatrist who oversaw the patient interview. In the general staff meeting, a second rating was completed separately by other psychiatrists present, after hearing the case details. Despite the presence of anchors, the IRR between the two raters was low (0.35–0.64) for all items except delusions (0.74). The authors concluded that general implementation of the Dimensional Assessment in clinical practice should be done with caution, and that assessors must be trained before use [23].

Despite its obvious problems, the loss of the GAF score left clinicians without a severity scale that could be easily implemented, required minimal training, and whose psychometric properties are known. There is no perfect solution to this problem, but one option that best satisfies these criteria exists in the form of the Clinical Global Impressions (CGI) scales, devised in 1976 for psychopharmacology research (Box 5.2) [24]. The two scales (the CGI-severity [CGI-S] and CGI-improvement [CGI-I]) have obvious face validity, take only 1–2 minutes to complete, and are in the public domain [25]. Unlike the GAF, which generated confusion by conflating function and severity, the CGI assessments are based on severity, or changes in severity. Experience with the population in question is a prerequisite, but this aspect is possibly one of its strengths – it only relies on an adequate level of clinical judgment [26]. Issues of interrater reliability will exist for any instrument used outside of research trials, yet a review noted that "The CGI-S and CGI-I scales offer a readily understood, practical measurement tool that can easily be administered by a clinician in a busy clinical practice setting" [27]. The CGI-S is presently in use for admission and discharge ratings of psychiatric inpatients at some academic and community hospitals as a replacement for the GAF. Although the CGI scales are easily comprehended and scored, training can help to reduce variance in scoring, and this has been demonstrated in the context of industry-sponsored research studies [28]. With increasing use, disorder-specific guidance has also been published for use in conditions such as bipolar disorder and schizophrenia, providing further context for scoring these patient populations [29, 30].

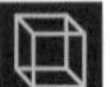

Box 5.2 What Is the CGI?

The Clinical Global Impressions (CGI) Scale is a standardized assessment tool to rate symptom severity and change over time, developed in 1976 [24]. The CGI Scale is widely used in clinical psychopharmacology trials, primarily in two forms: CGI-S (severity) and CGI-I (improvement). (An Efficacy Index was also created, but is not commonly used in recent decades.)

CGI-S (Severity)	CGI-I (Improvement)
1. Normal	1. Very much improved
2. Borderline mentally ill, not at all ill	2. Much improved
3. Mildly ill	3. Minimally improved
4. Moderately ill	4. No change
5. Markedly ill	5. Minimally worse
6. Severely ill	6. Much worse
7. Among the most extremely ill patients	7. Very much worse

Advantages

a Requires 1–2 minutes to complete.

b Instrument is in the public domain, has been used in psychopharmacology trials worldwide, and has been translated into multiple languages.

c Ratings are easily understood by all clinical personnel.

d The CGI-S can be performed without prior knowledge of the patient's condition (e.g. for newly admitted inpatients, or when patients or providers change settings).

e A symptom reduction of 20% corresponds to a rating of minimally improved on the CGI-I scale [31].

f Analyses of antipsychotic research data sets indicate strong correlation between changes in CGI-S and CGI-I and symptom changes using gold standard rating scales (PANSS, BPRS).

Issues

a The CGI-I requires knowledge of the patient's prior impression, and the rating may be difficult to move over time.

b CGI-S might best be performed at the beginning and end of a drug trial, and not at frequent intervals between (< 1 week).

c Ratings are dependent on the clinician's experience with that disorder. Example: a rating of 7 from a clinician who works with aggressive schizophrenia patients on an inpatient forensic unit may represent a different level of psychopathology than a rating of 7 from a clinician working primarily with schizophrenia outpatients.

d The data presented in Figure 5.5 show a strong linear association between CGI and PANSS ratings in a research setting when both were rated together by the same trained research personnel. Correlation between clinician ratings and trained raters is not known, nor between independent ratings of symptoms (by PANSS/BPRS) and CGI by separate raters. There may be other factors that require further study (ceiling effects, time effects, clinician expectation bias, etc.) [31, 25].

The value of CGI ratings is based on analyses of studies that correlate simultaneous symptom assessments (using PANSS or BPRS) and CGI ratings, with a total sample of nearly 6000 schizophrenia patients reported in some papers [31–33, 25]. As a matter of clinical use, the CGI-S has advantages when clinical personnel have equivalent levels of expertise with the severity range of schizophrenia patients in that setting, but where individual providers may not follow a patient throughout their course of treatment (e.g. the admitting psychiatrist is not the treating psychiatrist). The CGI-S can also be used when patients are moved between units or settings, as it does not require knowledge of interval change, and prior documentation is often sufficient to estimate prior severity. However, for the purpose of assessing early improvement, a symptom reduction of 20% corresponds neatly to a rating of **minimally improved** on the CGI-I scale, a 1-point change (Figure 5.5) [31]. Those who appear less than minimally improved at week 2 of oral antipsychotic therapy are thus unlikely to be responders without further assessment and changes in treatment (e.g. dose increase, etc.). When the CGI-S is used, a 20% decrease in the PANSS corresponds to less than a 1-point change. The impression that a patient improved one CGI-S point is associated with 30% symptom reduction (Figure 5.6) [25]. Were this assessment performed after 2 weeks of oral antipsychotic treatment, a 1-point CGI-S reduction would be associated

Figure 5.5 A PANSS reduction of 20% corresponds to a rating of minimally improved on the CGI-improvement (CGI-I) scale [31]

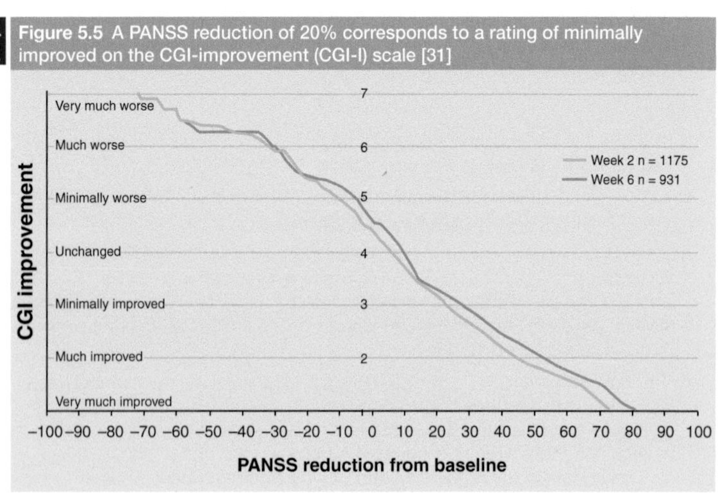

(Adapted from: S. Leucht, J. M. Kane, W. Kissling, *et al.* [2005]. What does the PANSS mean? *Schizophr Res*, 79, 231–238.)

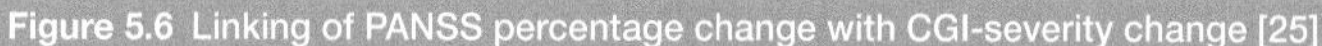

Figure 5.6 Linking of PANSS percentage change with CGI-severity change [25]

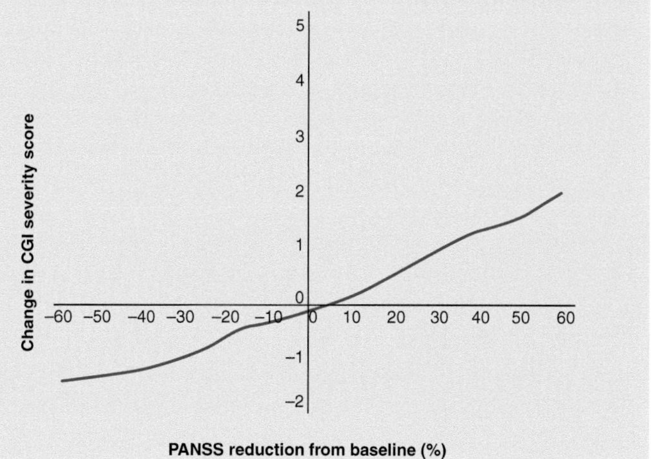

(Adapted from: S. Leucht, J. M. Kane, E. Etschel, *et al.* [2006]. Linking the PANSS, BPRS, and CGI: Clinical implications. *Neuropsychopharmacology*, 31, 2318–2325.)

with a favorable prognosis of an eventual meaningful clinical response (i.e. 50% reduction in global symptoms), since they had achieved ≥ 20% early improvement. The CGI scales provide a means of codifying the severity assessment that every clinician routinely performs in their own mind, and for communicating this information in objective language. They are not substitutes for detailed documentation of patient symptom dimensions, and should be considered as one of many perspectives on treatment response when caring for complex patients with schizophrenia.

C Modifying the 2-Week Rule for Long-Acting Injectable (LAI) Antipsychotics

Long-acting injectable (LAI) antipsychotics have a broad range of kinetics, and these correlate with time to steady state or therapeutic levels (see Chapter 1, Table 1.2 for the kinetic parameters of commonly used LAIs). The failure to load or initiate an LAI properly due to miscalculations about dose or early injection frequency can translate to subtherapeutic levels in the early weeks or months of treatment [34, 35]. Furthermore, some LAIs do not have an injectable initiation regimen or cannot be loaded (e.g. aripiprazole monohydrate, risperidone microspheres), so plasma levels early in treatment will be largely dependent on adherence with oral bridging therapy. The 2-week rule was derived from studies of acutely exacerbated schizophrenia patients; when treating that patient group, clinicians should preferentially consider starting an LAI that can be loaded (e.g. most first-generation antipsychotics, paliperidone palmitate, olanzapine pamoate) or has an initiation regimen (aripiprazole lauroxil), and thereby avoid the need for prolonged oral coverage. Decision making becomes greatly simplified when the question of oral adherence is removed, as lower than expected plasma levels will be attributed only to biological variability [10]. Population differences in cytochrome P450 (CYP) enzyme activities are an important source of variability, but even for a medication with limited phase I metabolism – paliperidone – there is a four-fold interindividual difference in dose-adjusted serum levels due to factors such as age, gender and body mass index [36, 37].

The initiation or loading process depends on the LAI, and this information is provided in detail in each relevant chapter of this handbook. The goal of loading an LAI is to achieve clinically relevant plasma levels within days or weeks, instead of in months (Figure 5.7, Figure 5.8). Although levels after loading may still be 25%–33%

Figure 5.7 Plasma fluphenazine levels during weekly loading with 50 mg [38]

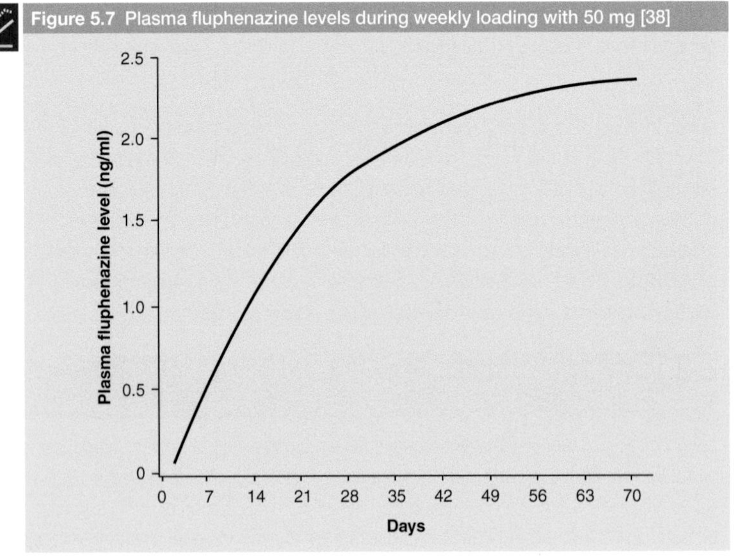

(Adapted from: M. W. Jann, L. Ereshefsky, and S. R. Saklad [1985]. Clinical pharmacokinetics of the depot antipsychotics. *Clin Pharmacokinet*, 10, 315–333.)

Figure 5.8 Plasma aripiprazole levels following an initiation regimen of 675 mg IM aripiprazole lauroxil nanocrystal (AL_{NC}), a single 30 mg oral dose, and simultaneous administration of 882 mg IM aripiprazole lauroxil [45]

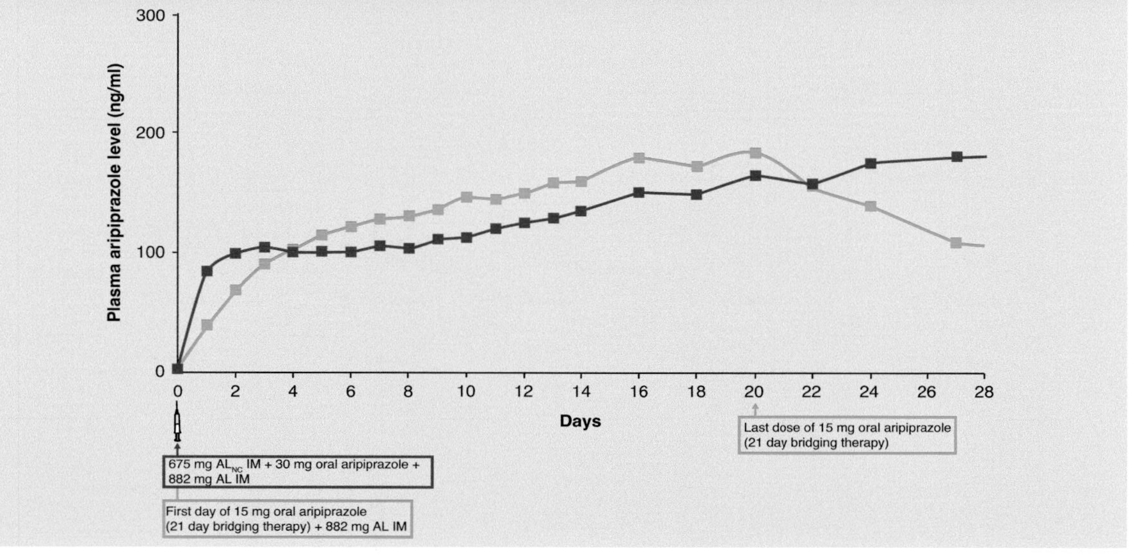

(Adapted from: R. Jain, J. M. Meyer, A. Y. Wehr, *et al*. [2020]. Size matters: The importance of particle size in a newly developed injectable formulation for the treatment of schizophrenia. *CNS Spectr*, 25, 323–330.)

below those at steady state [38–41], the therapeutic effect should increasingly be evident over the first month of treatment. Except for the 8-week formulation of aripiprazole lauroxil (1064 mg), the first maintenance LAI dose is typically due 4–5 weeks after the loading process is started, and this represents a useful juncture at which to reassess the patient, ideally supplemented with a trough plasma level drawn 1h–72h before the injection. In a perfect world, this plasma level result would be available to help to inform the maintenance dose. However, for patients exhibiting at least minimal improvement (i.e. 20% or more decrease in symptoms, or a CGI-I change of at least 1 point), there is less urgency, and one can choose a dose estimated to maintain the current plasma level, knowing that the level may increase over the next weeks and months as steady state is reached.

When patients have a less than minimal response, a decision must be made about going to higher drug dosages, or, when not possible, switching from a partial agonist (aripiprazole) to a full antagonist to achieve greater reduction in D_2 neurotransmission. If no plasma level result is available, this decision will be based on clinical judgment, the same method used for over 50 years since the invention of LAI antipsychotics [42]. Once the plasma level is reported, one of two conclusions will be reached: (a) this is a kinetic failure as evidenced by an unexpectedly low level; (b) the patient is a nonresponder at that plasma level, but achieves the expected antipsychotic concentration for the given dose [10]. For nonresponding patients who metabolize the medication as expected and are willing to take an oral medication reliably, one can add increasing doses of the oral counterpart of the LAI while continuing the LAI at a stable dose, and eventually consolidate all of the antipsychotic into the LAI using the trough plasma level drawn 1h–72h before the next maintenance LAI dose to help make this transition [43]. If use of oral supplementation is not realistic and the patient is not an ultrarapid metabolizer, continue to monitor and reassess at monthly intervals after dosage increases. If the antipsychotic must be changed to one using a different CYP pathway, track plasma levels of the new antipsychotic at periodic intervals as described above. It is very important to note that patients transitioning from an LAI formulation of aripiprazole may not see benefit from a D_2 antagonist antipsychotic despite levels above the therapeutic threshold for the latter, due to the high affinity for and occupancy of the D_2 receptor by aripiprazole [44]. As aripiprazole levels slowly diminish over weeks, the new antipsychotic will have greater access to the D_2 receptor, and its full antipsychotic potential will be seen. Avoid excessively high loading dosages of the D_2 antagonist in an attempt to override LAI aripiprazole; given the long half-life of LAI antipsychotics, the patient might experience an extended period of severe akathisia, dystonia or parkinsonism once aripiprazole levels drop significantly.

How to Use the Therapeutic Threshold to Titrate Antipsychotics Based on Response and Levels

As discussed in Chapter 2, plasma levels below the therapeutic threshold decrease chances of response. When a patient exhibits early improvement to a given oral antipsychotic dose by week 2, the clinician has the luxury of time to allow for further response and to obtain a 12h trough level quantifying the exposure for that dose. For those who lack early improvement at week 2, or 2 weeks following a dose increase, plasma levels are critical to deciphering the role of nonadherence or kinetic issues in inadequate response [8]. As noted in Chapter 4, the dictum "**one level is not enough**" applies in these situations when the patient is not responding and the plasma level is markedly below that expected based on concentration/dose correlations, and adjusting for the presence of any inducers [46]. (See discussion in Chapter 4 about use of the metabolic ratio of risperidone or clozapine to their respective metabolites, and genetic testing, to diagnose kinetic failures.) With a second plasma level, one can now look for variations that suggest poor adherence, or the absence of significant variations that suggest a kinetic issue due to ultrarapid metabolism, or, rarely, poor absorption.

For adherent inadequate responders who metabolize medications as expected but whose level is below the therapeutic threshold, the course of action involves a straightforward series of steps that will result in significant antipsychotic response, or termination of that antipsychotic trial after reaching a well-defined clinical endpoint (Box 5.3). At some point, more is not always better [15], but, in the absence of limiting adverse effects, further antipsychotic titration is warranted unless one reaches the point of futility, or local formulary regulations discourage or prohibit use of higher dosages [47]. As noted above, data examined from 1-year follow-up of 132 first-episode schizophrenia patients noted that those who fail to achieve approximately 50% symptomatic improvement starting with week 6 are at greater relapse risk. This 50% improvement corresponds to a 2.5-point reduction in CGI-I from baseline, or a 1.5-point reduction in CGI-S from baseline [31, 25].

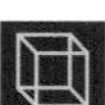

Box 5.3 Response to Inadequate Improvement after 2 Weeks of an Oral Dose (or Longer for an LAI or When Treating First-Episode Patients)

a When plasma levels are below the therapeutic threshold:

- **i** First, rule out adherence or kinetic issues if the drug concentration is more than 30% below that expected for the dose (see Chapter 3).
- **ii** If no tolerability issues exist, a dose increase is warranted to get into the therapeutic range. Where an individual patient might respond (if

they respond at all) is unknown, but the first step is to get beyond the minimum therapeutic threshold.

b When plasma levels are above the therapeutic threshold but less than minimal response occurs after 2 weeks following a dosage increase (or longer for an LAI or when treating first-episode patients), continue titration with reassessment **until one of 4 clinical endpoints is reached:**

Endpoint 1: Substantial improvement in psychotic symptoms is achieved

Endpoint 2: The patient is experiencing intolerable adverse effects

Endpoint 3: The point of futility has been reached with respect to trough plasma antipsychotic levels

Endpoint 4: Local or national formulary guidelines preclude use of higher dosages

Stopping an antipsychotic before one of those endpoints is reached deprives the patient of a full trial of that medication and may result in unnecessary switching. There may be compelling reasons why one does not complete an antipsychotic trial (e.g. a symptomatic patient refuses to continue with the medication titration despite the absence of adverse effects), but this should not be listed in the chart as a "**failure**" of that particular medication. Instead, document the reason the trial was not completed, the maximum plasma level attained and for how long, and note that this was an incomplete trial.

How to Use the Point of Futility to Titrate Antipsychotics Based on Response and Levels

When a patient fails to improve with ongoing titration, it is important to explore all reasons for antipsychotic nonresponse and not immediately assume the patient is treatment-resistant (Box 5.4). A failure to address substance use, untreated mania, or significant psychosocial stressors can limit the effectiveness of any antipsychotic trial. When adverse effects are not limiting, ongoing titration with plasma level confirmation is the most evidence-based plan of action until one reaches the point of futility. As discussed here and in Chapter 2, there is a subgroup of patients for whom adverse effects may not limit ongoing antipsychotic titration, even when the antipsychotic is a potent first-generation D_2 antagonist. The classic 1968 trifluoperazine titration study by Professor George Simpson illustrates this point, as it explored the range of doses which achieved a predefined level of neurological adverse effects (e.g. parkinsonism, akathisia, dystonia) (Table 5.3) [48]. The study was eventually terminated as one subject (# 5) had reached 480 mg/d of trifluoperazine (equivalent to 192 mg/d of haloperidol), yet had one of the lowest neurological adverse effect ratings. In

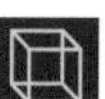

Box 5.4 Clinical Issues to Consider When Patients Fail to Improve Despite Antipsychotic Titration and Higher Plasma Antipsychotic Levels

a **The incorrect diagnosis:** Patients with schizophrenia spectrum disorders might be assigned a schizophrenia diagnosis based on the persistence of positive psychosis symptoms, but a review of past history suggests that there may be a bipolar diathesis, and the more appropriate diagnosis is schizoaffective disorder, bipolar type. Antipsychotics have antimanic properties, but do not have the same pharmacology as first-line mood stabilizers, which act at numerous second messenger intracellular pathways [52, 53]. While neurovegetative symptoms of mania appear improved with antipsychotics, other untreated aspects of mania will continue to drive positive psychotic symptoms and ongoing acts of impulsivity. This phenomenon was noted by the famous Danish physician Mogens Schou, who described it eloquently in the sixth edition of his guide to lithium treatment: "An experienced patient, who during previous manias had first tried a neuroleptic and then lithium, reported that during treatment with the former he felt as if the gas pedal and the brake were pressed down at the same time. With lithium it was as if the ignition had been switched off" [54]. If there is any suspicion that there is an element of mania, the following steps should be undertaken:

i Antidepressants must be discontinued as their presence may continue to exacerbate the psychotic and mood symptoms even in the presence of a mood stabilizer. If there is a kinetic impact from the loss of CYP inhibition, then the appropriate antipsychotic dosage adjustments should be made. Once positive psychosis symptoms are controlled, depressive symptoms can be managed with agents less likely to induce hypomania or a mixed state.

ii The patient should be mood stabilized with lithium or divalproex (or valproate), with preference given to lithium for those with adequate baseline renal function (eGFR ≥ 75 ml/min) due to its superior antisuicide and neuroprotective properties [53]. An initial target serum level is the upper end of the maintenance range: 1.0 mEq/l for lithium, 100 μg/ml for valproate. Higher levels used for acute mania can be considered.

iii For patients where there is more doubt about the presence of a bipolar diathesis, an empiric lithium or valproate trial can be considered. In patients with schizophrenia without a bipolar diathesis, lithium is not effective at improving core psychotic symptoms [55], and any evidence suggesting adjunctive valproate is effective is entirely based on open-label trials with a high risk of bias [56]. These agents may reduce aggression in non-bipolar patients but not other manifestations of schizophrenia, so the lack of substantial improvement should be considered as evidence against there being a bipolar diathesis.

b **The presence of substance use, whether persistent or episodic** [57]

c **Ongoing significant psychosocial stressors:** Stress increases dopamine release in patients with schizophrenia spectrum disorders, and in individuals at high risk for schizophrenia, in a manner distinct from that seen in healthy volunteers [58]. This observation gave rise to the methylphenidate challenge as a predictor of schizophrenia relapse. Stable patients who experienced greater activation by the dopamine reuptake inhibitor methylphenidate were at greater relapse risk in the following year [59]. It is also the basis for research noting that some schizophrenia patients living in homes with high levels of emotional expressivity have greater relapse risk during periods of undermedication [60–62]. Inquiry into sources of stress should be sought and addressed as much as possible to minimize their effects on psychosis symptoms.

d. Treatment-resistant schizophrenia: One-third or more of schizophrenia patients are treatment resistant, and their response rate to nonclozapine antipsychotics is < 5%, or 7%–9% for high-dose olanzapine [63, 11]. Reaching the point of futility for an antipsychotic with moderate or high D_2 antagonism is a signal that this patient is most likely treatment resistant. For treatment-resistant patients, the response rate to clozapine is 50% on average. Once patients have reached the point of futility, other evidence-based adjunctive strategies (e.g. ECT) must be considered [64, 11, 65–67].

Table 5.3 Results of a controlled titration study in which schizophrenia patients were started on trifluoperazine 15 mg/d without antiparkinsonian treatment, and advanced by 10 mg per week until they reached a predefined level of neurological adverse effects [48]

Patient	Age (years)	Length of hospitalization (years)	Maximum daily trifluoperazine dose (mg)	Degree of psychiatric improvement	Maximum neurological rating	Weight change (lbs)
1	35	16	30	–	3.0	–5
2	52	31	150	–	1.2	5
3	52	27	100	0	1.5	–3
4	23	6	220	+	1.1	25
5	**30**	**11**	**480**	**+**	**0.4**	**30**
6	41	23	100	±	1.1	10
7	51	14	20	+	3.1	10
8	57	16	30	+++	2.0	12
9	42	11	40	±	2.0	12
10	55	32	60	+	2.0	6
Mean	**43.8**	**18.7**	**123**		**1.74**	**10.2**

Comments

1 Despite reaching a trifluoperazine dose of 480 mg/d (equivalent to 192 mg/d haloperidol), patient **5** exhibited a low level of neurological adverse effects, with limited psychiatric benefit. Unfortunately, he did gain a substantial amount of weight (30 lbs).

2 This controlled titration trial is the best illustration of the need to utilize the point of futility. A fraction of schizophrenia patients may never experience dose-limiting adverse effects of D_2 antagonism, so further titration beyond certain evidence-based plasma level thresholds is fruitless, and exposes the patient to other adverse effects (e.g. sedation, weight gain, orthostasis, anticholinergic effects) with < 5% chance of improvement.

well-studied medications, the point of futility can clearly be defined based on < 5% probability of response to higher plasma levels. For fluphenazine, this occurs at 4.0 ng/ml, as seen in Figure 5.9 [49]. Unlike treatment with clozapine, clinical efficacy for D_2 antagonist antipsychotics correlates highly with striatal D_2 occupancy, and results from the Simpson study and other sources indicate that certain patients can tolerate plasma levels associated with ≥ 90% D_2 occupancy. In the case of fluphenazine, a level of 2.23 ng/ml generates 89% occupancy, and 4.4 ng/ml 96% occupancy, but those same imaging studies also found individuals with levels ranging from 6.13 ng/ml to 16.19 ng/ml [50, 51]. For D_2 antagonists, the futility point typically occurs when D_2 occupancy is 90%–95%, while for clozapine the limiting factor is the burden of other (non-dopamine) related adverse effects.

Plasma antipsychotic level and not dose is the best proxy for central nervous system activity, and high doses are sometimes needed to achieve the necessary level for patients with kinetic factors that contribute to lower levels, including ultrarapid metabolizers, or when use of CYP inducers is unavoidable. The case

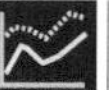

Figure 5.9 Estimated probability of improvement in the absence of disabling adverse effects based on plasma fluphenazine level [49]

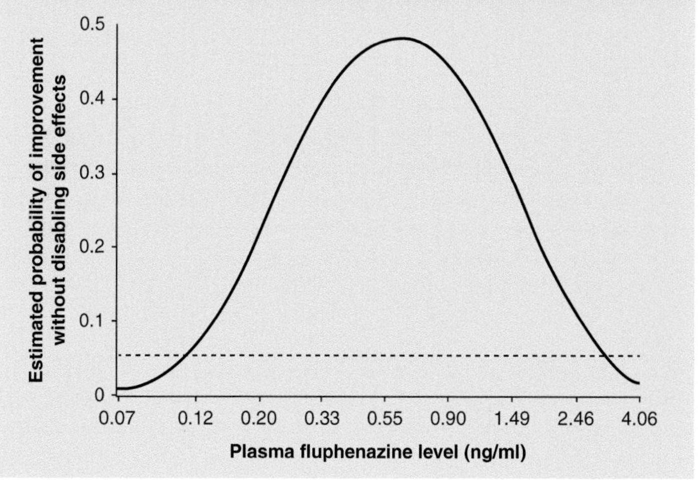

(Adapted from: K. K. Midha, J. W. Hubbard, S. R. Marder, *et al.* (1994). Impact of clinical pharmacokinetics on neuroleptic therapy in patients with schizophrenia. *J Psychiatry Neurosci*, 19, 254–264.)

documentation should always note that this patient's antipsychotic therapy is being guided by the plasma level, how those levels correlate with the literature, and the clinical response (symptoms and adverse effects) from ongoing titration [47]. The concept of the point of futility evolved based on treating schizophrenia spectrum patients in a forensic inpatient facility with a high prevalence of treatment resistance or impulsive aggression. It must be acknowledged that there is limited prospective, double-blind data supporting high dose exposure, particularly with inpatient populations [68, 69]. Due to unfounded fears about clozapine, or lack of knowledge, some clinicians may unfortunately and inappropriately resort to high-dose antipsychotics in lieu of starting clozapine, despite little chance of successful response [70, 71]. In an effort to limit this practice, certain institutional or national formularies deter prescribers from exceeding licensed dosages [47]. When permissible, the decision to pursue dosages above licensed maxima for management of the positive symptoms of schizophrenia (or for aggression) can reasonably be considered in the following circumstances:

a There are no dose-limiting adverse effects, and the plasma level is below the point of futility [10]. This will be especially true when the patient is a kinetic failure due to lower than expected plasma levels and the absence of known inducers of drug metabolism, and nonadherence has been ruled out with two or more plasma levels on the same dose with a limited coefficient of variation (e.g. < 30%).
b Other causes of treatment resistance have been ruled out (Box 5.4).
c Use of clozapine is precluded due to extremely poor patient cooperation with oral antipsychotics and the unavailability of intramuscular clozapine, there are difficulties in patient cooperation with ANC determination (despite the use of point-of-care ANC devices) [72], or the rare presence of certain medical conditions (e.g. pre-existing congestive heart failure with low ejection fraction).

Once the point of futility is reached, there is no compelling medical argument that can be made for exceeding this plasma level, bearing in mind that normal fluctuations in plasma levels may at times generate results above this limit. This will typically be the case for a patient whose average plasma level is very close to the point of futility (e.g. a mean plasma clozapine level of 985 ng/ml). As discussed in Chapter 3, the response to a level beyond the point of futility will depend on the context and the patient assessment (see Chapter 3, Box 3.1).

Ongoing Treatment Beyond the Acute Episode

Once a patient responds to a particular antipsychotic plasma level, the dose–response curve for that individual is now established. While clinical and imaging data provide plasma level guidance based on analysis of large samples, outliers exist who respond below the typical response threshold, or very close to the point of futility. Responders below the response threshold are particularly more common with LAI use [73]. The purpose of ongoing plasma level monitoring during oral antipsychotic treatment is to make sure a patient does not fall significantly below the plasma level which their brain needs for optimal response and stability [74]. While nonadherence is often signaled by plasma levels more than 30% below the established baseline (assuming other causes of low levels have been ruled out), when that might translate into relapse cannot be predicted: some patients may only tolerate levels within a narrow range (± 15%) and experience symptomatic exacerbation below that window; other patients may be minimally symptomatic for extended periods of time (weeks or months) with no antipsychotic present [75]. Regular plasma level monitoring of oral antipsychotic therapy is one of the evidence-based methods for tracking adherence to forestall prolonged periods of undertreatment that increase relapse risk [74].

For long-acting injectable (LAI) antipsychotics, one purpose of ongoing monitoring during the first year of treatment relates to plasma level "creep" that occurs due to the long time to steady state and saturation of tissue compartments that translates into higher plasma levels [76, 38]. Unlike oral antipsychotic therapy, the purpose of regular plasma level monitoring in the first year of LAI treatment is not adherence tracking, but to head off tolerability complaints from rising levels by making timely dosing adjustments. The other purpose is to permit appropriate dosing adjustments when CYP inhibitors or inducers are added for long-term treatment (14 days and longer). Newly approved LAIs present the CYP dosing adjustment considerations as part of the product information [77–82].

Summary Points

a Clinicians should understand the basis of the 2-week rule covering oral antipsychotic treatment of acutely symptomatic schizophrenia patients, and how this can be modified for first-episode patients, or for those on LAI antipsychotics.

b Symptom improvement as noted by a CGI-I change of 1 point equates to a 20% decrease in symptoms. A severity score decrease in CGI-S of 1 point equates to a 30% decrease in symptoms.

c An antipsychotic trial should only be terminated when one of four hard clinical endpoints is met: (1) Substantial improvement in psychotic symptoms is achieved; (2) The patient is experiencing intolerable adverse effects; (3) The point of futility has been reached with respect to trough plasma antipsychotic levels; (4) Local or national formulary guidelines preclude use of higher dosages.

d Plasma level monitoring of oral antipsychotic therapy is necessary beyond the acute episode to track adherence and minimize relapse risk. For LAI antipsychotics, checking levels during the first year permits dosing adjustments as levels slowly rise to steady state.

References

1. **Gorwood, P., Bayle, F., Vaiva, G., *et al.* (2013).** Is it worth assessing progress as early as week 2 to adapt antidepressive treatment strategy? Results from a study on agomelatine and a global meta-analysis. *Eur Psychiatry*, 28, 362–371.
2. **Leucht, S., Busch, R., Hamann, J., *et al.* (2005).** Early-onset hypothesis of antipsychotic drug action: A hypothesis tested, confirmed and extended. *Biol Psychiatry*, 57, 1543–1549.
3. **Agid, O., Kapur, S., Arenovich, T., *et al.* (2003).** Delayed-onset hypothesis of antipsychotic action: A hypothesis tested and rejected. *Arch Gen Psychiatry*, 60, 1228–1235.
4. **Younis, I. R., Gopalakrishnan, M., Mathis, M., *et al.* (2020).** Association of end point definition and randomized clinical trial duration in clinical trials of schizophrenia medications. *JAMA Psychiatry*, 77, 1064–1071.
5. **Vyas, P., Hwang, B. J., and Brasic, J. R. (2019).** An evaluation of lumateperone tosylate for the treatment of schizophrenia. *Expert Opin Pharmacother*, 30, 1–7.
6. **Meyer, J. M. (2020).** Lumateperone for schizophrenia. *Curr Psychiatr*, 19, 33–39.
7. **Samara, M. T., Leucht, C., Leeflang, M. M., *et al.* (2015).** Early improvement as a predictor of later response to antipsychotics in schizophrenia: A diagnostic test review. *Am J Psychiatry*, 172, 617–629.
8. **McCutcheon, R., Beck, K., D'Ambrosio, E., *et al.* (2018).** Antipsychotic plasma levels in the assessment of poor treatment response in schizophrenia. *Acta Psychiatr Scand*, 137, 39–46.
9. **Kylleso, L., Smith, R. L., Karlstad, O., *et al.* (2020).** Undetectable or subtherapeutic serum levels of antipsychotic drugs preceding switch to clozapine. *NPJ Schizophr*, 6, 17.
10. **Meyer, J. M. (2014).** A rational approach to employing high plasma levels of antipsychotics for violence associated with schizophrenia: Case vignettes. *CNS Spectr*, 19, 432–438.
11. **Meyer, J. M. and Stahl, S. M. (2019).** *The Clozapine Handbook*. Cambridge: Cambridge University Press.
12. **Conley, R. R., Carpenter, W. T., Jr., and Tamminga, C. A. (1997).** Time to clozapine response in a standardized trial. *Am J Psychiatry*, 154, 1243–1247.
13. **Haddad, P. M. and Correll, C. U. (2018).** The acute efficacy of antipsychotics in schizophrenia: A review of recent meta-analyses. *Ther Adv Psychopharmacol*, 8, 303–318.
14. **Loebel, A., Silva, R., Goldman, R., *et al.* (2016).** Lurasidone dose escalation in early nonresponding patients with schizophrenia: A randomized, double-blind, placebo-controlled study. *J Clin Psychiatry*, 77, 1672–1680.
15. **Giegling, I., Drago, A., Schafer, M., *et al.* (2010).** Interaction of haloperidol plasma level and antipsychotic effect in early phases of acute psychosis treatment. *J Psychiatr Res*, 44, 487–492.
16. **Schennach, R., Riesbeck, M., Mayr, A., *et al.* (2013).** Should early improvement be re-defined to better predict the maintenance of response in first-episode schizophrenia patients? *Acta Psychiatr Scand*, 127, 474–481.
17. **Siwek, M., Dudek, D., Rybakowski, J., *et al.* (2009).** Mood Disorder Questionnaire – characteristic and indications. *Psychiatr Pol*, 43, 287–299.
18. **Overall, J. E. and Gorham, D. R. (1962).** The Brief Psychiatric Rating Scale. *Psychol Rep*, 10, 799–812.
19. **Kay, S. R., Fiszbein, A., and Opler, L. A. (1987).** The positive and negative syndrome scale (PANSS) for schizophrenia. *Schizophr Bull*, 13, 261–276.
20. **American Psychiatric Association (2013).** *Diagnostic & Statistical Manual of Mental Disorders: Fifth Edition*. Washington, DC: American Psychiatric Press, Inc.
21. **Ritsner, M. S., Mar, M., Arbitman, M., *et al.* (2013).** Symptom severity scale of the DSM5 for schizophrenia, and other psychotic disorders: Diagnostic validity and clinical feasibility. *Psychiatry Res*, 208, 1–8.

22. **Park, S. C., Lee, K. U., and Choi, J. (2016).** Factor structure of the clinician-rated Dimensions of Psychosis Symptom Severity in patients with schizophrenia. *Psychiatry Investig*, 13, 253–254.
23. **Berendsen, S., van der Veen, N. M., van Tricht, M. J., *et al.* (2020).** Psychometric properties of the DSM-5 Clinician-Rated Dimensions of Psychosis Symptom Severity. *Schizophr Res*, 216, 416–421.
24. **Guy, W. (1976).** Clinical Global Impressions (028-CGI). In *ECDEU Assessment Manual for Psychopharmacology – Revised* (DHEW Publication ADM76-338). Rockville, MD: US Department of Health, Education, and Welfare: Public Health Service, Alcohol, Drug Abuse, and Mental Health Administration, NIMH Psychopharmacology Research Branch, Division of Extramural Research Programs, pp. 218–222.
25. **Leucht, S., Kane, J. M., Etschel, E., *et al.* (2006).** Linking the PANSS, BPRS, and CGI: Clinical implications. *Neuropsychopharmacology*, 31, 2318–2325.
26. **Mortimer, A. M. (2007).** Symptom rating scales and outcome in schizophrenia. *Br J Psychiatry Suppl*, 50, s7–14.
27. **Busner, J. and Targum, S. D. (2007).** The clinical global impressions scale: Applying a research tool in clinical practice. *Psychiatry (Edgmont)*, 4, 28–37.
28. **Targum, S. D., Busner, J., and Young, A. H. (2008).** Targeted scoring criteria reduce variance in global impressions. *Hum Psychopharmacol*, 23, 629–633.
29. **Spearing, M. K., Post, R. M., Leverich, G. S., *et al.* (1997).** Modification of the Clinical Global Impressions (CGI) Scale for use in bipolar illness (BP): The CGI-BP. *Psychiatry Res*, 73, 159–171.
30. **Haro, J. M., Kamath, S. A., Ochoa, S., *et al.* (2003).** The Clinical Global Impression-Schizophrenia scale: A simple instrument to measure the diversity of symptoms present in schizophrenia. *Acta Psychiatr Scand Suppl*, 16–23.
31. **Leucht, S., Kane, J. M., Kissling, W., *et al.* (2005).** What does the PANSS mean? *Schizophr Res*, 79, 231–238.
32. **Leucht, S., Kane, J. M., Kissling, W., *et al.* (2005).** Clinical implications of Brief Psychiatric Rating Scale scores. *Br J Psychiatry*, 187, 366–371.
33. **Leucht, S. and Engel, R. R. (2006).** The relative sensitivity of the Clinical Global Impressions Scale and the Brief Psychiatric Rating Scale in antipsychotic drug trials. *Neuropsychopharmacology*, 31, 406–412.
34. **Marder, S. R., Aravagiri, M., Wirshing, W. C., *et al.* (2002).** Fluphenazine plasma level monitoring for patients receiving fluphenazine decanoate. *Schizophr Res*, 53, 25–30.
35. **Hough, D., Gopal, S., Vijapurkar, U., *et al.* (2010).** Paliperidone palmitate maintenance treatment in delaying the time-to-relapse in patients with schizophrenia: A randomized, double-blind, placebo-controlled study. *Schizophr Res*, 116, 107–117.
36. **Samtani, M. N., Vermeulen, A., and Stuyckens, K. (2009).** Population pharmacokinetics of intramuscular paliperidone palmitate in patients with schizophrenia: A novel once-monthly, long-acting formulation of an atypical antipsychotic. *Clin Pharmacokinet*, 48, 585–600.
37. **Helland, A. and Spigset, O. (2017).** Serum concentrations of paliperidone after administration of the long-acting injectable formulation. *Ther Drug Monit*, 39, 659–662.
38. **Jann, M. W., Ereshefsky, L., and Saklad, S. R. (1985).** Clinical pharmacokinetics of the depot antipsychotics. *Clin Pharmacokinet*, 10, 315–333.
39. **Wei, F. C., Jann, M. W., Lin, H. N., *et al.* (1996).** A practical loading dose method for converting schizophrenic patients from oral to depot haloperidol therapy. *J Clin Psychiatry*, 57, 298–302.
40. **Altamura, A. C., Sassella, F., Santini, A., *et al.* (2003).** Intramuscular preparations of antipsychotics: Uses and relevance in clinical practice. *Drugs*, 63, 493–512.
41. **Pandina, G. J., Lindenmayer, J.-P., Lull, J., *et al.* (2010).** A randomized, placebo-controlled study to assess the efficacy and safety of 3 doses of paliperidone palmitate in adults with acutely

exacerbated schizophrenia [Erratum appears in *J Clin Psychopharmacol* 2010 Aug, 30(4), 364]. *J Clin Psychopharmacol*, 30, 235–244.

42. **Kurland, A. A. and Richardson, J. H. (1966).** A comparative study of two long acting phenothiazine preparations, fluphenazine-enanthate and fluphenazine-decanoate. *Psychopharmacologia*, 9, 320–327.

43. **Meyer, J. M. (2017).** Converting oral to long acting injectable antipsychotics: A guide for the perplexed. *CNS Spectr*, 22, 14–28.

44. **Takeuchi, H. and Remington, G. (2013).** A systematic review of reported cases involving psychotic symptoms worsened by aripiprazole in schizophrenia or schizoaffective disorder. *Psychopharmacology (Berl)*, 228, 175–185.

45. **Jain, R., Meyer, J. M., Wehr, A. Y., *et al.* (2020).** Size matters: The importance of particle size in a newly developed injectable formulation for the treatment of schizophrenia. *CNS Spectr*, 25, 323–330.

46. **Meyer, J. M. (2020).** Monitoring and improving antipsychotic adherence in outpatient forensic diversion programs. *CNS Spectr*, 25, 136–144.

47. **Barnes, T. R., Drake, R., Paton, C., *et al.* (2020).** Evidence-based guidelines for the pharmacological treatment of schizophrenia: Updated recommendations from the British Association for Psychopharmacology. *J Psychopharmacol*, 34, 3–78.

48. **Simpson, G. M. and Kunz-Bartholini, E. (1968).** Relationship of individual tolerance, behavior and phenothiazine produced extrapyramidal system disturbance. *Dis Nerv System*, 29, 269–274.

49. **Midha, K. K., Hubbard, J. W., Marder, S. R., *et al.* (1994).** Impact of clinical pharmacokinetics on neuroleptic therapy in patients with schizophrenia. *J Psychiatry Neurosci*, 19, 254–264.

50. **Coppens, H. J., Slooff, C. J., Paans, A. M., *et al.* (1991).** High central D2-dopamine receptor occupancy as assessed with positron emission tomography in medicated but therapy-resistant schizophrenic patients. *Biological Psychiatry*, 29, 629–634.

51. **Nyberg, S., Dencker, S. J., Malm, U., *et al.* (1998).** D(2)- and 5-HT(2) receptor occupancy in high-dose neuroleptic-treated patients. *Int J Neuropsychopharmacol*, 1, 95–101.

52. **Du, J., Quiroz, J., Yuan, P., *et al.* (2004).** Bipolar disorder: Involvement of signaling cascades and AMPA receptor trafficking at synapses. *Neuron Glia Biol*, 1, 231–243.

53. **Meyer, J. M. (2018).** Pharmacotherapy of psychosis and mania. In L. L. Brunton, R. Hilal-Dandan, and B. C. Knollmann, eds., *Goodman & Gilman's The Pharmacological Basis of Therapeutics*, 13th edn. Chicago, IL: McGraw-Hill, pp. 279–302.

54. **Schou, M. (2004).** *Lithium Treatment of Mood Disorders*, 6th edn. Basel: S. Karger AG.

55. **Leucht, S., Helfer, B., Dold, M., *et al.* (2015).** Lithium for schizophrenia. *Cochrane Database Syst Rev*, 10, CD003834.

56. **Wang, Y., Xia, J., Helfer, B., *et al.* (2016).** Valproate for schizophrenia. *Cochrane Database Syst Rev*, 11, CD004028.

57. **Weibell, M. A., Hegelstad, W. T. V., Auestad, B., *et al.* (2017).** The effect of substance use on 10-year outcome in first-episode psychosis. *Schizophr Bull*, 43, 843–851.

58. **Mizrahi, R., Addington, J., Rusjan, P. M., *et al.* (2012).** Increased stress-induced dopamine release in psychosis. *Biol Psychiatry*, 71, 561–567.

59. **Lieberman, J. A., Alvir, J., Geisler, S., *et al.* (1994).** Methylphenidate response, psychopathology and tardive dyskinesia as predictors of relapse in schizophrenia. *Neuropsychopharmacology*, 11, 107–118.

60. **Vaughn, C. E., Snyder, K. S., Jones, S., *et al.* (1984).** Family factors in schizophrenic relapse: Replication in California of British research on expressed emotion. *Arch Gen Psychiatry*, 41, 1169–1177.

61. **Nuechterlein, K. H., Snyder, K. S., Dawson, M. E., *et al.* (1986).** Expressed emotion, fixed-dose fluphenazine decanoate maintenance, and relapse in recent-onset schizophrenia. *Psychopharmacol Bull*, 22, 633–639.

62. **Hogarty, G. E., McEvoy, J. P., Munetz, M., *et al.* (1988).** Dose of fluphenazine, familial expressed emotion, and outcome in schizophrenia: Results of a two-year controlled study. *Arch Gen Psychiatry*, 45, 797–805.
63. **Howes, O. D., McCutcheon, R., Agid, O., *et al.* (2017).** Treatment-resistant schizophrenia: Treatment Response and Resistance in Psychosis (TRRIP) working group consensus guidelines on diagnosis and terminology. *Am J Psychiatry*, 174, 216–229.
64. **Siskind, D. J., Lee, M., Ravindran, A., *et al.* (2018).** Augmentation strategies for clozapine refractory schizophrenia: A systematic review and meta-analysis. *Aust N Z J Psychiatry*, 52, 751–767.
65. **Sinclair, D. J. M., Zhao, S., Qi, F., *et al.* (2019).** Electroconvulsive therapy for treatment-resistant schizophrenia. *Schizophr Bull*, 45, 730–732.
66. **Wagner, E., Lohrs, L., Siskind, D., *et al.* (2019).** Clozapine augmentation strategies – a systematic meta-review of available evidence. Treatment options for clozapine resistance. *J Psychopharmacol*, 269881118822171.
67. **Youn, T., Jeong, S. H., Kim, Y. S., *et al.* (2019).** Long-term clinical efficacy of maintenance electroconvulsive therapy in patients with treatment-resistant schizophrenia on clozapine. *Psychiatry Research*, 273, 759–766.
68. **Huang, C. C., Gerhardstein, R. P., Kim, D. Y., *et al.* (1987).** Treatment-resistant schizophrenia: Controlled study of moderate- and high-dose thiothixene. *Int Clin Psychopharmacol*, 2, 69–75.
69. **Kelly, D. L., Richardson, C. M., Yang, Y., *et al.* (2006).** Plasma concentrations of high-dose olanzapine in a double-blind crossover study. *Hum Psychopharmacol*, 21, 393–398.
70. **Cohen, D. (2014).** Prescribers fear as a major side-effect of clozapine. *Acta Psychiatr Scand*, 130, 154–155.
71. **Gee, S., Vergunst, F., Howes, O., *et al.* (2014).** Practitioner attitudes to clozapine initiation. *Acta Psychiatr Scand*, 130, 16–24.
72. **Kelly, D., Glassman, M., Mackowick, M., *et al.* (2020).** 09.1. Satisfaction with using a novel fingerstick for absolute neutrophil count (ANC) at the point of treatment in patients treated with clozapine. *Schizophr Bull*, 46, S20–S21.
73. **Baldelli, S., Clementi, E., and Cattaneo, D. (2018).** Can we rely on AGNP therapeutic targets also for LAI antipsychotics? *Pharmacopsychiatry*, 51, 270–271.
74. **Melkote, R., Singh, A., Vermeulen, A., *et al.* (2018).** Relationship between antipsychotic blood levels and treatment failure during the Clinical Antipsychotic Trials of Intervention Effectiveness (CATIE) study. *Schizophr Res*, 201, 324–328.
75. **Branchey, M. H., Branchey, L. B., and Richardson, M. A. (1981).** Effects of neuroleptic adjustment on clinical condition and tardive dyskinesia in schizophrenic patients. *Am J Psychiatry*, 138, 608–612.
76. **Ereshefsky, L., Saklad, S. R., Jann, M. W., *et al.* (1984).** Future of depot neuroleptic therapy: Pharmacokinetic and pharmacodynamic approaches. *J Clin Psychiatry*, 45, 50–59.
77. **Indivior Inc. (2019).** Perseris package insert. North Chesterfield.
78. **Janssen Pharmaceuticals Inc. (2019).** Invega Sustenna package insert. Janssen Pharmaceuticals, Inc., Titusville, NJ.
79. **Alkermes Inc. (2020).** Aristada package insert. Walltham MA.
80. **Eli Lilly and Company (2020).** Relprevv package insert. Indianapolis, IN.
81. **Janssen Pharmaceuticals Inc. (2020).** Risperdal Consta package insert. Titusville, NJ.
82. **Otsuka America Pharmaceutical Inc. (2020).** Abilify Maintena package insert. Rockville, MD.

6 Important Concepts about First-Generation Antipsychotics

QUICK CHECK

PRINCIPLES

- First-generation antipsychotics (FGAs) provide an inexpensive method of delivering D_2 antagonism.
- Many FGAs have extensive plasma level data, and several have multiple formulations including long-acting injectable (LAI) preparations.
- Certain FGA LAIs can be loaded, and this shortens the time to reach therapeutic plasma levels, and the time to steady state.
- Dosing of potent D_2 receptor antagonists should initially be modest, with titration proceeding based on response and plasma levels.
- The development of akathisia must be considered if a patient develops dysphoric affect or overt clinical worsening on higher dosages, even if the more overt objective aspects of akathisia are not evident.

Why Use a First-Generation Antipsychotic?

First-generation antipsychotics (FGAs) have no unique therapeutic benefit compared to newer antipsychotics, but their utility derives from the fact that they are inexpensive, that multiple formulations exist including long-acting injectable (LAI) preparations, and that there is an extensive trove of plasma level studies for the more commonly used medications [1–5]. Large randomized trials such as the UK Cost Utility of the Latest Antipsychotic Drugs in Schizophrenia Study (CUtLASS-1) (n = 227) found that there was no disadvantage over 1 year of treatment in terms of quality of life, symptoms, or associated costs of care when using FGAs, compared to second-generation antipsychotics (SGAs) (clozapine excepted) [6]. The CUtLASS-1 study results were generalizable to routine care due to the pragmatic design and broad inclusion criteria: DSM-IV schizophrenia, schizoaffective disorder, or delusional disorder; age 18 to 65 and at least 1 month since onset of psychotic symptoms; and psychiatrist electing to change the current FGA or SGA due to inadequate clinical response or intolerance [6]. The 2020 joint consensus paper from the Therapeutic Drug Monitoring (TDM) task force of the German Arbeitsgemeinschaft für Neuropsychopharmakologie und Pharmakopsychiatrie (AGNP) and the American Society for Clinical Psychopharmacology (ASCP) assigned a Level 1 recommendation (strongly recommended) for use of plasma level monitoring to six antipsychotics. Four of these are FGAs: fluphenazine, haloperidol, perazine, perphenazine [7].

In general, antipsychotics have comparable efficacy in adult schizophrenia patients who are not treatment resistant, but marked differences in tolerability [8, 9]. For treatment-resistant patients, the response rates to most antipsychotics are < 5%, for amisulpride and olanzapine < 10%, and for clozapine 40%–60% [10, 11]. Aside from the low-potency agent chlorpromazine, the dose-limiting adverse effects for most first-generation antipsychotics are usually neurological in nature (akathisia, parkinsonism, dystonia), but can also be related to hyperprolactinemia [8]. As recent studies have shown, many patients respond to modest FGA dosages, mitigating to some extent the risk of neurological adverse events [12]. Concerns about QT prolongation are confined to oral pimozide, thioridazine or chlorpromazine, intravenous haloperidol, overdose situations, and specific patients with histories of arrhythmias, electrolyte disturbances, use of multiple QT-prolonging medications, or a history of significant cardiovascular illnesses that markedly increase risk [12, 6, 13]. In 2020, clinicians from the US Association of Medicine and Psychiatry developed expert consensus guidelines for ECG monitoring in patients with medical and psychiatric comorbidities prescribed medications with potential for QTc prolongation [13]. Aside from intravenous use, the mean increase in QTc was 4–9 msec for haloperidol, comparable to that for lurasidone (5 msec), olanzapine (6 msec), risperidone (10 msec), and well below the highest-risk antipsychotics pimozide (19–24 msec) and thioridazine (28–37 msec) [13]. The authors constructed a risk assessment tool to determine those unusual circumstances when a baseline ECG should be performed even when not mandated by local prescribing guidelines.

Parkinsonism and dystonia are rarely overlooked, but early manifestations of akathisia may be confined to dysphoric affect or symptomatic worsening without obvious objective or subjective restlessness [14]. When clinicians are considering further titration of FGAs in search of greater response, they should be watchful for dysphoric affect or symptomatic worsening in addition to monitoring for the traditional signs of akathisia, parkinsonism and dystonia [2, 5]. If a patient on an oral FGA experiences akathisia or its psychiatric sequelae (dysphoric affect, symptom exacerbation) following a dose increase, immediate dose reduction back to the prior tolerated dose is warranted, with consideration of brief exposure to adjunctive medications (e.g. clonazepam, propranolol, mirtazapine [if no history of mania]) until resolved [15]. Dose reduction is also recommended when managing parkinsonism, and strong consideration should be given to using amantadine in lieu of anticholinergic medications (e.g. benztropine, biperiden, diphenhydramine, trihexyphenidyl) to avoid the cognitive dysfunction from central nervous system anticholinergic burden [16–18]. Prolonged use of adjunctive medications will be needed if akathisia or other neurological adverse effects develop during LAI FGA treatment, and these adjunctive agents should be withdrawn slowly over 2–4 weeks once the adverse effect abates. The next LAI injection will need to be delayed until complete resolution of the adverse effect without the need for adjunctive medication. One can estimate the new LAI maintenance dose using the plasma level obtained during the period when akathisia, parkinsonism, or dystonia were at their greatest severity, and from a level drawn after the neurological symptoms resolved.

Efficacy-related reasons to use an FGA include the need for greater D_2 antagonism, and the availability of an LAI formulation for nonadherent individuals. Despite higher risk for neurological adverse effects from potent D_2 blockade, FGAs (excluding chlorpromazine) have low risk for metabolic dysfunction, are not strongly anticholinergic, are nonsedating, and have lower rates of hyperprolactinemia compared to the three most offending agents: amisulpride, risperidone, and its metabolite 9-OH risperidone (also known as paliperidone) [19, 8].

B Converting between Different First-Generation Antipsychotics

Oral dose equivalency analyses have been performed using a variety of methods (Table 6.1), and can be helpful in converting between antipsychotics for schizophrenia patients who are not treatment resistant [20]. As with all meta-analyses, these dose conversion estimates are guides – individual differences in drug metabolism, concurrent medications, and inherent tolerability greatly influence the extent to which one antipsychotic can be substituted for another. Once a switch is made, one should

Table 6.1 Oral dose equivalency of commonly used first- and second-generation antipsychotics in acute schizophrenia [24, 20]

Medication	Oral equivalent (mg)
First generation	
Haloperidol	1.00
Fluphenazine	1.25
Trifluoperazine	2.50
Perphenazine	3.75
Thiothixene	3.75
Zuclopenthixol	3.75
Loxapine	12.5
Chlorpromazine	37.5
Second generation	
Amisulpride	82.4
Aripiprazole	1.82
Brexpiprazole	0.53
Cariprazine	1.21
Lurasidone	23.2
Risperidone	1.00
Olanzapine	2.15
Ziprasidone	29.5

Comments

[a] Clozapine dose equivalencies are not provided as the primary use is for treatment-resistant schizophrenia and there are no equivalent medications [11].

[b] Quetiapine dose equivalents are not provided as both naturalistic and clinical trials data raise concerns about efficacy as monotherapy for schizophrenia [25, 26]. When used at doses > 400 mg/d for schizophrenia treatment, quetiapine also has substantial metabolic adverse effects [27, 28].

Note: Other antipsychotic dose equivalencies for antipsychotics not listed here can be calculated using a spreadsheet developed by Professor Stefan Leucht and colleagues [20]. The results are reported based on a variety of methods (e.g. minimum effective dose, 95% effective dose, etc.) and the spreadsheet can be downloaded from their website:

www.cfdm.de/media/doc/Antipsychotic%20dose%20conversion%20calculator.xls

always use the principles outlined in Chapter 4 (i.e. the 2-week rule, and its modified versions for first-episode patients or those on LAIs) to monitor treatment.

Dose conversion guidelines for LAIs are a bit more problematic, in part due to the widely varying kinetic properties of these formulations, and whether the data are derived from steady state plasma levels. For example, the estimated steady state plasma level for paliperidone palmitate from three long-term studies (n = 69) is calculated to be 0.1645 x the monthly dose, using the American dosages which are based on the molecular weight of paliperidone + palmitate. (To convert paliperidone palmitate to paliperidone dosing, multiply by 25/39 [i.e. 0.641]: thus, 234 mg/month of paliperidone palmitate equals 150 mg/month of paliperidone) [21]. Using the highest monthly dose of paliperidone palmitate (234 mg), the steady state level should be 38.5 ng/ml, equivalent to 5.5 mg/d of oral risperidone [22]. Oral risperidone and oral haloperidol have similar milligram potency, based on extensive comparative studies [20], so one would expect that 234 mg/month of paliperidone palmitate would be comparable to approximately 5 mg/d of oral haloperidol. However, the LAI conversion formula from the 2020 meta-analysis generates an oral haloperidol equivalent dose of 7.9 mg/d [20]. The other question when switching any antipsychotic is one of efficacy: can a patient maintained on an FGA LAI be switched to a less potent D_2 antagonist (olanzapine risperidone, paliperidone) or to a partial agonist (aripiprazole)? This depends on the patient's inherent need for D_2 antagonism for psychiatric stability as estimated from the FGA plasma level at steady state and the relevant imaging literature [23]. Fortunately, all FGAs have identical mechanisms of action, so conversion between FGA LAI preparations can be guided by the current plasma level and its associated level of D_2 antagonism. This information can then be used to estimate the therapeutically equivalent plasma level of the next FGA LAI to generate a similar amount of D_2 occupancy (Box 6.1). From that estimated plasma level, one can calculate the dose of the new FGA LAI (see individual antipsychotic chapters in this handbook). If the prior LAI is at steady state, there is no need to load the new LAI since the slow decay in plasma levels for the first antipsychotic will overlap with the slow climb to steady state for the second FGA. Over many months, the second FGA will be the only antipsychotic present, and one can adjust the LAI dosages based on clinical response and the plasma levels.

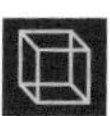

Box 6.1 Switching between Long-Acting Injectable First-Generation Antipsychotics: Estimating Dose Equivalency from Plasma Levels and D_2 Occupancy

Method: Obtain a steady state trough plasma level for the current LAI 1h–72h before the next dose. From that level, estimate the D_2 receptor occupancy for the current FGA (see individual antipsychotic chapters in this handbook), and find the plasma level of the new FGA which provides a comparable level of D_2 blockade. Use this information to estimate the dose of the new FGA LAI.

Example 1: A patient on haloperidol decanoate 250 mg/month has a steady state plasma level of 5.8 ng/ml, but is developing site reactions to the sesame oil vehicle. The treating clinician wishes to switch the patient to zuclopenthixol decanoate which uses a coconut oil diluent. What is a comparable zuclopenthixol decanoate dose?

a The D_2 occupancy for a haloperidol level of 5.8 ng/ml is approximately 90% (Figure 6.1) [29, 30].

b The estimated zuclopenthixol plasma level to achieve 90% D_2 occupancy is 10 ng/ml (Figure 6.2) [31].

c According to the manufacturer's labeling, the average steady state preinjection trough plasma level for zuclopenthixol decanoate 200 mg every 2 weeks is approximately 10 ng/ml [32]. Maximum plasma levels are reached 3–7 days following each injection, very similar to that with haloperidol decanoate, so zuclopenthixol decanoate 200 mg can be started in lieu of haloperidol decanoate. Loading will not be required since haloperidol decanoate is at steady state and will provide ongoing D_2 antagonism for many weeks until zuclopenthixol is at steady state [33, 34].

Example 2: A Norwegian patient on perphenazine decanoate 162 mg/3 weeks has a steady state trough plasma level of 6.0 nmol/l, but is moving to the United Kingdom where this product is not available. What monthly dose of haloperidol decanoate might be a reasonable substitute?

a The D_2 occupancy for a perphenazine level of 6.0 nmol/l is approximately 80% (Figure 6.3) [35].

b The estimated haloperidol plasma level to achieve 80% D_2 occupancy is approximately 3.5 ng/ml (Figure 6.1) [31]. This plasma level corresponds to an oral haloperidol dose of 4.5 mg/d.

c The oral to LAI dose conversion formula for haloperidol decanoate indicates that 20 times the oral dose is the monthly maintenance LAI dose – in this case, that would be 90 mg/month [36]. Haloperidol decanoate is commonly available as 100 mg/ml, so the decision was made to try 100 mg/month initially. Maximum plasma levels of haloperidol are reached on average 7 days following each injection, very similar to that with perphenazine decanoate [37], so haloperidol decanoate 100 mg can be started in lieu of perphenazine decanoate. Loading will not be required since perphenazine decanoate is at steady state and will provide ongoing D_2 antagonism for many weeks until haloperidol is at steady state [38].

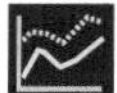

Figure 6.1 Fitted D_2 receptor occupancy curve for haloperidol [29]

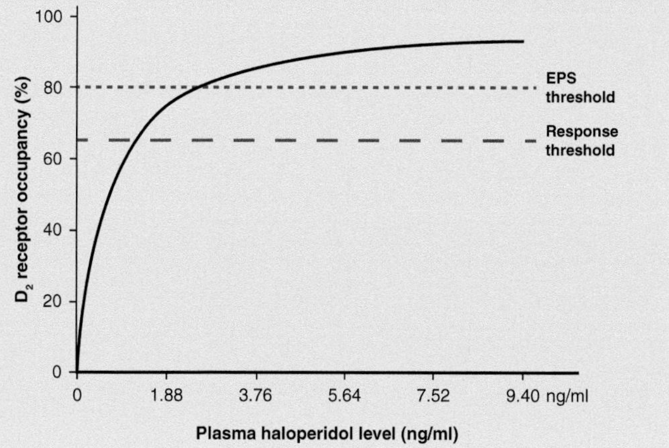

(Adapted from: R. Regenthal, U. Kunstler, U. Junhold, *et al*. [1997]. Haloperidol serum concentrations and D2 dopamine receptor occupancy during low-dose treatment with haloperidol decanoate. *Int Clin Psychopharmacol*, 12, 255–261.)

Figure 6.2 Fitted D_2 receptor occupancy curve for zuclopenthixol [31]

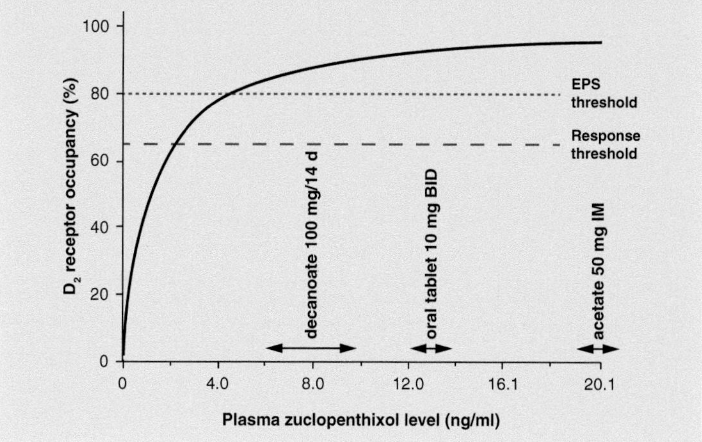

(Adapted from: S. Nyberg, L. Farde, A. Bartfai, A., *et al*. [1995]. Central D2 receptor occupancy and effects of zuclopenthixol acetate in humans. *Int Clin Psychopharmacol*, 10, 221–227.)

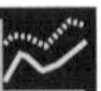

Figure 6.3 Fitted D_2 receptor occupancy curve for perphenazine [35]

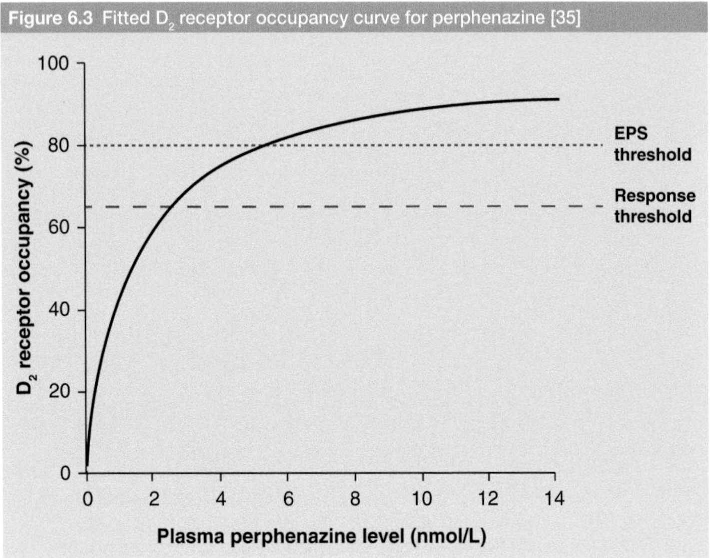

(Adapted from: M. Talvik, A. L. Nordstrom, N. E. Larsen, *et al*. [2004]. A cross-validation study on the relationship between central D2 receptor occupancy and serum perphenazine concentration. *Psychopharmacology*, 175, 148–153.)

References

1. **Van Putten, T., Marder, S. R., and Mintz, J. (1985).** Plasma haloperidol levels: Clinical response and fancy mathematics. *Arch Gen Psychiatry*, 42, 835–838.
2. **Van Putten, T., Marder, S. R., Wirshing, W. C., *et al.* (1991).** Neuroleptic plasma levels. *Schizophr Bull*, 17, 197–216.
3. **Midha, K. K., Hubbard, J. W., Marder, S. R., *et al.* (1994).** Impact of clinical pharmacokinetics on neuroleptic therapy in patients with schizophrenia. *J Psychiatry Neurosci*, 19, 254–264.
4. **de Oliveira, I. R., de Sena, E. P., Pereira, E. L., *et al.* (1996).** Haloperidol blood levels and clinical outcome: A meta-analysis of studies relevant to testing the therapeutic window hypothesis. *J Clin Pharm Ther*, 21, 229–236.
5. **Ulrich, S., Wurthmann, C., Brosz, M., *et al.* (1998).** The relationship between serum concentration and therapeutic effect of haloperidol in patients with acute schizophrenia. *Clin Pharmacokinet*, 34, 227–263.
6. **Jones, P. B., Barnes, T. R. E., Davies, L., *et al.* (2006).** Randomized controlled trial of the effect on quality of life of second- vs first-generation antipsychotic drugs in schizophrenia: Cost Utility of the Latest Antipsychotic Drugs in Schizophrenia Study (CUtLASS 1). *Arch Gen Psychiatry*, 63, 1079–1087.
7. **Schoretsanitis, G., Kane, J. M., Correll, C. U., *et al.* (2020).** Blood levels to optimize antipsychotic treatment in clinical practice: A joint consensus statement of the American Society of Clinical Psychopharmacology (ASCP) and the Therapeutic Drug Monitoring (TDM) Task Force of the Arbeitsgemeinschaft für Neuropsychopharmakologie und Pharmakopsychiatrie (AGNP). *J Clin Psychiatry*, 81, https://doi.org/10.4088/JCP.4019cs13169.
8. **Huhn, M., Nikolakopoulou, A., Schneider-Thoma, J., *et al.* (2019).** Comparative efficacy and tolerability of 32 oral antipsychotics for the acute treatment of adults with multi-episode schizophrenia: A systematic review and network meta-analysis. *Lancet*, 394, 939–951.
9. **Pillinger, T., McCutcheon, R. A., Vano, L., *et al.* (2020).** Comparative effects of 18 antipsychotics on metabolic function in patients with schizophrenia, predictors of metabolic dysregulation, and association with psychopathology: A systematic review and network meta-analysis. *Lancet Psychiatry*, 7, 64–77.
10. **Kahn, R. S., Winter van Rossum, I., Leucht, S., *et al.* (2018).** Amisulpride and olanzapine followed by open-label treatment with clozapine in first-episode schizophrenia and schizophreniform disorder (OPTiMiSE): A three-phase switching study. *Lancet Psychiatry*, 5, 797–807.
11. **Meyer, J. M. and Stahl, S. M. (2019).** *The Clozapine Handbook*. Cambridge: Cambridge University Press.
12. **Lieberman, J. A., Stroup, T. S., McEvoy, J. P., *et al.* (2005).** Effectiveness of antipsychotic drugs in patients with chronic schizophrenia. *N Engl J Med*, 353, 1209–1223.
13. **Xiong, G. L., Pinkhasov, A., Mangal, J. P., *et al.* (2020).** QTc monitoring in adults with medical and psychiatric comorbidities: Expert consensus from the Association of Medicine and Psychiatry. *J Psychosom Res*, 135, 110138.
14. **Van Putten, T., Marder, S. R., Mintz, J., *et al.* (1992).** Haloperidol plasma levels and clinical response: A therapeutic window relationship. *Am J Psychiatry*, 149, 500–505.
15. **Salem, H., Nagpal, C., Pigott, T., *et al.* (2017).** Revisiting antipsychotic-induced akathisia: Current issues and prospective challenges. *Curr Neuropharmacol*, 15, 789–798.
16. **Vinogradov, S., Fisher, M., Warm, H., *et al.* (2009).** The cognitive cost of anticholinergic burden: Decreased response to cognitive training in schizophrenia. *Am J Psychiatry*, 166, 1055–1062.
17. **Ang, M. S., Abdul Rashid, N. A., Lam, M., *et al.* (2017).** The impact of medication anticholinergic burden on cognitive performance in people with schizophrenia. *J Clin Psychopharmacol*, 37, 651–656.

18. **Eum, S., Hill, S. K., Rubin, L. H., *et al.* (2017).** Cognitive burden of anticholinergic medications in psychotic disorders. *Schizophr Res*, 190, 129–135.
19. **Meyer, J. M. and Koro, C. E. (2004).** The effects of antipsychotic therapy on serum lipids: A comprehensive review. *Schizophr Res*, 70, 1–17.
20. **Leucht, S., Crippa, A., Siafis, S., *et al.* (2020).** Dose-response meta-analysis of antipsychotic drugs for acute schizophrenia. *Am J Psychiatry*, 177, 342–353.
21. **Schoretsanitis, G., Spina, E., Hiemke, C., *et al.* (2018).** A systematic review and combined analysis of therapeutic drug monitoring studies for long-acting paliperidone. *Expert Rev Clin Pharmacol*, 11, 1237–1253.
22. **de Leon, J., Wynn, G., and Sandson, N. B. (2010).** The pharmacokinetics of paliperidone versus risperidone. *Psychosomatics*, 51, 80–88.
23. **Covell, N. H., McEvoy, J. P., Schooler, N. R., *et al.* (2012).** Effectiveness of switching from long-acting injectable fluphenazine or haloperidol decanoate to long-acting injectable risperidone microspheres: An open-label, randomized controlled trial. *J Clin Psychiatry*, 73, 669–675.
24. **Leucht, S., Samara, M., Heres, S., *et al.* (2016).** Dose equivalents for antipsychotic drugs: The DDD method. *Schizophr Bull*, 42 Suppl 1, S90–94.
25. **Asmal, L., Flegar, S. J., Wang, J., *et al.* (2013).** Quetiapine versus other atypical antipsychotics for schizophrenia. *Cochrane Database Syst Rev*, CD006625.
26. **Vanasse, A., Blais, L., Courteau, J., *et al.* (2016).** Comparative effectiveness and safety of antipsychotic drugs in schizophrenia treatment: A real-world observational study. *Acta Psychiatr Scand*, 134, 374–384.
27. **Meyer, J. M., Davis, V. G., Goff, D. C., *et al.* (2008).** Change in metabolic syndrome parameters with antipsychotic treatment in the CATIE Schizophrenia Trial: Prospective data from phase 1. *Schizophr Res*, 101, 273–286.
28. **Meyer, J. M. (2010).** Antipsychotics and metabolics in the post-CATIE era. *Curr Top Behav Neurosci*, 4, 23–42.
29. **Regenthal, R., Kunstler, U., Junhold, U., *et al.* (1997).** Haloperidol serum concentrations and D2 dopamine receptor occupancy during low-dose treatment with haloperidol decanoate. *Int Clin Psychopharmacol*, 12, 255–261.
30. **Fitzgerald, P. B., Kapur, S., Remington, G., *et al.* (2000).** Predicting haloperidol occupancy of central dopamine D2 receptors from plasma levels. *Psychopharmacology*, 149, 1–5.
31. **Nyberg, S., Farde, L., Bartfai, A., *et al.* (1995).** Central D2 receptor occupancy and effects of zuclopenthixol acetate in humans. *Int Clin Psychopharmacol*, 10, 221–227.
32. **Lundbeck Australia (2013).** Clopixol, Clopixol Acuphase, Clopixol Depot package insert. North Ryde, NSW, Australia.
33. **Chang, W. H., Lin, S. K., Juang, D. J., *et al.* (1993).** Prolonged haloperidol and reduced haloperidol plasma concentrations after decanoate withdrawal. *Schizophr Res*, 9, 35–40.
34. **Nyberg, S., Farde, L., and Halldin, C. (1996).** Long-time persistence of D2 dopamine receptor occupancy after discontinuation of haloperidol decanoate. *Schizophr Res*, 18, 199–200.
35. **Talvik, M., Nordstrom, A. L., Larsen, N. E., *et al.* (2004).** A cross-validation study on the relationship between central D2 receptor occupancy and serum perphenazine concentration. *Psychopharmacology*, 175, 148–153.
36. **Ereshefsky, L., Toney, G., Saklad, S. R., *et al.* (1993).** A loading-dose strategy for converting from oral to depot haloperidol. *Hosp Community Psychiatry*, 44, 1155–1161.
37. **Taylor, D. (2009).** Psychopharmacology and adverse effects of antipsychotic long-acting injections: A review. *Br J Psychiatry Suppl*, 52, S13–19.
38. **Dencker, S. J., Giös, I., Mårtensson, E., *et al.* (1994).** A long-term cross-over pharmacokinetic study comparing perphenazine decanoate and haloperidol decanoate in schizophrenic patients. *Psychopharmacology (Berl)*, 114, 24–30.

7 Haloperidol and Haloperidol Decanoate

QUICK CHECK

PRINCIPLES

- Haloperidol provides an inexpensive method of delivering D_2 antagonism, with extensive plasma level data, and multiple formulations including a long-acting injectable (LAI) preparation (haloperidol decanoate).
- A method for quickly loading haloperidol decanoate has been confirmed based on plasma levels: 3 weekly injections (days 1, 8, 15) of 10 times the daily oral dose generates a plasma level after the third injection comparable to that on the oral dose. Maintenance injections start 2 weeks after the third loading injection and are 20 times the daily oral dose.

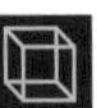

InfoBox Oral Haloperidol Plasma Level Essentials

Oral dose correlation (bedtime dosing, 12h trough)	Level of evidence	Therapeutic threshold	Level of evidence	Point of futility	Level of evidence
10 mg = 7.8 ng/ml [1, 2, 3] **Multiply oral dose by 0.78** (see Table 7.1 for effects of CYP inhibitors/inducers on this relationship)	**High**	2 ng/ml [4, 3, 5]	**High**	18 ng/ml [1, 6]	**High**

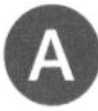

Basic Pharmacokinetic Information for Oral and Long-Acting Injectable Haloperidol

Haloperidol is among the most extensively studied of all antipsychotics. By 1996, 18 fixed-dose haloperidol trials were in the literature [7, 8], and a 1998 paper noted that 50 studies had been published on haloperidol plasma levels, though many had significant methodological limitations [9]. This clinical database has been supplemented by numerous single photon (SPECT) and, later, Positron Emission Tomography (PET) imaging studies of dopamine D_2 receptor occupancy, starting in 1988 [10–12, 1]. Haloperidol was assigned a Level 1 recommendation (strongly

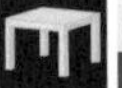

Table 7.1 Oral haloperidol kinetic facts [14]

Basic facts	Inhibition effects	Induction effects
US FDA approval: Apr. 12, 1967 Absolute oral bioavailability: 60% $T_{1/2}$ 24 (12–36) hours T_{max} 2–6 hours Metabolism: Primarily CYP 2D6, also CYP 3A4 and CYP 1A2 **Formulations:** Tablets, oral solution (also acute intramuscular)	No active metabolites [9] Strong CYP 2D6 inhibitors increase exposure 25%–50% [15] Strong CYP 1A2 inhibitors increase exposure on average 62.5% (range 48%–79%) [15] Strong 3A4 inhibitors increase exposure 17% [15] Individuals with only one functional 2D6 gene experience two-fold greater trough serum levels. Those with no functioning alleles 3–4-fold higher [16, 17]	Carbamazepine, phenobarbital, or phenytoin decrease mean plasma levels by 40%–72% [18, 15, 19] Rifampin decreases plasma haloperidol levels by a mean of 70% [20] Discontinuation of carbamazepine results in a 2–5-fold increase in plasma levels [21, 22]

recommended) for use of plasma level monitoring in the 2020 consensus paper authored jointly by the Therapeutic Drug Monitoring (TDM) task force of the German Arbeitsgemeinschaft für Neuropsychopharmakologie und Pharmakopsychiatrie (AGNP) and the American Society for Clinical Psychopharmacology (ASCP) [13].

B Essential Information for Oral and Long-Acting Injectable Haloperidol

1 Essential Oral Haloperidol Information

Detecting adherence with no established plasma level baseline requires a knowledge of the expected plasma level for a given dose. The oral haloperidol concentration–dose relationship presented in the InfoBox is based on results from multiple studies, and assumes that the patient is an extensive metabolizer at relevant CYP enzymes, and is not exposed to CYP inhibitors or inducers [1, 2, 3]. To achieve a plasma level of 2.0 ng/ml (the response threshold), the expected dose required will be almost exactly 2.5 mg QHS. Although many clinicians are trained using haloperidol in 5 mg increments, this is a very potent D_2 antagonist and it is easy to exceed a patient's tolerability threshold [23]. A starting dose of 2.5 mg QHS, and incremental increases of 2.5 mg QHS for nonresponders ought to be considered, since many will respond to levels from 2 to 5 ng/ml [4, 24]. Recalling that a 10 mg QHS dose equals a plasma level of 7.8 ng/ml will be useful to understanding the loading regimen for haloperidol decanoate, and for deciding when to suspect nonadherence in a newly treated patient on oral haloperidol until a second level can be drawn.

2 Essential Long-Acting Injectable Haloperidol Information

Haloperidol decanoate is solubilized in sesame oil, an aspect of this formulation that presents a higher risk for injection site reactions than seen with water-based injectables, and which also requires a specific injection technique [14]. The time to maximal drug levels (T_{max}) is approximately 6 days on average (Table 7.2, Figure 7.1), which lends itself to loading as a means of quickly achieving therapeutic plasma levels and decreasing the time to steady state [25]. Although the half-life with repeated use is 3 weeks, this is sufficiently long to support a 4-week injection cycle. The disconnect between peripheral kinetics and central nervous system response is due to the slow decay of peripheral plasma levels and even slower attenuation of D_2 receptor occupancy [26–28]. To minimize patient discomfort, the maximum injection volume for oil-based depot antipsychotics is 3 ml. As the most common formulation used is 100 mg/ml, monthly doses > 300 mg are divided evenly into injections administered 2 weeks apart. (A 50 mg/ml formulation also exists.)

Table 7.2 Haloperidol decanoate essentials

Vehicle	Concentration	Dosage	T_{max} (days)	$T_{1/2}$ (days) multiple dosing	Able to be loaded	Maintenance dose: oral equivalence
Sesame oil	50 mg/ml 100 mg/ml (max injection volume 3 ml)	25–300 mg/ 4 weeks Max: 300 mg/ 2 weeks	3–9	21	Yes	Monthly dose = 20 times the daily oral dose

(For further reading about use of LAI antipsychotics, please see the comprehensive edited book ***Antipsychotic Long-Acting Injections***, now in its 2nd edition [29]).

Various oral conversion formulas were developed once it became apparent that the optimal monthly dose during early treatment is 20 times the prior stable oral dose [30, 31]. The formula that provides the most rapid and equivalent conversion from a known oral dose, with limited or no need for oral bridging therapy, is based on detailed plasma level data from a trial in which patients were stabilized on 10 mg/d of oral haloperidol (Figure 7.2). Oral haloperidol was abruptly stopped at the time of the first of three weekly haloperidol decanoate injections, each of which was 10 times the oral dose (100 mg) [2]. As expected, the mean plasma levels on 10 mg/d were almost exactly 7.8 ng/ml (7.95 ± 4.94 ng/ml). One week after the third loading injection, the mean plasma haloperidol levels were comparable to 10 mg oral haloperidol (7.79 ± 4.79 ng/ml) without use of any oral haloperidol. Levels during the week following the first injection and abrupt discontinuation of oral haloperidol were 55% lower than the baseline, suggesting that oral supplementation with 50% of the prior dose may be needed in more symptomatic patients **for the first week only,** to maintain psychiatric stability [25]. Maintenance dosing starts 2 weeks after the third loading injection using 20 times the oral dose. If the calculated monthly dose exceeds 300 mg, it must be divided evenly into injections administered every 2 weeks.

The Therapeutic Threshold for Haloperidol

1 Clinical Evidence for a Therapeutic Threshold

Clinical evidence, especially from fixed-dose, prospective, randomized trials, is the most important tool we have for estimation of plasma level response thresholds (see Chapter 2). In 1996, a meta-analysis of haloperidol response was performed that included only fixed-dose (or fixed plasma level range) studies of adult schizophrenia patients who underwent a pre-treatment washout period, who were not treatment resistant, and for which individual patient level data were available [8]. From the 18 relevant studies, a threshold level of 4 ng/ml was suggested, based on a statistical

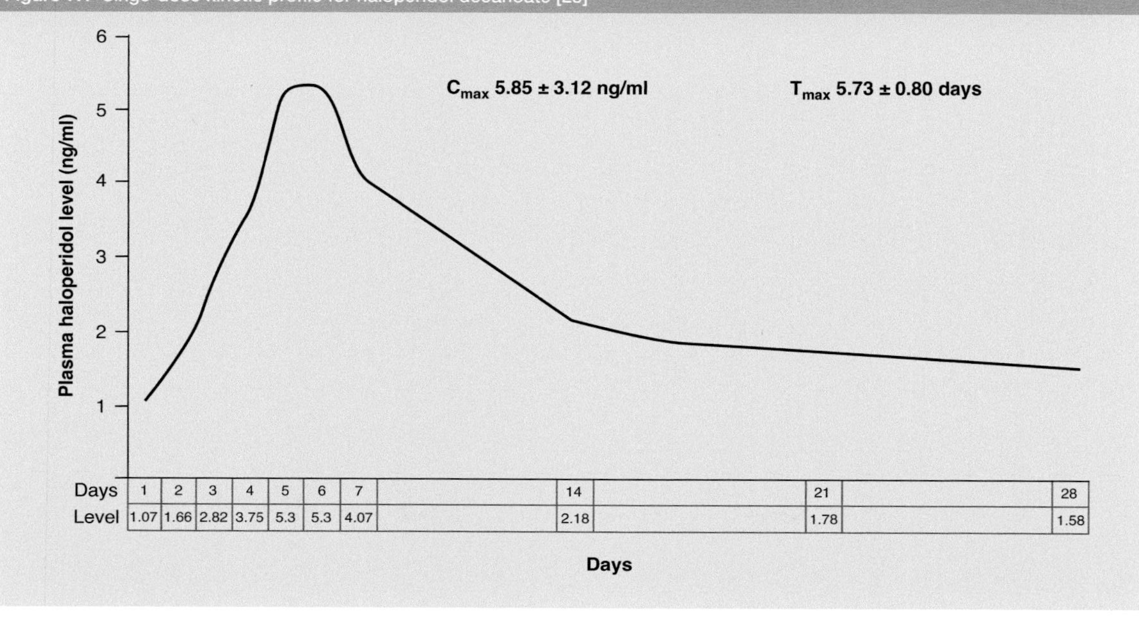

Figure 7.1 Singe-dose kinetic profile for haloperidol decanoate [25]

(Adapted from: J. M. Meyer [2017]. Converting oral to long acting injectable antipsychotics: A guide for the perplexed. *CNS Spectr*, 22, 14–28.)

Figure 7.2 Plasma haloperidol levels during 100 mg loading study [32]

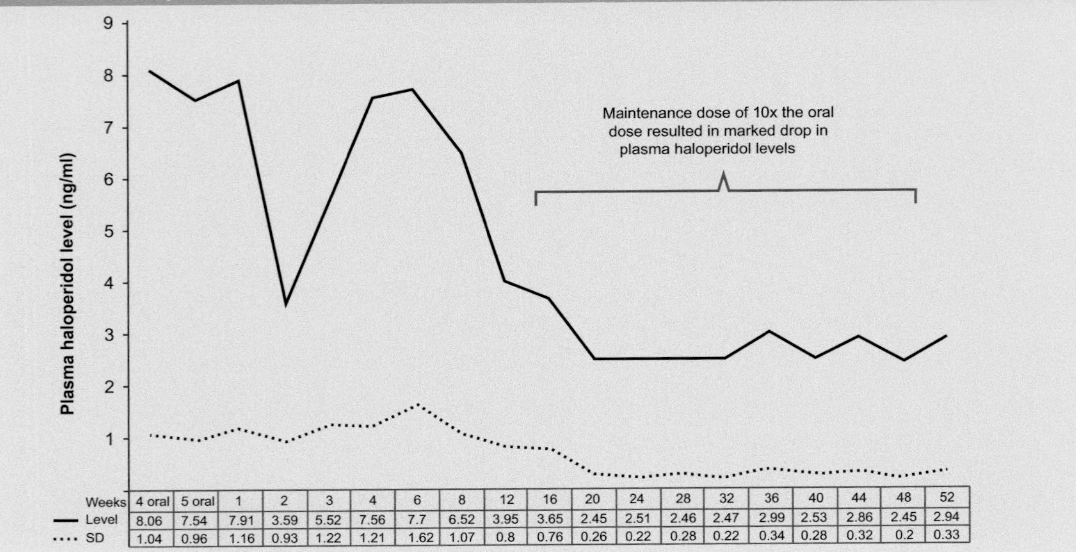

Weeks	4 oral	5 oral	1	2	3	4	6	8	12	16	20	24	28	32	36	40	44	48	52
— Level	8.06	7.54	7.91	3.59	5.52	7.56	7.7	6.52	3.95	3.65	2.45	2.51	2.46	2.47	2.99	2.53	2.86	2.45	2.94
···· SD	1.04	0.96	1.16	0.93	1.22	1.21	1.62	1.07	0.8	0.76	0.26	0.22	0.28	0.22	0.34	0.28	0.32	0.2	0.33

Implications

a 100 mg (i.e. 10x the oral dose) loaded weekly for 3 weeks provides coverage equal to 10 mg/d.

b However, oral coverage of 5 mg (i.e. half the oral dose) is needed during the first 1–2 weeks to maintain levels comparable to 10 mg/d before the first injection.

c The maintenance dose of 200 mg/4 wks (i.e. 20x the oral dose) should start 2 weeks after the third loading injection to achieve levels comparable to 10 mg/d oral. Levels should be checked periodically during the first 6–8 months due to level creep as tissue compartments become saturated.

d Steady state is reached by the fourth month of treatment when haloperidol decanoate is not loaded. As with all LAI injectables, monthly or bimonthly monitoring of plasma antipsychotic levels in the first year can help detect level creep and forestall tolerability issues due to supratherapeutic levels.

(Adapted from: M. W. Jann, F. C. Wei, H. N. Lin, *et al.* [1996]. Haloperidol and reduced haloperidol plasma concentrations after a loading dose regimen with haloperidol decanoate. *Prog Neuropsychopharmacol Biol Psychiatry*, 20, 73–86.)

analysis that defined three clusters: < 4 ng/ml; 4–26 ng/ml; and > 26 ng/ml. This was followed in 1998 by an examination of 35 clinical trials (including a wider variety of study designs) that arrived at a threshold of 5.6 ng/ml [9]. Over time, the proposed threshold level has dropped, based on re-examination of the lower ranges in large, fixed-dose studies. In the largest of these trials (n = 69), the proportion of responders in the range of 2–5 ng/ml was 43%, compared to 9% for levels < 2 ng/ml [33]. This paper concluded by suggesting 2 ng/ml as the response threshold, and the authors provided the following detail: "Patients with plasma levels of 1.8, 1.5, 1.6, 1.1, 1.1, and 1.4 ng/ml all improved (with the Clinical Global Impressions-Improvement [CGI-I] scale as the criterion) as their plasma levels rose above 2.0 ng/ml (the plasma levels at which improvement occurred were 2.9, 2.6, 2.1, 2.2, 2.0, and 6.7 ng/ml, respectively). One man with a plasma level of 1.8 ng/ml improved remarkably." The 2 ng/ml threshold from that 1992 paper corresponds closely to the result of a 2013 analysis matching the modeled kinetics of oral haloperidol and changes in Positive and Negative Syndrome Scale (PANSS) scores from 473 subjects [34]. A nonlinear mixed-effects modeling approach was used, combined with bootstrapping and simulation-based methods for model evaluation. From this approach, the recommended plasma haloperidol level to achieve a 30% reduction in PANSS score from baseline was 2.7 ng/ml. Lastly, there is a receiver operating characteristic (ROC) analysis from a fixed-dose study of 34 schizophrenia patients which found that a plasma level of 2.0 ng/ml best separated true responders from false positives [35]. As noted in Chapter 2, ROC analysis is ideal for establishing a cutpoint below which the proportion of false positives is higher; however, the level chosen (2.0 ng/ml) had 100% specificity but only 52% sensitivity, and thus may not have optimally balanced those two parameters [36]. The 2020 AGNP/ASCP consensus paper proposes a 1.0 ng/ml threshold, but unfortunately there is limited clinical data to suggest response to levels under 2.0 ng/ml. As noted above, it is convenient that the dose required for a steady state 12h trough level of 2.0 ng/ml is 2.5 mg QHS. This starting dose should be considered for less severely ill patients, or when treating first-episode schizophrenia patients who tend to be more sensitive to dopamine antagonism and respond to lower plasma levels and dosages [37, 38].

2 Imaging Evidence for a Therapeutic Threshold

The technology, kinetics, and binding specificity of ligands developed for D_2 occupancy imaging improved throughout the 1990s, and the heterogeneity of reported results for receptor occupancy studies lessened markedly, especially as newer studies used PET imaging instead of SPECT [39]. A 2000 PET imaging trial by investigators in Toronto,

Canada, studied 21 adult schizophrenia patients (mean age 29.8 years) to calculate haloperidol D_2 receptor occupancy using a plasma haloperidol level of 0.40 ng/ml as the EC_{50} (i.e. the concentration which achieves 50% receptor occupancy) [39]. Scans were performed at trough plasma levels (12h post-dose) and at steady state. This study calculated that a plasma haloperidol level of 1 ng/ml would result in 70% D_2 receptor occupancy, a level modestly lower than the value of 1.4 ng/ml in a smaller (n = 8) and older cohort (mean age 40.5 years) (Figure 7.3) [5]. More recent PET data from healthy male volunteers (n = 8) randomized to one of three oral haloperidol doses for 7 days (0.5 mg, 1 mg, 3 mg) arrived at EC_{50} plasma levels of 0.791 ng/ml and 0.650 ng/ml in the putamen and caudate nucleus respectively [40]. Using an average of those two striatal EC_{50} values, a level of 1.68 ng/ml would achieve 70% D_2 receptor occupancy, and 1.34 ng/ml 65% occupancy [40]. That imaging studies suggest a level slightly over 1 ng/ml could be therapeutic might be one factor in the AGNP/ASCP choice of 1 ng/ml as the threshold plasma haloperidol level, but clinical trials consistently find lack of response for levels < 2 ng/ml among exacerbated

Figure 7.3 Fitted D_2 occupancy curve for plasma haloperidol levels [5]

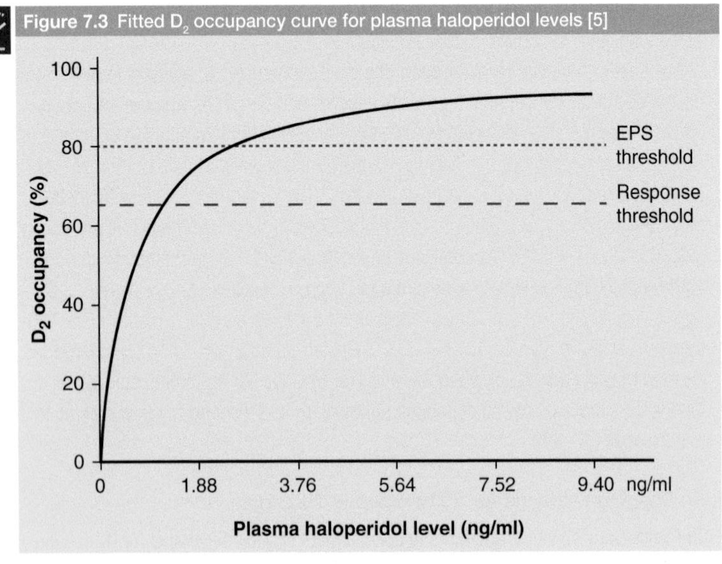

(Adapted from: R. Regenthal, U. Kunstler, U. Junhold, *et al.* [1997]. Haloperidol serum concentrations and D2 dopamine receptor occupancy during low-dose treatment with haloperidol decanoate. *Int Clin Psychopharmacol*, 12, 255–261.)

patients not experiencing their first episode of schizophrenia [33, 9]. It is for this reason that the clinical trial data are given greater weight, but this can be revised if results from future studies, especially in first-episode patients, provide corroborating evidence for lower values. To emphasize the point made in Chapter 2, the therapeutic threshold represents an initial target in nonresponders. Once above that threshold, further titration should be considered for nonresponse after 2 weeks of oral therapy (or 4 weeks after commencement of a haloperidol decanoate loading regimen) using the principles discussed in Chapter 5.

The Point of Futility for Haloperidol

1 Clinical Evidence for a Point of Futility

The level where an average patient might respond or achieve the maximum symptom reduction is important, but the question of futility revolves around when further titration should stop for nonresponders in the absence of dose-limiting side effects [24]. Given its high D_2 affinity, haloperidol titration in many instances will end at one of the hard clinical endpoints (intolerability) due to neurological adverse effects [33], or the unpleasant, dysphoric subjective experience associated with excessive D_2 blockade ***for that patient*** (see Chapter 5 for discussion of clinical endpoints) [41, 42]. Defining the upper limit using the concept of the point of futility addresses a question of paramount importance when managing a more severely ill schizophrenia spectrum population, and, as noted in Chapter 2, creates an easily understood unified concept: **further titration beyond this point is of limited value with an estimated < 5% chance of response; however, assuming tolerability, there is no inherent unusual safety concern in exploring plasma levels up to that point** [6]. The AGNP/ASCP consensus paper presents both a therapeutic reference range and a laboratory alert level, but this dual system may be confusing to those who do not thoroughly understand the differentiation between these two, and it may potentially discourage providers from further titration when there is evidence to support efficacy above the reference range – again assuming tolerability [13].

There is no question that diminishing tolerability is a significant factor in defining haloperidol's upper therapeutic range, with various papers suggesting upper limits ranging from 12 ng/ml to 40 ng/ml depending on the sample chosen, definitions of response, and mathematical choices in calculating the upper limit [8]. For many patients, more haloperidol may not necessarily generate greater symptomatic improvement [24], with maximal symptom reduction estimated to occur around 10 ng/ml based on a meta-analysis of 35 studies [9]. When tolerability is not limiting, the choice of a point of futility requires inference from response rates at higher plasma haloperidol levels, and the proportion expected to tolerate those levels. Analyses of this type are exceedingly rare, but fortunately were published for fluphenazine, another high-potency first-generation antipsychotic. Plasma fluphenazine levels as high as 16.2 ng/ml are described in the literature, reflecting the reality that some patients may not develop intolerable neurological adverse effects from high levels of D_2 occupancy [43, 44], yet the probability of response for levels > 4.0 ng/ml is < 5% (Figure 7.4). This is the point of futility for fluphenazine titration in nonresponders [6]. Based solely on naturalistic outcomes in forensic inpatients with schizophrenia spectrum disorders, a point of futility for haloperidol of 30 ng/ml has been proposed [6, 45], but this initial estimate deserves further review.

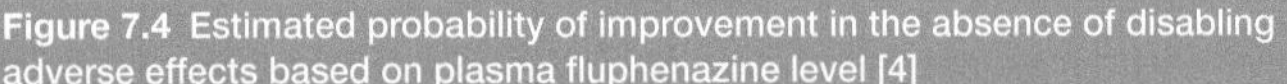
Figure 7.4 Estimated probability of improvement in the absence of disabling adverse effects based on plasma fluphenazine level [4]

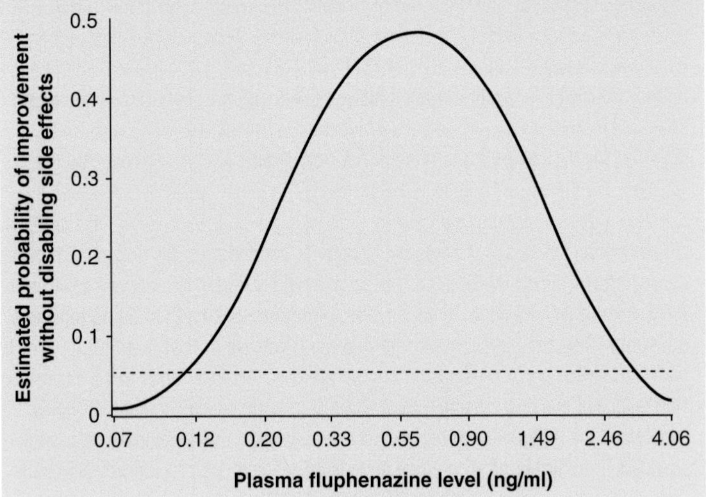

(Adapted from: K. K. Midha, J. W. Hubbard, S. R. Marder, *et al.* [1994]. Impact of clinical pharmacokinetics on neuroleptic therapy in patients with schizophrenia. *J Psychiatry Neurosci*, 19, 254–264.)

As nearly every study agrees, very few patients will tolerate plasma haloperidol levels above 18 ng/ml, with approximately 90% of patients developing intolerable adverse effects at that level (Figure 7.5) [4]. The question is: When tolerability is not limiting, when is the expectation of treatment response under 5%? Using

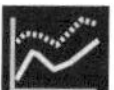

Figure 7.5 Plasma haloperidol levels and proportion of patients with intolerable adverse effects [4]

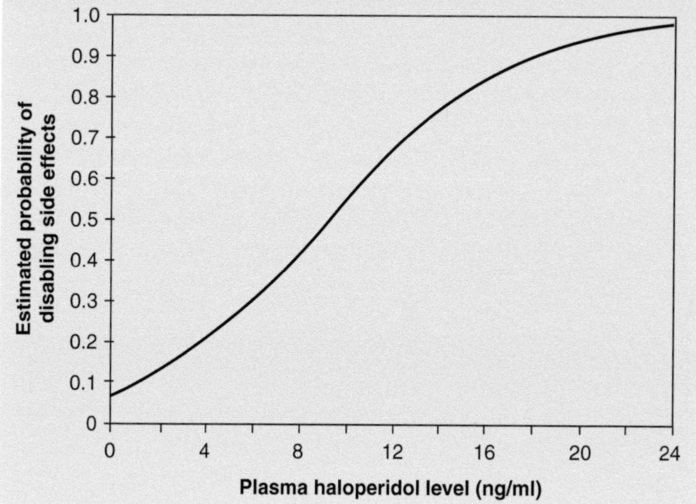

(Adapted from: K. K. Midha, J. W. Hubbard, S. R. Marder, *et al.* [1994]. Impact of clinical pharmacokinetics on neuroleptic therapy in patients with schizophrenia. *J Psychiatry Neurosci*, 19, 254–264.)

30% symptom reduction as the response criterion, the 1996 analysis of 18 fixed-dose studies found sufficient patient level data in 11 trials to classify responders, and reported a response rate of 69% (116/69) in the window of 4–26 ng/ml [8]. Interestingly, the response rate was still 53% (67/127) for levels > 26 ng/ml [8]. The high response rate for levels > 26 ng/ml may be related to the choice of 30% symptom reduction as the response criterion, as opposed to the more stringent but clinically meaningful 50% reduction used to arrive at the 2-week rule [46]. The exhaustive 1998 meta-analysis of optimal haloperidol plasma level ranges from 35 acute schizophrenia trials also used an empirically derived score to filter out lower-quality trials; however, their analysis did not focus on the proportion of responders within the proposed range (5.6–16.9 ng/ml), but differences in extent of symptom reduction compared to those outside of the range [9]. Given these limitations in the literature, findings from the fluphenazine analysis are instructive as it shares identical pharmacodynamic properties with haloperidol. For fluphenazine, the point of futility occurs close to where the 90% intolerability curve meets the 90% responder curve (Figure 7.6) [4]. The 90% intolerability line for haloperidol can be drawn at 18 ng/ml (Figure 7.5), but the 90% response level is less clear. The largest fixed-dose trial found that, for a mean plasma level 15.2 ± 2.7 ng/ml, the proportion of patients rated as much improved or very much improved on the CGI-I scale was 38% [33]. As discussed in Chapter 5, this represents a 2–3-point improvement on the CGI-I and corresponds to a PANSS reduction of 40%–50% [47]. When presented graphically, no patients with more than minimal response in positive psychosis symptoms had plasma levels > 18 ng/ml (Figure 7.7). This information combined with the 90% tolerability threshold of 18 ng/ml suggests that a point of futility for plasma haloperidol levels of 18 ng/ml is a reasonable choice.

Figure 7.6 Estimated probability of response (dotted line) or disabling adverse effects (bold line) based on plasma fluphenazine level [4]

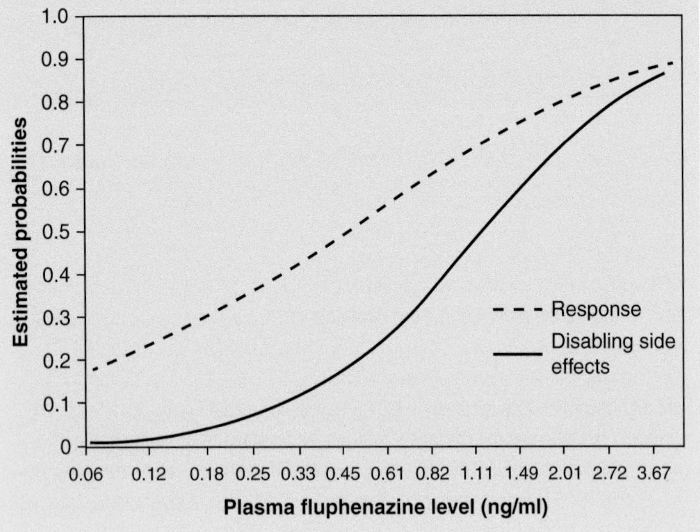

(Adapted from: K. K. Midha, J. W. Hubbard, S. R. Marder, *et al*. [1994]. Impact of clinical pharmacokinetics on neuroleptic therapy in patients with schizophrenia. *J Psychiatry Neurosci*, 19, 254–264.)

Figure 7.7 Relationship between plasma haloperidol level and change in BPRS psychosis factor scores for 69 male schizophrenia patients [33]

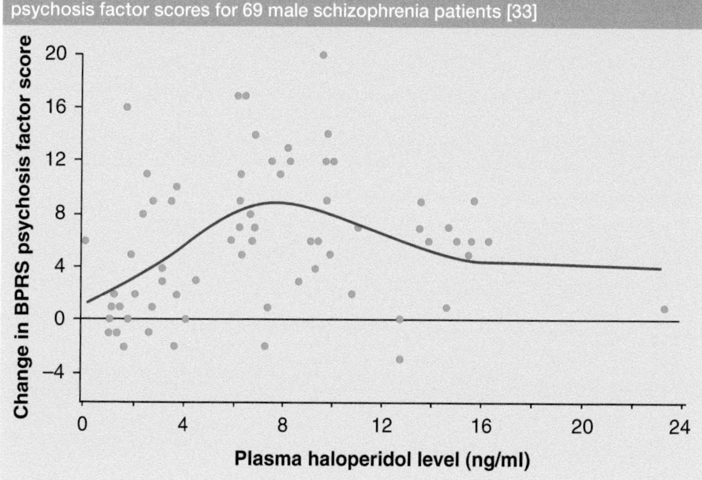

(Adapted from: T. Van Putten, S. R. Marder, J. Mintz, *et al.* [1992]. Haloperidol plasma levels and clinical response: A therapeutic window relationship. *Am J Psychiatry*, 149, 500–505.)

2 Imaging Evidence for a Point of Futility

Tolerability decreases when D_2 receptor occupancy exceeds 80% for dopamine antagonists, so the proposed "sweet spot" of D_2 receptor occupancy ranges from 65% to 80% [42]. The 1998 meta-analysis of 35 haloperidol trials suggested a plasma level "sweet spot" of 10 ng/ml [9], but the expected D_2 receptor occupancy for this level is 96% using the equation from the 2000 Toronto PET study [39]. This estimated D_2 occupancy for 10 ng/ml from the Toronto data is also consistent with that depicted in Figure 7.3, where a level of 9.4 ng/ml already exceeds 90% occupancy [5]. That plasma levels predicted to exceed 80% D_2 blockade are tolerable to a large group of patients is illustrated by adverse effect data from the pivotal risperidone trial [48]. This study used haloperidol 20 mg/d as a comparator, a dose estimated to have a mean 12h trough plasma level of 15.6 ng/ml and 98% D_2 receptor occupancy, yet less than 50% of patients in that treatment arm required antiparkinsonian medication [48]. The other confusing aspect of the imaging data is that a plasma haloperidol level around

1.6 ng/ml should generate 80% D_2 blockade [39, 5], yet clinical studies indicate that levels < 2 ng/ml are usually subtherapeutic [3]. When there is a discrepancy between clinical and imaging studies, greater weight should be given to the clinical data, as clinical judgment and plasma levels have proven to be reliable guides to response and tolerability decisions with haloperidol therapy.

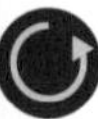

Summary Points

a The correlation between haloperidol plasma levels and schizophrenia response has been widely studied. The suggested therapeutic response threshold is 2 ng/ml, and the point of futility is 18 ng/ml. The 2020 AGNP/ASCP consensus paper strongly recommends plasma level monitoring.

b The oral haloperidol concentration–dose relationship is well established: 10 mg at bedtime = 7.80 ng/ml (12h trough).

c The monthly maintenance dose of haloperidol decanoate during the early months of treatment is 20 times the daily oral dose. Three weekly injections (day 1, 8, 15) of 10 times the oral dose generate a plasma level after the third injection comparable to that with the daily oral dose. Maintenance injections start 2 weeks after the third loading injection. Levels should be checked periodically during the first 6–8 months due to level creep as tissue compartments become saturated.

References

1. **Van Putten, T., Marder, S. R., Wirshing, W. C., *et al.* (1991).** Neuroleptic plasma levels. *Schizophr Bull*, 17, 197–216.
2. **Wei, F. C., Jann, M. W., Lin, H. N., *et al.* (1996).** A practical loading dose method for converting schizophrenic patients from oral to depot haloperidol therapy. *J Clin Psychiatry*, 57, 298–302.
3. **Kapur, S., Zipursky, R., Roy, P., *et al.* (1997).** The relationship between D2 receptor occupancy and plasma levels on low dose oral haloperidol: A PET study. *Psychopharmacology*, 131, 148–152.
4. **Midha, K. K., Hubbard, J. W., Marder, S. R., *et al.* (1994).** Impact of clinical pharmacokinetics on neuroleptic therapy in patients with schizophrenia. *J Psychiatry Neurosci*, 19, 254–264.
5. **Regenthal, R., Kunstler, U., Junhold, U., *et al.* (1997).** Haloperidol serum concentrations and D2 dopamine receptor occupancy during low-dose treatment with haloperidol decanoate. *Int Clin Psychopharmacol*, 12, 255–261.
6. **Meyer, J. M. (2014).** A rational approach to employing high plasma levels of antipsychotics for violence associated with schizophrenia: Case vignettes. *CNS Spectr*, 19, 432–438.
7. **Van Putten, T. and Marder, S. R. (1986).** Variable dose studies provide misleading therapeutic windows. *J Clin Psychopharmacol*, 6, 55–56.
8. **de Oliveira, I. R., de Sena, E. P., Pereira, E. L., *et al.* (1996).** Haloperidol blood levels and clinical outcome: A meta-analysis of studies relevant to testing the therapeutic window hypothesis. *J Clin Pharm Ther*, 21, 229–236.
9. **Ulrich, S., Wurthmann, C., Brosz, M., *et al.* (1998).** The relationship between serum concentration and therapeutic effect of haloperidol in patients with acute schizophrenia. *Clin Pharmacokinet*, 34, 227–263.
10. **Dahl, S. G. (1988).** Pharmacokinetics of neuroleptic drugs and the utility of plasma level monitoring. *Psychopharmacol Ser*, 5, 34–46.
11. **Farde, L., Wiesel, F. A., Halldin, C., *et al.* (1988).** Central D2-dopamine receptor occupancy in schizophrenic patients treated with antipsychotic drugs. *Arch Gen Psychiatry*, 45, 71–76.
12. **Smith, M., Wolf, A. P., Brodie, J. D., *et al.* (1988).** Serial [18F]N-methylspiroperidol PET studies to measure changes in antipsychotic drug D-2 receptor occupancy in schizophrenic patients. *Biol Psychiatry*, 23, 653–663.
13. **Schoretsanitis, G., Kane, J. M., Correll, C. U., *et al.* (2020).** Blood levels to optimize antipsychotic treatment in clinical practice: A joint consensus statement of the American Society of Clinical Psychopharmacology (ASCP) and the Therapeutic Drug Monitoring (TDM) Task Force of the Arbeitsgemeinschaft für Neuropsychopharmakologie und Pharmakopsychiatrie (AGNP). *J Clin Psychiatry*, 81, https://doi.org/10.4088/JCP.4019cs13169.
14. **Meyer, J. M. (2018).** Pharmacotherapy of psychosis and mania. In L. L. Brunton, R. Hilal-Dandan, and B. C. Knollmann, eds., *Goodman & Gilman's The Pharmacological Basis of Therapeutics*, 13th edn. Chicago, IL: McGraw-Hill, pp. 279–302.
15. **Kudo, S. and Ishizaki, T. (1999).** Pharmacokinetics of haloperidol: An update. *Clin Pharmacokinet*, 37, 435–456.
16. **Suzuki, A., Otani, K., Mihara, K., *et al.* (1997).** Effects of the CYP2D6 genotype on the steady-state plasma concentrations of haloperidol and reduced haloperidol in Japanese schizophrenic patients. *Pharmacogenetics*, 7, 415–418.
17. **Panagiotidis, G., Arthur, H. W., Lindh, J. D., *et al.* (2007).** Depot haloperidol treatment in outpatients with schizophrenia on monotherapy: Impact of CYP2D6 polymorphism on pharmacokinetics and treatment outcome. *Ther Drug Monit*, 29, 417–422.
18. **Fast, D. K., Jones, B. D., Kusalic, M., *et al.* (1986).** Effect of carbamazepine on neuroleptic plasma levels and efficacy. *Am J Psychiatry*, 143, 117–118.

19. **Spina, E. and Perucca, E. (2002).** Clinical significance of pharmacokinetic interactions between antiepileptic and psychotropic drugs. *Epilepsia*, 43 Suppl2, 37–44.
20. **Mylan Institutional LLC (2019).** Haloperidol package insert. Rockford, IL.
21. **Jann, M. W., Fidone, G. S., Hernandez, J. M., *et al.* (1989).** Clinical implications of increased antipsychotic plasma concentrations upon anticonvulsant cessation. *Psychiatry Res*, 28, 153–159.
22. **Raitasuo, V., Lehtovaara, R., and Huttunen, M. O. (1994).** Effect of switching carbamazepine to oxcarbazepine on the plasma levels of neuroleptics: A case report. *Psychopharmacology (Berl)*, 116, 115–116.
23. **Kapur, S. and Seeman, P. (2001).** Does fast dissociation from the dopamine d(2) receptor explain the action of atypical antipsychotics? A new hypothesis. *Am J Psychiatry*, 158, 360–369.
24. **Giegling, I., Drago, A., Schafer, M., *et al.* (2010).** Interaction of haloperidol plasma level and antipsychotic effect in early phases of acute psychosis treatment. *J Psychiatr Res*, 44, 487–492.
25. **Meyer, J. M. (2017).** Converting oral to long acting injectable antipsychotics: A guide for the perplexed. *CNS Spectr*, 22, 14–28.
26. **Chang, W. H., Lin, S. K., Juang, D. J., *et al.* (1993).** Prolonged haloperidol and reduced haloperidol plasma concentrations after decanoate withdrawal. *Schizophr Res*, 9, 35–40.
27. **Harasko-van der Meer, C., Brucke, T., Wenger, S., *et al.* (1993).** Two cases of long term dopamine D2 receptor blockade after depot neuroleptics. *J Neural Transm*, 94, 217–221.
28. **Kurose, S., Mimura, Y., Uchida, H., *et al.* (2020).** Dissociation in pharmacokinetic attenuation between central dopamine D_2 receptor occupancy and peripheral blood concentration of antipsychotics: A systematic review. *J Clin Psychiatry*, 81, 19r13113.
29. **Haddad, P., Lambert, T., and Lauriello, J., eds. (2016).** *Antipsychotic Long-Acting Injections*, 2nd edn. New York: Oxford University Press.
30. **Deberdt, R., Elens, P., Berghmans, W., *et al.* (1980).** Intramuscular haloperidol decanoate for neuroleptic maintenance therapy: Efficacy, dosage schedule and plasma levels. An open multicenter study. *Acta Psychiatr Scand*, 62, 356–363.
31. **Ereshefsky, L., Toney, G., Saklad, S. R., *et al.* (1993).** A loading-dose strategy for converting from oral to depot haloperidol. *Hosp Community Psychiatry*, 44, 1155–1161.
32. **Jann, M. W., Wei, F. C., Lin, H. N., *et al.* (1996).** Haloperidol and reduced haloperidol plasma concentrations after a loading dose regimen with haloperidol decanoate. *Prog Neuropsychopharmacol Biol Psychiatry*, 20, 73–86.
33. **Van Putten, T., Marder, S. R., Mintz, J., *et al.* (1992).** Haloperidol plasma levels and clinical response: A therapeutic window relationship. *Am J Psychiatry*, 149, 500–505.
34. **Pilla Reddy, V., Kozielska, M., Johnson, M., *et al.* (2013).** Population pharmacokinetic–pharmacodynamic modeling of haloperidol in patients with schizophrenia using positive and negative syndrome rating scale. *J Clin Psychopharmacol*, 33, 731–739.
35. **Van Putten, T., Marder, S. R., May, P. R., *et al.* (1985).** Plasma levels of haloperidol and clinical response. *Psychopharmacol Bull*, 21, 69–72.
36. **Marder, S. R., Davis, J. M., and Janicak, P. G., eds. (1993).** *Clinical Use of Neuroleptic Plasma Levels.* Washington, DC: American Psychiatric Press Inc.
37. **Kapur, S., Zipursky, R., Jones, C., *et al.* (2000).** Relationship between dopamine D(2) occupancy, clinical response, and side effects: A double-blind PET study of first-episode schizophrenia. *Am J Psychiatry*, 157, 514–520.
38. **Merlo, M. C., Hofer, H., Gekle, W., *et al.* (2002).** Risperidone, 2 mg/day vs. 4 mg/day, in first-episode, acutely psychotic patients: Treatment efficacy and effects on fine motor functioning. *J Clin Psychiatry*, 63, 885–891.
39. **Fitzgerald, P. B., Kapur, S., Remington, G., *et al.* (2000).** Predicting haloperidol occupancy of central dopamine D2 receptors from plasma levels. *Psychopharmacology*, 149, 1–5.

40. **Lim, H. S., Kim, S. J., Noh, Y. H., *et al.* (2013).** Exploration of optimal dosing regimens of haloperidol, a D2 antagonist, via modeling and simulation analysis in a D2 receptor occupancy study. *Pharm Res*, 30, 683–693.

41. **de Haan, L., van Bruggen, M., Lavalaye, J., *et al.* (2003).** Subjective experience and D2 receptor occupancy in patients with recent-onset schizophrenia treated with low-dose olanzapine or haloperidol: A randomized, double-blind study. *Am J Psychiatry*, 160, 303–309.

42. **Veselinović, T., Scharpenberg, M., Heinze, M., *et al.* (2019).** Dopamine D2 receptor occupancy estimated from plasma concentrations of four different antipsychotics and the subjective experience of physical and mental well-being in schizophrenia: Results from the randomized NeSSy Trial. *J Clin Psychopharmacol*, 39, 550–560.

43. **Simpson, G. M. and Kunz-Bartholini, E. (1968).** Relationship of individual tolerance, behavior and phenothiazine produced extrapyramidal system disturbance. *Dis Nerv System*, 29, 269–274.

44. **Nyberg, S., Dencker, S. J., Malm, U., *et al.* (1998).** D(2)- and 5-HT(2) receptor occupancy in high-dose neuroleptic-treated patients. *Int J Neuropsychopharmacol*, 1, 95–101.

45. **Meyer, J. M. (2020).** Monitoring and improving antipsychotic adherence in outpatient forensic diversion programs. *CNS Spectr*, 25, 136–144.

46. **Samara, M. T., Leucht, C., Leeflang, M. M., *et al.* (2015).** Early improvement as a predictor of later response to antipsychotics in schizophrenia: A diagnostic test review. *Am J Psychiatry*, 172, 617–629.

47. **Leucht, S., Kane, J. M., Etschel, E., *et al.* (2006).** Linking the PANSS, BPRS, and CGI: Clinical implications. *Neuropsychopharmacology*, 31, 2318–2325.

48. **Marder, S. R. and Meibach, R. C. (1994).** Risperidone in the treatment of schizophrenia. *Am J Psychiatry*, 151, 825–835.

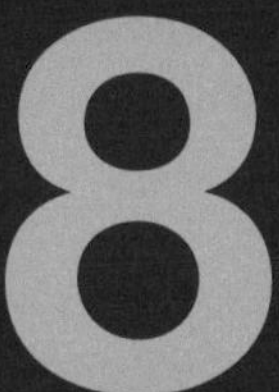

Fluphenazine and Fluphenazine Decanoate

QUICK CHECK

PRINCIPLES

- Fluphenazine provides an inexpensive method of delivering D_2 antagonism, with extensive plasma level data and a long-acting injectable (LAI) preparation (fluphenazine decanoate).
- Three weekly injections of fluphenazine decanoate 50 mg generate a plasma level after the third injection that is slightly above the therapeutic threshold (1.09 ng/ml). Maintenance injections start 2 weeks after the third loading injection, and a dose of 25 mg every 2 weeks is associated with trough levels of 1.0–1.2 ng/ml.

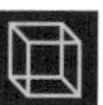

InfoBox Oral Fluphenazine Plasma Level Essentials

Oral dose correlation (bedtime dosing, 12h trough)	Level of evidence	Therapeutic threshold	Level of evidence	Point of futility	Level of evidence
Smokers: 10 mg = 0.6 ng/ml [1, 2] Nonsmokers: 10 mg = 0.8 ng/ml [3] Unknown smoking status: 10 mg = 1.0 ng/ml [4] **Multiply oral dose by 0.06 (smoker)** *OR* **0.08 – 0.10 (nonsmoker, unsure)** (see Table 8.1 for effects of CYP inhibitors/inducers on this relationship)	Moderate	1.0 ng/ml [5, 2]	High	4.0 ng/ml [6]	High

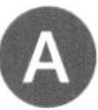

Basic Pharmacokinetic Information for Oral and Long-Acting Injectable Fluphenazine

As with many first-generation antipsychotics (FGAs), fluphenazine has no unique therapeutic benefit compared to other D_2 antagonists, but does have multiple formulations including a long-acting injectable (LAI), and an extensive database of plasma level information [1–2, 5–12]. The cytochrome P450 pathways and effects of inhibitors and inducers are less well studied than for other FGAs, and there are fewer studies on oral dose–concentration relationships which account for confounding issues such as smoking [3]. Nonetheless, there are a small number of double-blind, randomized fixed-dose studies that provide correlations between plasma levels and clinical response [13]. Unlike haloperidol, there are surprisingly few Positron Emission Tomography (PET) imaging studies of dopamine D_2 receptor occupancy, and none with subjects whose plasma levels are close to the response threshold, so inferences about the response threshold and point of futility are almost exclusively based on clinical data [14, 15]. Fluphenazine was assigned a Level 1 recommendation (strongly recommended) for use of plasma level monitoring in the 2020 consensus paper authored jointly by the Therapeutic Drug Monitoring (TDM) task force of the German Arbeitsgemeinschaft für Neuropsychopharmakologie und Pharmakopsychiatrie (AGNP) and the American Society for Clinical Psychopharmacology (ASCP) [16].

Table 8.1 Oral fluphenazine kinetic facts

Basic facts	Inhibition effects	Induction effects
US FDA approval: Aug. 24, 1960 $T_{1/2}$ 13 (6–20) hours [17] Absolute oral bioavailability: 2.7–3.4% [18]* T_{max} 2.4 (1–7) hours Metabolism: Multiple CYP pathways, particularly CYP 1A2 and CYP 2D6 **Formulations:** Tablets, oral solution (also acute intramuscular)	There are two active metabolites, 7-OH fluphenazine and fluphenazine-N-oxide, but their CNS exposure is only 11% of the CNS fluphenazine exposure based on striatal levels [19] 26 patients on fluphenazine decanoate were randomized to adjunctive fluoxetine (a strong CYP 2D6 inhibitor) 20 mg/d or placebo for 6 weeks. In the 15 patients on fluoxetine, the mean serum fluphenazine levels increased by 65% ± 85%, while the change on placebo (n = 11) was 11% ± 50%. This result fell short of statistical significance (p = 0.08) [20] Impact of strong CYP 1A2 inhibitors not studied – recommend rechecking plasma fluphenazine levels if co-prescribed any strong CYP 1A2 or CYP 2D6 inhibitor for more than 14 days	Smoking increases clearance 62% [3] There is one case report of plasma fluphenazine level increasing from 0.60 ng/ml to 1.17 ng/ml after carbamazepine 800 mg/d was discontinued in a patient on fluphenazine decanoate 37.5 mg/week [21]

* The absolute oral bioavailability of fluphenazine is extremely low (2.7–3.4%) [18]. The acute intramuscular IM preparation (concentration 2.5 mg/ml) is estimated to provide at least 4 times the bioavailable drug, so initial acute IM doses should be no greater than 0.5 ml (1.25 mg IM, equal to 5 mg oral) [22]. In a study examining the now abandoned practice of rapid neuroleptization, a median dose of 15 IM in the first 24 hours resulted in significantly higher rates of neurological adverse effects than a median oral dose of 7.5 mg in the first 24 hours, and with no difference in response trajectory or extent of response by day 7 [22].

Essential Information for Oral and Long-Acting Injectable Fluphenazine

1 Essential Oral Fluphenazine Information

Detecting adherence with no established plasma level baseline requires a knowledge of the expected plasma level for a given dose. The oral fluphenazine concentration–dose relationship presented in the InfoBox is based on results from a small number of studies, with a 10 mg bedtime dose expected to generate plasma levels in the range of 0.6–1.0 ng/ml, with lower values expected in smokers [1–2]. While lower plasma levels in smokers indicate that cytochrome P450 (CYP) 1A2 is involved in fluphenazine metabolism, there is no kinetic data about changes in levels following smoking cessation, or kinetic interaction studies with strong CYP 1A2 inhibitors (e.g. ciprofloxacin, fluvoxamine). The one study with a strong CYP 2D6 inhibitor fluoxetine showed a modest effect in patients on fluphenazine decanoate [20]. Given this paucity of drug–drug kinetic information, one should avoid use of strong CYP inhibitors if possible. If not possible and the patient requires a strong CYP inhibitor for 14 days or more, levels should be checked weekly for the first 3 weeks until they are at steady state, and fluphenazine dosages adjusted accordingly. As with many phenothiazines, absolute oral bioavailability of fluphenazine is extremely low (2.7–3.4%) [18]. This is of practical importance since the acute intramuscular (IM) solution (2.5 mg/ml) is estimated to provide at least four times the systemic exposure on a milligram basis compared to the oral, so acute IM dosages should be 25% that of oral dosing initially (e.g. 1.25 mg IM, approximately equal to 5 mg oral) [22].

2 Essential Long-Acting Injectable Fluphenazine Information

Fluphenazine decanoate is solubilized in sesame oil, an aspect of this formulation that presents a higher risk for injection site reactions than seen with water-based injectables, and which also requires a specific injection technique. The time to maximal plasma levels (T_{max}) is extremely short, and is measured in hours not days, occurring at 20–24 hours on average (Table 8.2, Figure 8.1). This short T_{max} must be appreciated when starting patients with unknown tolerance for D_2 blockade, as more sensitive individuals may experience abrupt onset of neurological adverse effects during the first 48 hours of treatment as levels peak. Despite the short T_{max}, the steady state half-life is at least 2 weeks with repeated dosing. Once at steady state, the dosing interval can be extended to 3 weeks in some patients due to the slow decay in plasma levels and even slower attenuation of D_2 receptor occupancy [23–26]. One loading study with detailed plasma level data has been published, and loading is the optimal strategy to quickly achieve therapeutic plasma levels that are close to those at steady state [27]. As seen in Figure 8.2, after three weekly injections of 50 mg (days 0, 7, 14), the mean plasma level on day 17.5 was 1.09 ng/ml, above the therapeutic threshold. For first-episode or less severely ill schizophrenia patients, lower dosages can certainly be used [7]. As is true for all oil-based depot antipsychotics, the maximum injection volume is 3 ml to minimize patient discomfort. In most countries, the only formulation is 25 mg/ml, so doses above 75 mg every 2 weeks should be evenly split into weekly dosages. There is a 100 mg/ml form available in Canada and the UK, but this should be used very carefully as it shares the same kinetic characteristics, with peak plasma levels occuring within 24 hours of injection [28].

Table 8.2 Fluphenazine decanoate essentials

Vehicle	Concentration	Dosage	T_{max} (days)	$T_{1/2}$ (days) multiple dosing	Able to be loaded	Maintenance dose: oral equivalence
Sesame oil	25 mg/ml[a] (max injection volume 3 ml)	12.5–75 mg/2 weeks **Max:** 75 mg/ week	0.3–1.5 days	14	Yes	See Section B, 2: "Essential Long-Acting Injectable Fluphenazine Information"

[a] May also be available as 100 mg/ml in some countries (e.g. Canada, UK).

(For further reading about use of LAI antipsychotics, please see the comprehensive edited book ***Antipsychotic Long-Acting Injections***, now in its 2nd edition [29])

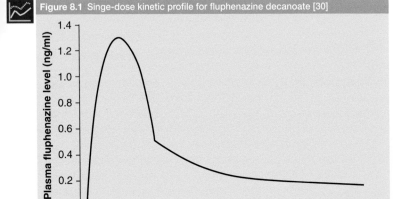

Figure 8.1 Singe-dose kinetic profile for fluphenazine decanoate [30]

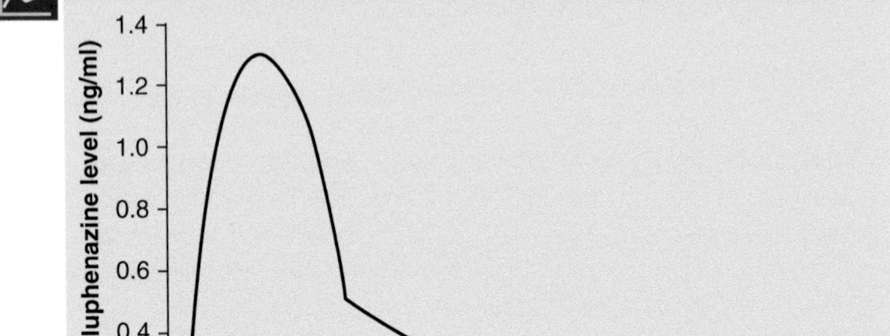

(Adapted from: L. Ereshefsky and C. A. Mascarenas [2003]. Comparison of the effects of different routes of antipsychotic administration on pharmacokinetics and pharmacodynamics. *J Clin Psychiatry*, 64, 18–23.)

Unlike for haloperidol decanoate, there is no single, well-tested conversion formula that emerged for transitioning from oral to LAI fluphenazine [31]. For those stabilized on oral fluphenazine, a 12h trough plasma level is the best guide to loading and

Figure 8.2 Plasma levels from weekly 50 mg injections of fluphenazine decanoate [7]

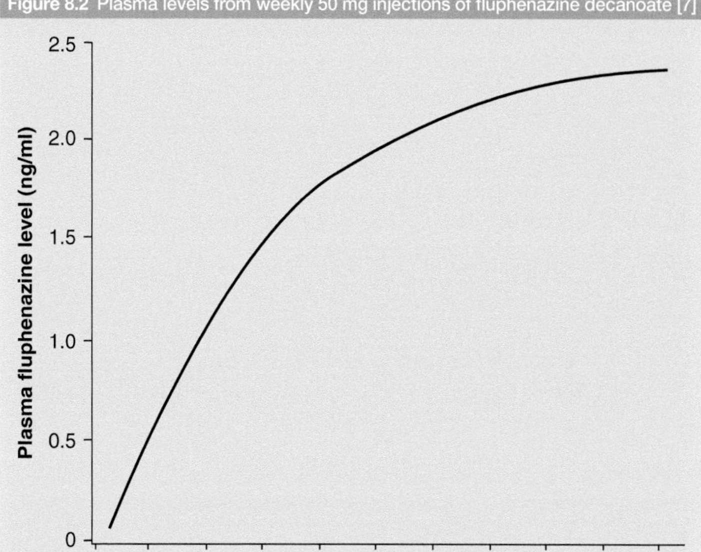

(Adapted from: M. W. Jann, L. Ereshefsky, and S. R. Saklad [1985]. Clinical pharmacokinetics of the depot antipsychotics. *Clin Pharmacokinet*, 10, 315–333.)

maintenance strategies. Using the levels documented with weekly injections of 50 mg (Figure 8.2), one can adjust the loading dose accordingly. Longer-term data (Figures 8.3a, 8.3b) also indicate that a 25 mg injection every 2 weeks achieves a steady state level of approximately 1.0–1.2 ng/ml, with brief peaks in the 24 hours following each injection [32, 5]. Consistent with these results, a 1-year study of fluphenazine decanoate 12.5 mg every 2 weeks noted mean trough plasma levels in the range of 0.44–0.50 ng/ml at the 6-month and 12-month time points [11]. While plasma levels on 12.5 mg biweekly are below the therapeutic threshold, some patients may do well on LAI fluphenazine at these levels [33, 24, 34]. Once loaded, levels should be checked periodically during the first 6–8 months due to level creep as tissue compartments become saturated (Figure 8.3a and 8.3b) [5].

Figure 8.3a Plasma fluphenazine levels over the 2- week dosing interval in patients on fluphenazine decanoate 25 mg for 3 months [32]

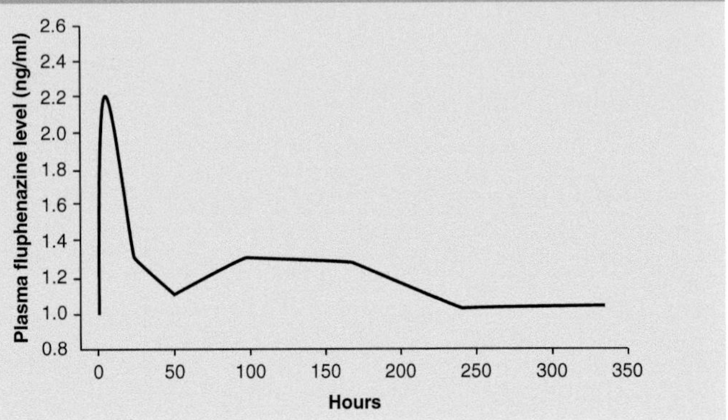

(Adapted from: W. M. Glazer [1988]. Fluphenazine decanoate: Its steady-state pharmacologic profile and relationship to tardive dyskinesia. *Schizophr Res*, 1, 425–429.)

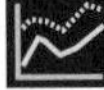

Figure 8.3b Steady state occurs after 12 weeks of treatment with fluphenazine decanoate, with possible level creep at later time points. Data from patients on 25 mg every 2 weeks [5]

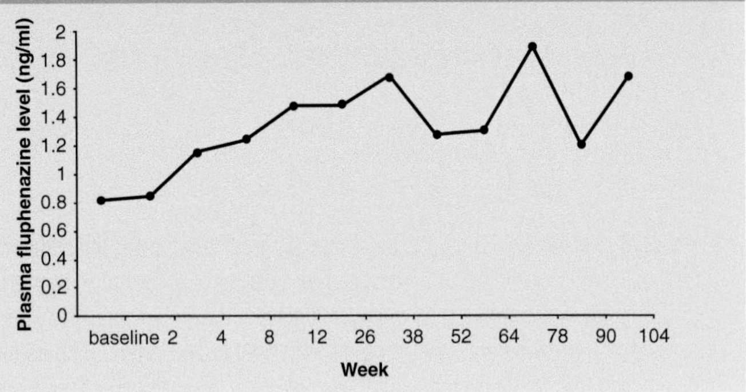

(Adapted from: S. R. Marder, K. K. Midha, T. Van Putten, *et al.* [1991]. Plasma levels of fluphenazine in patients receiving fluphenazine decanoate: Relationship to clinical response. *Br J Psychiatry*, 158, 658–665.)

Implications

a Steady state is reached by the fourth month of treatment when fluphenazine decanoate is not loaded.

b As with all LAI injectables, monthly or bimonthly monitoring of plasma antipsychotic levels in the first year can help detect level creep and forestall tolerability issues due to supratherapeutic levels.

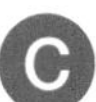

The Therapeutic Threshold for Fluphenazine

1 Clinical Evidence for a Therapeutic Threshold

Clinical evidence, especially from fixed-dose, prospective, randomized trials, is the most important tool we have for estimation of plasma level response thresholds (see Chapter 2), but the small number of fixed-dose fluphenazine trials suffer from methodological issues (e.g. open label, lack of rater blinding to dose, small sample sizes in certain dosing arms, etc.) [4]. Marder's comprehensive 1993 book ***Clinical Use of Neuroleptic Plasma Levels*** noted that only two of the five fixed-dose studies had interpretable data, and this did not yield sufficient patient level information to create a receiver operating characteristic (ROC) curve. A subsequent fixed-dose open-label trial was published in 1994 examining outcomes in 36 first-episode schizophrenia patients assigned to 20 mg/d, with response defined by the clinical global impressions (CGI) improvement score [4]. As only one dose was studied, and the sample size was modest, this trial may have lacked the statistical power to detect any differences in the mean steady state fluphenazine level (drawn at weeks 3 and 4) between responders (n = 13; 2.17 ± 1.15 ng/ml) and nonresponders (n = 13; 1.73 ± 0.75 ng/ml). The following year, a team led by investigators at the Medical College of Pennsylvania published results from a randomized, double-blind, fixed-dose, 4-week trial of three doses (10 mg/d, 20 mg/d, 30 mg/d) in 72 inpatients (68% male, mean age 28.7 ± 7.0 years), data that provided the most methodologically rigorous estimate for a response threshold [2]. The study utilized a 40% or greater reduction in Brief Psychiatric Rating Scale (BPRS) score as the response definition, and plasma levels were obtained as 12h troughs. Using the 40% BPRS improvement cutoff, 55% (42/76) met response criteria. There was no correlation between plasma level and symptom improvement among nonresponders, but ROC analysis for responders calculated a plasma level threshold of 0.97 ng/ml, with 77% specificity and 65% sensitivity (p = 0.006) [2]. The positive predictive value of the 0.97 ng/ml threshold is 72.2%.

A response threshold near 1.0 ng/ml is also supported by other clinical data. A 2-year randomized fluphenazine decanoate trial found that mean plasma levels below 0.9 ng/ml at 9 months discriminated between those who did and did not relapse by study end (Figure 8.4) [5]. Another large, randomized fixed-dose study of 72 inpatients from a team at the Veterans Affairs Medical Center (VAMC) in West Los Angeles found that the odds of significant improvement without "disabling" adverse effects were optimal at levels slightly under 0.9 ng/ml (Figure 8.5) [13, 6].

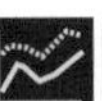

Figure 8.4 Distribution of plasma fluphenazine levels drawn at 9 months in patients who exacerbated (mean 0.51 ± 0.36 ng/ml) and those who did not (mean 1.59 ± 1.27 ng/ml) in a 2-year fluphenazine decanoate trial (p = 0.001) [5]

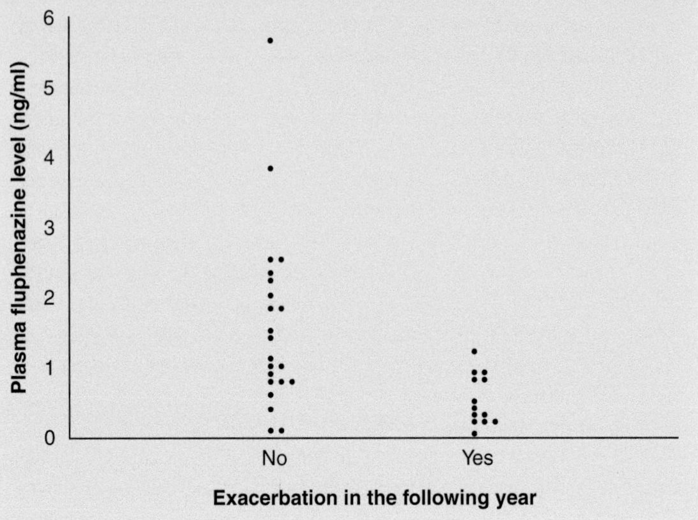

(Adapted from: S. R. Marder, K. K. Midha, T. Van Putten, *et al.* [1991]. Plasma levels of fluphenazine in patients receiving fluphenazine decanoate: Relationship to clinical response. *Br J Psychiatry*, 158, 658–665.)

Some patients may respond to levels well below 0.9 ng/ml, but for nonresponders a response threshold of approximately 1.0 ng/ml is a reasonable target.

2 Imaging Evidence for a Therapeutic Threshold

Fluphenazine has extremely limited D_2 receptor occupancy data, and none at plasma levels under 2.0 ng/ml (Table 8.3). An extensive 2011 systematic review of the correlation between antipsychotic plasma levels and D_2 receptor occupancy does not include fluphenazine [35]. The extent of the PET imaging data is presented in Table 8.3 from studies focusing on higher dose usage [14, 15]. While this information provides no insight into a response threshold, it will be useful when examining the point of futility.

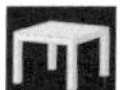

Table 8.3 D_2 occupancy and plasma fluphenazine levels

	Level (as reported)	Striatal occupancy
Nyberg 1998 [15]	2.23 ng/ml (5.1 nM)	89%
Coppens 1991 [14]	4.4 ng/ml (4.4 mcg/L)	92% R, 100% L
Coppens 1991 [14]	5.2 ng/ml (5.2 mcg/L)	100% R, 97% L
Nyberg 1998 [15]	6.13 ng/ml (14 nM)	91%
Nyberg 1998 [15]	7.88 ng/ml (18 nM)	92%
Nyberg 1998 [15]	16.19 ng/ml (37 nM)	97%
Nyberg 1998 [15]	11.38 ng/ml (26 nM)	96%

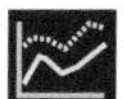

Figure 8.5 Estimated probability of improvement in the absence of disabling adverse effects based on plasma fluphenazine level [6]

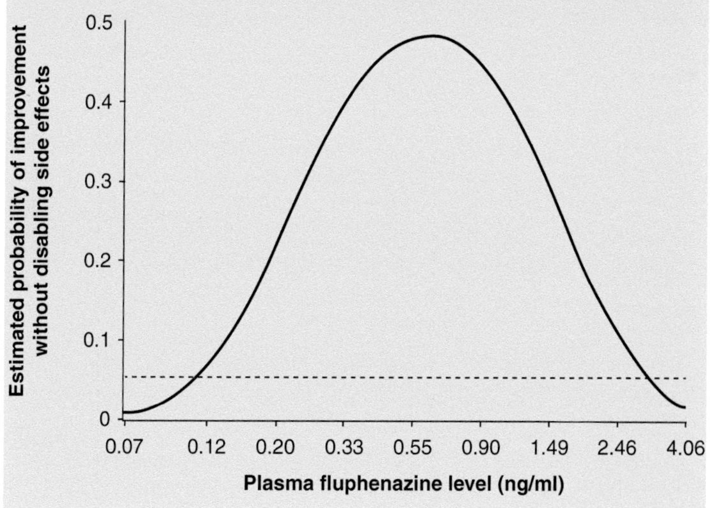

(Adapted from: K. K. Midha, J. W. Hubbard, S. R. Marder, *et al*. [1994]. Impact of clinical pharmacokinetics on neuroleptic therapy in patients with schizophrenia. *J Psychiatry Neurosci*, 19, 254–264.)

D The Point of Futility for Fluphenazine

1 Clinical Evidence for a Point of Futility

The plasma level where an average patient might achieve maximum symptom reduction is important, but the question of futility revolves around when further titration should stop for nonresponders in the absence of dose-limiting side effects [6]. Like most potent D_2 antagonists, fluphenazine titration will often end due to intolerable neurological adverse effects, or the unpleasant, dysphoric subjective experience associated with excessive D_2 blockade ***for that patient*** (see Chapter 5 for discussion of clinical endpoints) [13, 9]. Defining the point of futility addresses an important question for treating extremely ill schizophrenia patients, and creates an easily understood concept: further titration beyond this point is of limited value, with an estimated < 5% chance of response (Chapter 2). However, assuming tolerability, there is no inherent unusual safety concern in exploring plasma levels up to that point, with various papers suggesting upper limits as high as a fluphenazine level of 10 ng/ml [36, 37, 16]. Plasma fluphenazine levels as high as 27.9 ng/ml are described in the literature without the need for antiparkinsonian medication [10], reflecting the reality that some patients may not develop intolerable neurological adverse effects from extremely high levels of D_2 occupancy [38]. Nonetheless, the question is: At what point is the probability of response < 5%, assuming higher levels are tolerated? Figure 8.6 provides this information from the West Los Angeles VAMC study [13]. As one can see in this elegant graphic, the probability of response for levels > 4.0 ng/ml is < 5% – thus 4.0 ng/ml represents the point of futility [6]. A small fraction of patients will tolerate higher plasma fluphenazine levels, but pursuing this strategy in search of efficacy is not an evidence-based decision – those patients needs clozapine [39].

2 Imaging Evidence for a Point of Futility

Partial agonist antipsychotics (e.g. aripiprazole, cariprazine) require D_2 receptor occupancy levels ranging from 80 to 100% for efficacy, but D_2 antagonists incur an increasing risk for neurological adverse effects when occupancy exceeds 80% [40–43]. Given the paucity of imaging studies, fluphenazine's point of futility is best estimated based on clinical findings. Despite this, one can draw an important conclusion from the small number of imaging data points available: a plasma level above the point of futility (4.0 ng/ml) is associated with > 90% D_2 receptor occupancy. Higher plasma levels will almost saturate the D_2 receptor (Table 8.3) [14, 15]. This finding is consistent with the estimated D_2 occupancy from the clinically derived point of futility for the most widely studied FGA, haloperidol [44].

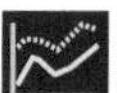

Figure 8.6 Estimated probability of response (dotted line) or disabling adverse effects (bold line) based on plasma fluphenazine level [6]

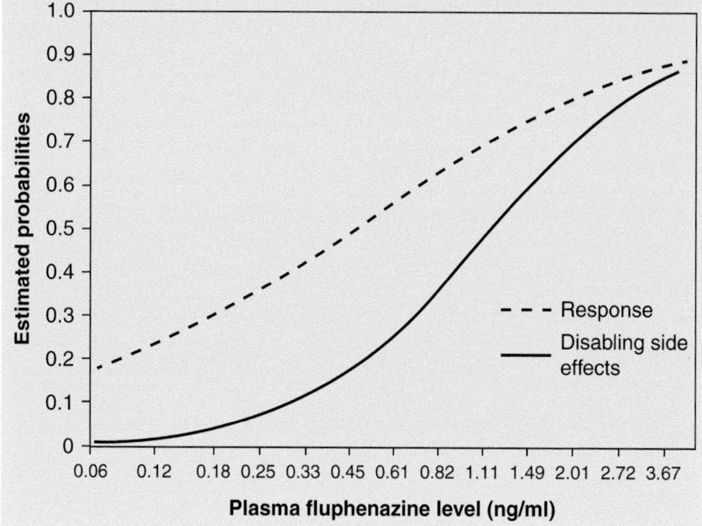

(Adapted from: K. K. Midha, J. W. Hubbard, S. R. Marder, *et al*. [1994]. Impact of clinical pharmacokinetics on neuroleptic therapy in patients with schizophrenia. *J Psychiatry Neurosci*, 19, 254–264.)

Summary Points

a The correlation between fluphenazine plasma levels and schizophrenia response has not been widely studied in fixed-dose, double-blind, randomized trials. From the largest and most rigorous studies, the suggested therapeutic response threshold is 1.0 ng/ml, and the point of futility is 4.0 ng/ml. The 2020 AGNP/ASCP consensus paper strongly recommends plasma level monitoring.

b The oral fluphenazine concentration–dose relationship is not as well established as for other first-generation antipsychotics (e.g. haloperidol) and may be influenced by smoking status. Thus, 10 mg at bedtime may be associated with a steady state 12h trough level of 0.60 ng/ml for smokers, or 0.8–1.0 ng/ml for nonsmokers or mixed groups.

c Fluphenazine decanoate has a very short T_{max} of 20–24 hours (i.e. 1 day). Three weekly fluphenazine decanoate loading injections of 50 mg (days 0, 7, 14) will generate a plasma level above the therapeutic threshold (mean level 1.09 ng/ml on day 17.5). For first-episode or less severely ill schizophrenia patients, lower dosages should be considered to avoid neurological adverse effects at peak plasma levels 24 h after the injection.

d A maintenance fluphenazine decanoate dose of 25 mg every 2 weeks will result in steady state levels of 1.0–1.2 ng/ml after 3 months of treatment. Levels should be checked periodically during the first 6–8 months due to level creep as tissue compartments become saturated. Dosages under 25 mg every 2 weeks, or extended dosing intervals (e.g. 3 weeks), may be therapeutic for some patients, but greater long-term relapse risk is seen for levels < 0.90 ng/ml.

References

1. **Dysken, M. W., Javaid, J. I., Chang, S. S., *et al.* (1981).** Fluphenazine pharmacokinetics and therapeutic response. *Psychopharmacology (Berl)*, 73, 205–210.
2. **Levinson, D. F., Simpson, G. M., Lo, E. S., *et al.* (1995).** Fluphenazine plasma levels, dosage, efficacy, and side effects. *Am J Psychiatry*, 152, 765–771.
3. **Ereshefsky, L., Jann, M. W., Saklad, S. R., *et al.* (1985).** Effects of smoking on fluphenazine clearance in psychiatric inpatients. *Biol Psychiatry*, 20, 329–332.
4. **Koreen, A. R., Lieberman, J., Alvir, J., *et al.* (1994).** Relation of plasma fluphenazine levels to treatment response and extrapyramidal side effects in first-episode schizophrenic patients. *Am J Psychiatry*, 151, 35–39.
5. **Marder, S. R., Midha, K. K., Van Putten, T., *et al.* (1991).** Plasma levels of fluphenazine in patients receiving fluphenazine decanoate: Relationship to clinical response. *Br J Psychiatry*, 158, 658–665.
6. **Midha, K. K., Hubbard, J. W., Marder, S. R., *et al.* (1994).** Impact of clinical pharmacokinetics on neuroleptic therapy in patients with schizophrenia. *J Psychiatry Neurosci*, 19, 254–264.
7. **Jann, M. W., Ereshefsky, L., and Saklad, S. R. (1985).** Clinical pharmacokinetics of the depot antipsychotics. *Clin Pharmacokinet*, 10, 315–333.
8. **Marder, S. R., Van Putten, T., Aravagiri, M., *et al.* (1989).** Plasma levels of parent drug and metabolites in patients receiving oral and depot fluphenazine. *Psychopharmacol Bull*, 25, 479–482.
9. **Van Putten, T., Marder, S. R., Wirshing, W. C., *et al.* (1991).** Neuroleptic plasma levels. *Schizophr Bull*, 17, 197–216.
10. **Miller, R. S., Peterson, G. M., McLean, S., *et al.* (1995).** Monitoring plasma levels of fluphenazine during chronic therapy with fluphenazine decanoate. *J Clin Pharm Ther*, 20, 55–62.
11. **Gitlin, M. J., Nuechterlein, K. H., Mintz, J., *et al.* (2000).** Fluphenazine levels during maintenance treatment of recent-onset schizophrenia: Relation to side effects, psychosocial function and depression. *Psychopharmacology*, 148, 350–354.
12. **Marder, S. R., Aravagiri, M., Wirshing, W. C., *et al.* (2002).** Fluphenazine plasma level monitoring for patients receiving fluphenazine decanoate. *Schizophr Res*, 53, 25–30.
13. **Van Putten, T., Aravagiri, M., Marder, S. R., *et al.* (1991).** Plasma fluphenazine levels and clinical response in newly admitted schizophrenic patients. *Psychopharmacol Bull*, 27, 91–96.
14. **Coppens, H. J., Slooff, C. J., Paans, A. M., *et al.* (1991).** High central D2-dopamine receptor occupancy as assessed with positron emission tomography in medicated but therapy-resistant schizophrenic patients. *Biol Psychiatry*, 29, 629–634.
15. **Nyberg, S., Dencker, S. J., Malm, U., *et al.* (1998).** D(2)- and 5-HT(2) receptor occupancy in high-dose neuroleptic-treated patients. *Int J Neuropsychopharmacol*, 1, 95–101.
16. **Schoretsanitis, G., Kane, J. M., Correll, C. U., *et al.* (2020).** Blood levels to optimize antipsychotic treatment in clinical practice: A joint consensus statement of the American Society of Clinical Psychopharmacology (ASCP) and the Therapeutic Drug Monitoring (TDM) Task Force of the Arbeitsgemeinschaft für Neuropsychopharmakologie und Pharmakopsychiatrie (AGNP). *J Clin Psychiatry*, 81, https://doi/10.4088/JCP.4019cs13169.
17. **Midha, K. K., Hawes, E. M., Hubbard, J. W., *et al.* (1988).** Variation in the single dose pharmacokinetics of fluphenazine in psychiatric patients. *Psychopharmacology (Berl)*, 96, 206–211.
18. **Koytchev, R., Alken, R. G., McKay, G., *et al.* (1996).** Absolute bioavailability of oral immediate and slow release fluphenazine in healthy volunteers. *Eur J Clin Pharmacol*, 51, 183–187.
19. **Aravagiri, M., Marder, S. R., Yuwiler, A., *et al.* (1995).** Distribution of fluphenazine and its metabolites in brain regions and other tissues of the rat. *Neuropsychopharmacology*, 13, 235–247.
20. **Goff, D. C., Midha, K. K., Sarid-Segal, O., *et al.* (1995).** A placebo-controlled trial of fluoxetine added to neuroleptic in patients with schizophrenia. *Psychopharmacology (Berl)*, 117, 417–423.

21. **Jann, M. W., Fidone, G. S., Hernandez, J. M., *et al.* (1989).** Clinical implications of increased antipsychotic plasma concentrations upon anticonvulsant cessation. *Psychiatry Res*, 28, 153–159.
22. **Coffman, J. A., Nasrallah, H. A., Lyskowski, J., *et al.* (1987).** Clinical effectiveness of oral and parenteral rapid neuroleptization. *J Clin Psychiatry*, 48, 20–24.
23. **Harasko-van der Meer, C., Brucke, T., Wenger, S., *et al.* (1993).** Two cases of long term dopamine D2 receptor blockade after depot neuroleptics. *J Neural Transm*, 94, 217–221.
24. **Carpenter, W. T., Jr., Buchanan, R. W., Kirkpatrick, B., *et al.* (1999).** Comparative effectiveness of fluphenazine decanoate injections every 2 weeks versus every 6 weeks. *Am J Psychiatry*, 156, 412–418.
25. **Taylor, D. (2009).** Psychopharmacology and adverse effects of antipsychotic long-acting injections: A review. *Br J Psychiatry Suppl*, 52, S13–19.
26. **Meyer, J. M. (2018).** Pharmacotherapy of psychosis and mania. In L. L. Brunton, R. Hilal-Dandan and B. C. Knollmann, eds., *Goodman & Gilman's The Pharmacological Basis of Therapeutics*, 13th edn. Chicago, IL: McGraw-Hill, pp. 279–302.
27. **Ereshefsky, L., Saklad, S. R., Jann, M. W., *et al.* (1984).** Future of depot neuroleptic therapy: Pharmacokinetic and pharmacodynamic approaches. *J Clin Psychiatry*, 45, 50–59.
28. **Bristol-Myers Squibb Company (2017).** Modecate Concentrate (Fluphenazine Decanoate injection, BP 100 mg/ml) product monograph. Montreal, Canada.
29. **Haddad, P., Lambert, T., and Lauriello, J., eds. (2016).** *Antipsychotic Long-Acting Injections*, 2nd edn. New York: Oxford University Press.
30. **Ereshefsky, L. and Mascarenas, C. A. (2003).** Comparison of the effects of different routes of antipsychotic administration on pharmacokinetics and pharmacodynamics. *J Clin Psychiatry*, 64, 18–23.
31. **Meyer, J. M. (2017).** Converting oral to long acting injectable antipsychotics: A guide for the perplexed. *CNS Spectr*, 22, 14–28.
32. **Glazer, W. M. (1988).** Fluphenazine decanoate: Its steady-state pharmacologic profile and relationship to tardive dyskinesia. *Schizophr Res*, 1, 425–429.
33. **Heresco-Levy, U., Greenberg, D., Lerer, B., *et al.* (1997).** Serum neuroleptic levels during reduced dose fluphenazine decanoate maintenance therapy. *Isr J Psychiatry Relat Sci*, 34, 281–289.
34. **Baldelli, S., Clementi, E., and Cattaneo, D. (2018).** Can we rely on AGNP therapeutic targets also for LAI antipsychotics? *Pharmacopsychiatry*, 51, 270–271.
35. **Uchida, H., Takeuchi, H., Graff-Guerrero, A., *et al.* (2011).** Predicting dopamine D2 receptor occupancy from plasma levels of antipsychotic drugs: A systematic review and pooled analysis. *J Clin Psychopharmacol*, 31, 318–325.
36. **Meyer, J. M. (2014).** A rational approach to employing high plasma levels of antipsychotics for violence associated with schizophrenia: Case vignettes. *CNS Spectr*, 19, 432–438.
37. **Meyer, J. M. (2020).** Monitoring and improving antipsychotic adherence in outpatient forensic diversion programs. *CNS Spectr*, 25, 136–144.
38. **Simpson, G. M. and Kunz-Bartholini, E. (1968).** Relationship of individual tolerance, behavior and phenothiazine produced extrapyramidal system disturbance. *Dis Nerv System*, 29, 269–274.
39. **Kane, J., Honigfeld, G., Singer, J., *et al.* (1988).** Clozapine for the treatment-resistant schizophrenic: A double-blind comparison with chlorpromazine. *Arch Gen Psychiatry*, 45, 789–796.
40. **Kapur, S. and Seeman, P. (2001).** Does fast dissociation from the dopamine d(2) receptor explain the action of atypical antipsychotics? A new hypothesis. *Am J Psychiatry*, 158, 360–369.
41. **Sparshatt, A., Taylor, D., Patel, M. X., *et al.* (2010).** A systematic review of aripiprazole – dose, plasma concentration, receptor occupancy, and response: Implications for therapeutic drug monitoring. *J Clin Psychiatry*, 71, 1447–1556.

42. **Seneca, N., Finnema, S. J., Laszlovszky, I., *et al.* (2011).** Occupancy of dopamine D(2) and D(3) and serotonin 5-HT(1)A receptors by the novel antipsychotic drug candidate, cariprazine (RGH-188), in monkey brain measured using positron emission tomography. *Psychopharmacology (Berl)*, 218, 579–587.
43. **Uchida, H., Takeuchi, H., Graff-Guerrero, A., *et al.* (2011).** Dopamine D2 receptor occupancy and clinical effects: A systematic review and pooled analysis. *J Clin Psychopharmacol*, 31, 497–502.
44. **Lim, H. S., Kim, S. J., Noh, Y. H., *et al.* (2013).** Exploration of optimal dosing regimens of haloperidol, a D2 antagonist, via modeling and simulation analysis in a D2 receptor occupancy study. *Pharm Res*, 30, 683–693.

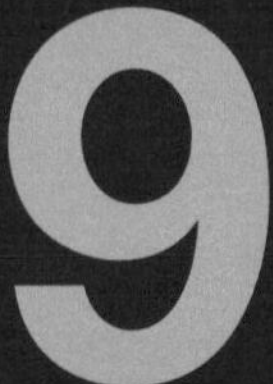

Perphenazine and Perphenazine Decanoate

QUICK CHECK

PRINCIPLES

- **Perphenazine provides an inexpensive method of delivering D_2 antagonism, with sufficient plasma level data to define a therapeutic threshold.**
- **A long-acting injectable (LAI) preparation (perphenazine decanoate) is available in certain countries (Belgium, Denmark, Finland, Iceland, The Netherlands, Norway, Portugal, Sweden).**

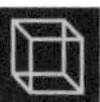

InfoBox Oral Perphenazine Plasma Level Essentials

Oral dose correlation (bedtime dosing, 12h trough)	Level of evidence	Therapeutic threshold	Level of evidence	Point of futility	Level of evidence
CYP 2D6 EM: 10 mg = 0.4 ng/ml [1] CYP 2D6 PM: 10 mg = 0.8 ng/ml [1] **Multiply oral dose by 0.04 (2D6 EM)** ***OR*** **0.08 (2D6 PM)** (see Table 9.1 for effects of CYP inhibitors/inducers on this relationship)	High	0.81 ng/ml	High	5.0 ng/ml	Moderate

CYP: cytochrome P450; EM: extensive metabolizer; PM: poor metabolizer

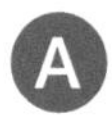

A Basic Pharmacokinetic Information for Oral and Long-Acting Injectable Perphenazine

As with many first-generation antipsychotics (FGAs), perphenazine has no unique therapeutic benefit compared to other D_2 antagonists, but does have a long-acting injectable (LAI) preparation available in certain parts of the world (Belgium, Denmark, Finland, Iceland, The Netherlands, Norway, Portugal, Sweden) and a large database of plasma level information. As the FGA arm of the Clinical Antipsychotic Trials of Intervention Effectiveness (CATIE) schizophrenia study, many clinicians came to appreciate that modest perphenazine dosages are effective, that perphenazine is associated with lower metabolic risk than many second-generation antipsychotics, and that perphenazine treatment is associated with less prolactin elevation than risperidone therapy [2, 3]. In the CATIE schizophrenia trial, the mean modal perphenazine dose was 20.8 mg/d, equal to 5.55 mg/d haloperidol, with only 8% experiencing extrapyramidal adverse effects on that dose [2]. Perphenazine's metabolic pathways and metabolite binding profiles are generally known, but some gaps exist in the literature regarding drug–drug interactions [1, 4–5]. The small number of double-blind, randomized fixed-dose trials (primarily of long-acting injectable perphenazine) and other controlled studies provide sufficient data to draw inferences about the response threshold [6–8]. There is surprisingly little Positron Emission Tomography (PET) imaging information on dopamine D_2 receptor occupancy, but the available data correlates with the response threshold derived from clinical studies, and provides insights into an estimated point of futility [9].

Table 9.1 Oral perphenazine kinetic facts

Basic facts	Inhibition effects	Induction effects
US FDA approval: Feb. 27, 1957 $T_{1/2}$ 9–12 hours [11] $T_{1/2}$ 9.9–18.8 hours (7-OH perphenazine) [11] Absolute oral bioavailability: 60% (40%–80%) [12] T_{max} 2.4 (1–7) hours [12] Metabolism: Multiple CYP pathways, primarily CYP 2D6 and, to a lesser extent, CYP 1A2, CYP 3A4 [13] **Formulations:** Tablets	CYP 2D6 converts perphenazine to active metabolites 7-OH perphenazine and the minimally active N-dealkylperphenazine. At steady state 7-OH perphenazine is present at a concentration 53% of that of perphenazine [4] CYP 2D6 PM experience approximately two-fold higher plasma levels of perphenazine [14, 3] Smokers have 33% faster clearance than nonsmokers [5] Paroxetine 20 mg/d for 10 days increased perphenazine C_{max} 2–13-fold in CYP 2D6 EMs (n = 8) [15]. Mean trough plasma levels are 2x higher in CYP 2D6 PM [1] Perphenazine is a moderate CYP 2D6 inhibitor [16]	No published data on interaction with carbamazepine, phenytoin, or phenobarbital

Perphenazine was assigned a Level 1 recommendation (strongly recommended) for use of plasma level monitoring in the 2020 consensus paper authored jointly by the Therapeutic Drug Monitoring (TDM) task force of the German Arbeitsgemeinschaft für Neuropsychopharmakologie und Pharmakopsychiatrie (AGNP) and the American Society for Clinical Psychopharmacology (ASCP) [10].

Essential Information for Oral and Long-Acting Injectable Perphenazine

1 Essential Oral Perphenazine Information

The oral perphenazine concentration–dose relationship presented in the InfoBox indicates that a 10 mg bedtime dose is expected to generate a 12h trough plasma level of 0.4 ng/ml [3]. Perphenazine is metabolized via a number of cytochrome P450 (CYP) pathways, with CYP 2D6 playing a more prominent role in humans than the other isoenzymes [3, 13, 5]. Those who are CYP 2D6 poor metabolizers will have two-fold higher levels for a given dose [1], while smokers are expected to have approximately 33% lower plasma levels [5]. The impact of smoking indicates involvement of CYP 1A2 in perphenazine's metabolism, but there is no data about changes in levels following smoking cessation, or kinetic interaction studies with strong CYP 1A2 inhibitors (e.g. ciprofloxacin, fluvoxamine). One-week pretreatment with paroxetine 20 mg/d (a strong CYP 2D6 inhibitor) did show a significant effect on the single-dose kinetics of perphenazine, with **peak** plasma levels increasing six-fold, but no levels were obtained after 8 hours [15]. Fortunately, another trial with patients on a variety of 2D6 inhibitors found that **trough** plasma levels were maximally increased two-fold [1]. If a strong 2D6 inhibitor must be used for ≥ 14 days, the perphenazine dose should be decreased by 50%, and a level rechecked at steady state approximately 1 week later. Further dosing adjustments may be necessary based on the new level, clinical response, and a prior baseline level (if available). *In vitro* data also support a role for CYP 3A4, but there is no information on interactions with strong 3A4 inhibitors or 3A4 inducers. Given this paucity of drug–drug kinetic information, one should avoid use of strong CYP 1A2 and 3A4 inhibitors, or 3A4 inducers, if possible. If not possible, and treatment with a strong CYP 1A2 or 3A4 inhibitor or 3A4 inducer is needed for ≥ 14 days, perphenazine levels should be checked weekly for the first 3 weeks until at steady state, and dosages adjusted accordingly. The absolute oral bioavailability of perphenazine is higher than for many other phenothiazines, with a 60% value commonly cited (range 40%–80%) [12, 17].

2 Essential Long-Acting Injectable Perphenazine Information

Perphenazine decanoate is solubilized in sesame oil, an aspect of this formulation that presents a higher risk for injection site reactions than seen with water-based injectables, and which also requires a specific injection technique. The time to maximal plasma levels (T_{max}) is approximately 7 days and the steady state half-life is 27 days with repeated dosing (Table 9.2) [6, 18]. For most patients, the dosing interval is 3–4 weeks, but 2-week intervals are occasionally used [19, 20]. As is true for all oil-based depot antipsychotics, the maximum injection volume is 3 ml to minimize patient discomfort. Unlike haloperidol, there is no well-established conversion formula

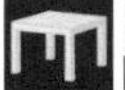

Table 9.2 Perphenazine decanoate essentials* [18, 22]

Vehicle	Concentration	Dosage	T_{max} (days)	$T_{1/2}$ (days) multiple dosing	Able to be loaded	Maintenance dose: oral equivalence
Sesame oil	108 mg/ml	27–216 mg/3–4 weeks **Max:** 216 mg/ 3 weeks	7	27	Yes	See Section B, 2: "Essential Long-Acting Injectable Perphenazine Information"

* Available in Belgium, Denmark, Finland, Iceland, The Netherlands, Norway, Portugal, Sweden

(For further reading about use of LAI antipsychotics, please see the comprehensive edited book ***Antipsychotic Long-Acting Injections***, now in its 2nd edition [26])

for transitioning from oral to LAI perphenazine [21]. For those stabilized on oral perphenazine, a 12h trough plasma level is the best guide to maintenance dosing. A 2004 imaging study found that the steady state level was 1.67 ± 1.15 ng/ml on an average dose of 154.8 ± 56.6 mg/month, but there were only six subjects [9]. A larger study of 20 stable schizophrenia patients on perphenazine decanoate examined the minimum level at which exacerbation occurred by gradually reducing the dose by 25% every 12 weeks [8]. Perphenazine decanoate was dosed every 2 weeks, so the correlations between dose and level at time of exacerbation reflect steady state. As seen in Figure 9.1, the correlation between dose and serum level was extremely high ($r = 0.87$, $p < 0.01$), and from this one can derive an equation to predict steady state levels from a dose administered every 4 weeks (Figure 9.1) [8]. The manufacturer recommends an aggressive loading schedule of 162–216 mg given on days 0, 7, and 21, but this may result in excessively high plasma levels [22]. In one fixed-dose trial, 52 adult patients were administered 108 mg on day 0 and 7, and serum levels were obtained on days 14 and 21 [23]. Unfortunately, the paper did not provide the levels on days 14 and 21, but the sum of those two levels (range 1.61–8.88 ng/ml), which the authors used to draw correlations about steady state levels. The authors noted that the ratio of the 14-day level to the 21-day level was 1.5, so from this one can estimate that the day 21 levels ranged from 0.645–3.55 ng/ml [23]. Some may experience neurological adverse effects from this dosing strategy as levels ≥ 2.42 ng/ml are associated with ≥ 80% D_2 occupancy [9], but this study provides an estimate of the exposure from this loading regimen. For first-episode patients, less severely ill schizophrenia patients, or patients who have a history of sensitivity to D_2 antagonism, administering these dosages 2 weeks apart should be considered to avoid neurological adverse effects at peak plasma levels 7 days after the injection. If loaded with at least two injections in the first month, steady state is usually achieved by 12 weeks [24], but levels should be checked periodically during the first 6–8 months due to level creep as tissue compartments become saturated [25].

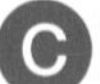

C The Therapeutic Threshold for Perphenazine

1 Clinical Evidence for a Therapeutic Threshold

Clinical evidence, especially from fixed-dose, prospective, randomized trials, is the most important tool we have for estimation of plasma level response thresholds (see Chapter 2), but this type of data is almost nonexistent for perphenazine. There were, however, a large number of prospective and naturalistic studies performed in the 1970s and 1980s that arrived at similar conclusions: plasma levels below 0.81 ng/ml (2 nmol/l) were unlikely to be therapeutic [27–29]. This threshold was then tested

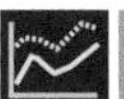

Figure 9.1 Serum level results from a long-term dose reduction study (n = 20) show a strong linear correlation between steady state perphenazine level and perphenazine decanoate dose [8]

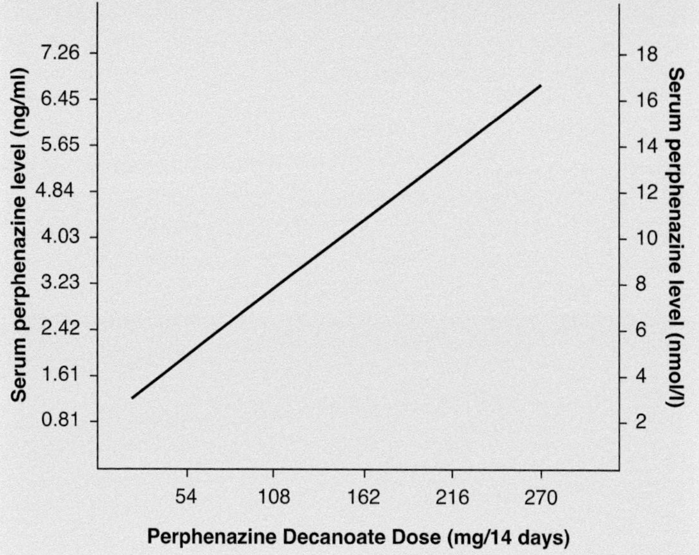

From this data one can estimate the steady state level for perphenazine decanoate administered every 4 weeks using the following formula:

Steady state level (ng/ml) = (4-week dose in mg) x 0.0104 + 0.962

Example: Patient on 108 mg/4 weeks should have a steady state level calculated as follows:

(108 x 0.0104) + 0.962 = 2.09 ng/ml

(Adapted from: K. Kistrup, J. Gerlach, T. Aaes-Jorgensen, *et al*. [1991]. Perphenazine decanoate and cis(z)-flupentixol decanoate in maintenance treatment of schizophrenic outpatients: serum levels at the minimum effective dose. *Psychopharmacology*, 105, 42–48.)

in a naturalistic study of 228 adult inpatients (114 males, 114 females) suffering from an acute exacerbation of schizophrenia spectrum disorders, with oral perphenazine flexibly dosed by clinicians over 5 weeks or more (if necessary) [6]. Patients were classified as responders based on clinical criteria (significant improvement resulting in discharge), and the severity of neurological adverse effects was also rated. The response rate for those with levels < 0.81 ng/ml was 45%, compared to an 86%

response rate with levels in the range of 0.81–2.42 ng/ml (i.e. 2.0–6.0 nmol/l) [6]. Among the 21 nonresponders with suboptimal levels, 81% were clinically improved once trough perphenazine levels were raised above the threshold of 0.81 ng/ml. Although no receiver operating characteristic curves were generated from this older data, the consistency of results establishes that achieving plasma levels ≥ 0.81 ng/ml is a reasonable initial target for nonresponders.

2 Imaging Evidence for a Therapeutic Threshold

Perphenazine has extremely limited imaging data, but the one D_2 receptor occupancy PET study supports the clinical results. The fitted curve from a small group of stable schizophrenia patients on long-term perphenazine decanoate is illustrated in Figure 9.2 and indicates that a plasma level of 0.81 ng/ml corresponds to

Figure 9.2 Fitted D_2 occupancy curve for plasma perphenazine levels [9]

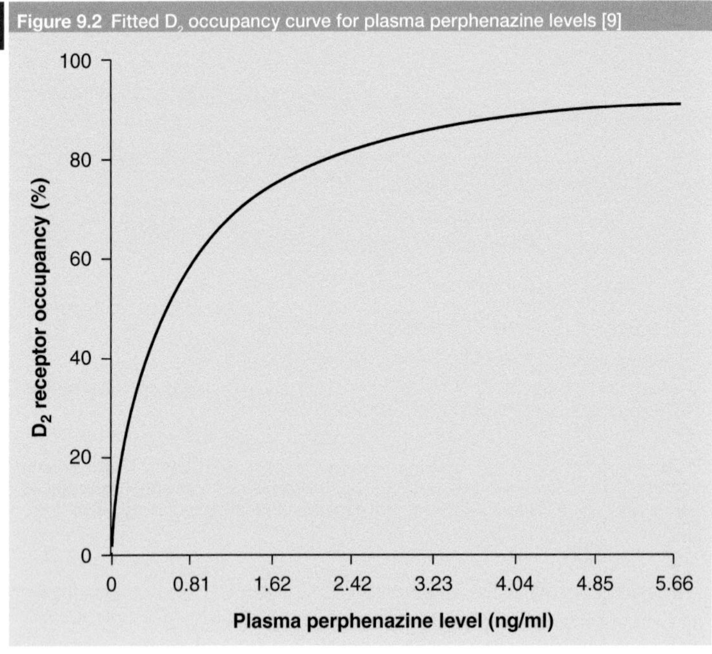

(Adapted from: M. Talvik, A. L. Nordstrom, N. E. Larsen, *et al*. [2004]. A cross-validation study on the relationship between central D2 receptor occupancy and serum perphenazine concentration. *Psychopharmacology*, 175, 148–153.)

approximately 65% receptor occupancy [9]. As discussed in Chapter 2, the imaging literature on D_2 antagonists has found that antipsychotic efficacy generally starts at 65% D_2 occupancy, implying that the clinically derived response threshold correlates well with the imaging data.

The Point of Futility for Perphenazine

1 Clinical Evidence for a Point of Futility

As with most potent D_2 antagonists, a perphenazine trial may be terminated due to neurological adverse effects, or the unpleasant, dysphoric subjective experience associated with excessive D_2 blockade ***for that patient*** (see Chapter 5 for discussion of clinical endpoints) [6]. Defining the point of futility addresses an important question for treating extremely ill schizophrenia patients, and creates an easily understood concept: further titration beyond this point is of limited value with an estimated < 5% chance of response (Chapter 2). From extremely well-studied D_2 antagonists such as haloperidol and fluphenazine, the point of futility typically appears when more than 90% of patients find treatment intolerable, and this correlates with > 90% D_2 receptor occupancy [30–32]. Clinical studies indicate that the risk for developing neurological adverse effects starts at a perphenazine level of 2.42 ng/ml (6 nmol/l), but there is no specific data indicating the point at which 90% or more of patients experience these adverse effects. In a large study of 228 adult inpatients discussed previously, only 50% of the 105 subjects with a mean level of 4.61 ng/ml (range 1.25–40.0 ng/ml) had neurological adverse effects [6]. There are reports of patients tolerating extremely high perphenazine levels without such adverse effects, but this is consistent with other literature indicating that a small proportion of individuals do not develop D_2-related adverse effects regardless of the dose or plasma level [33]. The plasma level at which the neurological adverse effect risk increases is reasonably clear, but there is insufficient clinical data to estimate where the point of futility will occur with higher plasma perphenazine levels.

2 Imaging Evidence for a Point of Futility

Given the inadequacies of the clinical data, one has to look at the plasma level associated with > 90% D_2 receptor occupancy to estimate a point of futility [9]. From the curve in Figure 9.2, this perphenazine plasma level is roughly between 4.84 and 5.24 ng/ml. As expected, a level associated with 90% receptor occupancy is higher than the mean 4.61 ng/ml level that generated a 50% rate of neurological adverse effects as noted above [6]. For patients who tolerate ongoing perphenazine titration, it seems reasonable to consider alternatives (e.g. clozapine) when the plasma level reaches the midpoint of this range (5.0 ng/ml) as further titration is unlikely to be tolerated or effective. The exact proportion of patients who might respond at a plasma level > 5.0 ng/ml without adverse effects is unknown, but conclusions gleaned from the haloperidol and fluphenazine trial data indicate that this probability is extremely small – most likely under 10%.

Summary Points

a The correlation between perphenazine plasma levels and schizophrenia response has not been widely studied in fixed-dose, double-blind, randomized trials. From the largest and most rigorous studies, the suggested therapeutic response threshold is 0.81 ng/ml. The point of futility can be estimated from PET studies, and is 5.0 ng/ml. The 2020 AGNP/ASCP consensus paper strongly recommends plasma level monitoring.

b The oral perphenazine concentration–dose relationship indicates that 10 mg at bedtime is associated with a steady state 12h trough level of 0.40 ng/ml for CYP 2D6 extensive metabolizers, or 0.8 ng/ml for CYP 2D6 poor metabolizers.

c Perphenazine decanoate has a T_{max} of 7 days, but no well-established conversion formula. Perphenazine decanoate loading injections of 108 mg given 1 week apart (days 0, 7) will generate a plasma level on day 21 in the range of 0.645–3.55 ng/ml. For first-episode patients, less severely ill schizophrenia patients, or patients who have a history of sensitivity to D_2 antagonism, administering these dosages 2 weeks apart should be considered to avoid neurological adverse effects at peak plasma levels 7 days after the injection.

d An equation was derived from a long-term study to predict the monthly maintenance level based on the perphenazine decanoate dose [8]: **Steady state level (ng/ml) = (4-week dose in mg) x 0.0104 + 0.962.** This is a rough estimate with a large degree of variation due to genetic factors (e.g. CYP 2D6 polymorphisms) and smoking status. Plasma levels should be checked every 1–2 months during the first 6–8 months as doses are adjusted, and also to monitor for level creep as tissue compartments become saturated.

References

1. **Linnet, K. and Wiborg, O. (1996).** Steady-state serum concentrations of the neuroleptic perphenazine in relation to CYP2D6 genetic polymorphism. *Clin Pharmacol Ther*, 60, 41–47.
2. **Lieberman, J. A., Stroup, T. S., McEvoy, J. P., *et al.* (2005).** Effectiveness of antipsychotic drugs in patients with chronic schizophrenia. *N Engl J Med*, 353, 1209–1223.
3. **Meyer, J. M., Davis, V. G., Goff, D. C., *et al.* (2008).** Change in metabolic syndrome parameters with antipsychotic treatment in the CATIE Schizophrenia Trial: prospective data from phase 1. *Schizophr Res*, 101, 273–286.
4. **Sweet, R. A., Pollock, B. G., Mulsant, B. H., *et al.* (2000).** Pharmacologic profile of perphenazine's metabolites. *J Clin Psychopharmacol*, 20, 181–187.
5. **Jin, Y., Pollock, B. G., Coley, K., *et al.* (2010).** Population pharmacokinetics of perphenazine in schizophrenia patients from CATIE: impact of race and smoking. *J Clin Pharmacol*, 50, 73–80.
6. **Hansen, L. B. and Larsen, N. E. (1985).** Therapeutic advantages of monitoring plasma concentrations of perphenazine in clinical practice. *Psychopharmacology (Berl)*, 87, 16–19.
7. **Mazure, C. M., Nelson, J. C., Jatlow, P. I., *et al.* (1990).** The relationship between blood perphenazine levels, early resolution of psychotic symptoms, and side effects. *J Clin Psychiatry*, 51, 330–334.
8. **Kistrup, K., Gerlach, J., Aaes-Jorgensen, T., *et al.* (1991).** Perphenazine decanoate and cis(z)-flupentixol decanoate in maintenance treatment of schizophrenic outpatients: serum levels at the minimum effective dose. *Psychopharmacology*, 105, 42–48.
9. **Talvik, M., Nordstrom, A. L., Larsen, N. E., *et al.* (2004).** A cross-validation study on the relationship between central D2 receptor occupancy and serum perphenazine concentration. *Psychopharmacology*, 175, 148–153.
10. **Schoretsanitis, G., Kane, J. M., Correll, C. U., *et al.* (2020).** Blood levels to optimize antipsychotic treatment in clinical practice: a joint consensus statement of the American Society of Clinical Psychopharmacology (ASCP) and the Therapeutic Drug Monitoring (TDM) Task Force of the Arbeitsgemeinschaft für Neuropsychopharmakologie und Pharmakopsychiatrie (AGNP). *J Clin Psychiatry*, 81, https://doi.org/10.4088/JCP.4019cs13169.
11. **Mylan Pharmaceuticals Inc. (2018).** Perphenazine package insert. Morgantown, WV.
12. **Patteet, L., Morrens, M., Maudens, K. E., *et al.* (2012).** Therapeutic drug monitoring of common antipsychotics. *Ther Drug Monit*, 34, 629–651.
13. **Olesen, O. V. and Linnet, K. (2000).** Identification of the human cytochrome P450 isoforms mediating in vitro N-dealkylation of perphenazine. *Br J Clin Pharmacol*, 50, 563–571.
14. **Dahl-Puustinen, M. L., Liden, A., Alm, C., *et al.* (1989).** Disposition of perphenazine is related to polymorphic debrisoquin hydroxylation in human beings. *Clin Pharmacol Ther*, 46, 78–81.
15. **Ozdemir, V., Naranjo, C. A., Herrmann, N., *et al.* (1997).** Paroxetine potentiates the central nervous system side effects of perphenazine: contribution of cytochrome P4502D6 inhibition in vivo. *Clin Pharmacol Ther*, 62, 334–347.
16. **Mulsant, B. H., Foglia, J. P., Sweet, R. A., *et al.* (1997).** The effects of perphenazine on the concentration of nortriptyline and its hydroxymetabolites in older patients. *J Clin Psychopharmacol*, 17, 318–321.
17. **Halayqa, M. and Domanska, U. (2014).** PLGA biodegradable nanoparticles containing perphenazine or chlorpromazine hydrochloride: effect of formulation and release. *Int J Mol Sci*, 15, 23909–23923.
18. **Taylor, D. (2009).** Psychopharmacology and adverse effects of antipsychotic long-acting injections: a review. *Br J Psychiatry Suppl*, 52, S13–19.

19. **Knudsen, P., Hansen, L. B., Auken, G., *et al.* (1985).** Perphenazine decanoate vs. perphenazine enanthate: efficacy and side effects in a 6 week double-blind, comparative study of 50 drug monitored psychotic patients. *Acta Psychiatr Scand Suppl*, 322, 15–28.
20. **Tuninger, E. and Levander, S. (1997).** Long-term outcome of depot neuroleptic maintenance treatment among chronic psychotic patients. *Acta Psychiatr Scand*, 96, 347–353.
21. **Meyer, J. M. (2017).** Converting oral to long acting injectable antipsychotics: a guide for the perplexed. *CNS Spectr*, 22, 14–28.
22. **Orion Pharma AB (2017).** Trilafon Dekanoat. Danderyd, Sweden.
23. **Larsen, N. E. and Hansen, L. B. (1989).** Prediction of the optimal perphenazine decanoate dose based on blood samples drawn within the first three weeks. *Ther Drug Monit*, 11, 642–646.
24. **Dencker, S. J., Giös, I., Mårtensson, E., *et al.* (1994).** A long-term cross-over pharmacokinetic study comparing perphenazine decanoate and haloperidol decanoate in schizophrenic patients. *Psychopharmacology (Berl)*, 114, 24–30.
25. **Marder, S. R., Midha, K. K., Van Putten, T., *et al.* (1991).** Plasma levels of fluphenazine in patients receiving fluphenazine decanoate: relationship to clinical response. *Br J Psychiatry*, 158, 658–665.
26. **Haddad, P., Lambert, T., and Lauriello, J., eds. (2016).** *Antipsychotic Long-Acting Injections*, 2nd edn. New York: Oxford University Press.
27. **Eggert Hansen, C., Rosted Christensen, T., Elley, J., *et al.* (1976).** Clinical pharmacokinetic studies of perphenazine. *Br J Clin Pharmacol*, 3, 915–923.
28. **Hansen, L. B. and Larsen, N. E. (1977).** Plasma concentrations of perphenazine and its sulphoxide metabolite during continuous oral treatment. *Psychopharmacology*, 53, 127–130.
29. **Hansen, L. B., Larsen, N. E., and Gulmann, N. (1982).** Dose–response relationships of perphenazine in the treatment of acute psychoses. *Psychopharmacology (Berl)*, 78, 112–115.
30. **Van Putten, T., Marder, S. R., Mintz, J., *et al.* (1992).** Haloperidol plasma levels and clinical response: a therapeutic window relationship. *Am J Psychiatry*, 149, 500–505.
31. **Midha, K. K., Hubbard, J. W., Marder, S. R., *et al.* (1994).** Impact of clinical pharmacokinetics on neuroleptic therapy in patients with schizophrenia. *J Psychiatry Neurosci*, 19, 254–264.
32. **Regenthal, R., Kunstler, U., Junhold, U., *et al.* (1997).** Haloperidol serum concentrations and D2 dopamine receptor occupancy during low-dose treatment with haloperidol decanoate. *Int Clin Psychopharmacol*, 12, 255–261.
33. **Simpson, G. M. and Kunz-Bartholini, E. (1968).** Relationship of individual tolerance, behavior and phenothiazine produced extrapyramidal system disturbance. *Dis Nerv System*, 29, 269–274.

10 Zuclopenthixol and Zuclopenthixol Decanoate; Flupenthixol and Flupenthixol Decanoate

QUICK CHECK

PRINCIPLES

- Where available, zuclopenthixol and flupenthixol provide an inexpensive method of delivering D_2 antagonism, with a modest amount of plasma level data to define a therapeutic threshold.
- The metabolism of zuclopenthixol is much better characterized than for flupenthixol. The early plasma level studies with oral flupenthixol are difficult to interpret due to the inclusion of the inactive *trans* isomer in reported levels. For these reasons, zuclopenthixol should be used in lieu of flupenthixol.
- A long-acting injectable (LAI) version of each antipsychotic (zuclopenthixol decanoate, flupenthixol decanoate) is available in certain countries (Australia, New Zealand, Canada, UK).

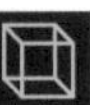

InfoBox Oral Zuclopenthixol and Flupenthixol Plasma Level Essentials

	Oral dose correlation (bedtime dosing, 12h trough)	Level of evidence	Therapeutic threshold	Level of evidence	Point of futility	Level of evidence
Zuclopenthixol	10 mg = 6.5 ng/ml [1] **Multiply oral dose by 0.65** (see Table 10.1 for effects of CYP inhibitors/ inducers on this relationship)	High	2.0 ng/ml [2, 3, 4]	Low	9.0 ng/ml [5]	Low
Flupenthixol	*Cis* only: 10 mg = 2.0 ng/ml [6] **Multiply oral dose by 0.20** (see Table 10.1 for effects of CYP inhibitors/ inducers on this relationship)	High	0.43 ng/ml [7, 8]	Low	3.0 ng/ml [7, 8]	Low

Basic Pharmacokinetic Information for Oral and Long-Acting Injectable Zuclopenthixol and Flupenthixol

As with many first-generation antipsychotics (FGAs), zuclopenthixol and flupenthixol have no unique therapeutic benefit compared to other D_2 antagonists, but have long-acting injectable (LAI) preparations available in certain parts of the world and a modest database of plasma level information. In addition to an LAI formulation, zuclopenthixol also has an injectable formulation (zuclopenthixol acetate) that provides therapeutic levels over several days, with a time to peak plasma levels (T_{max}) of 24–48 hours [1]. Zuclopenthixol and flupenthixol derive from clopenthixol, an antipsychotic developed by Lundbeck and approved in Europe and the UK in 1961 [9]. Subsequent research found that only the *cis* isomer was active, leading to the introduction of this isomer in purified form as zuclopenthixol in 1962. Flupenthixol is a halogenated modification of clopenthixol approved in 1965, with all of the antipsychotic activity also residing in the *cis* isomer [6]. Interestingly, the oral form of flupenthixol is a racemic mixture of the two isomers, but the depot, flupenthixol decanoate, is made only with the *cis* isomer [9]. This creates some confusion as the older literature was based on studies using the oral tablet, and those assays reflected the sum of both *cis* and *trans* isomers. In some papers the investigators attempted to calculate the *cis*-flupenthixol level by dividing the summed total level by 2, under the incorrect assumption that the two isomers are present in equal concentrations [10] (Figure 10.1). It was later discovered that at steady state the *trans* isomer is present at levels approximately two-fold higher than *cis* isomer levels, so dose–plasma level correlations and D_2 receptor occupancy data from studies that did not measure *cis*-flupenthixol levels specifically generated values that are 3 times higher than data derived from *cis*-flupenthixol exposure alone [6, 8]. Recent papers report level ranges from the *cis* isomer only [11], and the

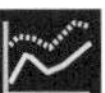

Figure 10.1 Distribution of steady state plasma *cis*-flupenthixol levels by oral dose, calculated as the summed total concentration of *cis* and *trans* isomers divided by 2 [10]

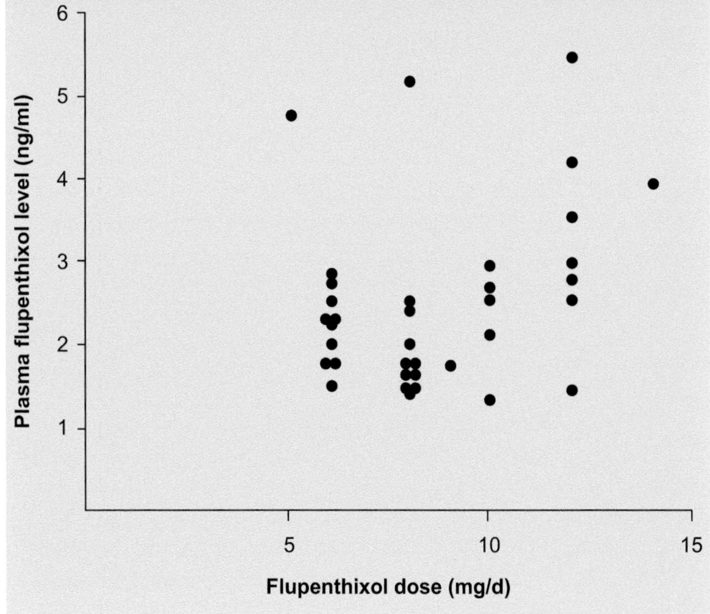

(Adapted from: A. E. Balant-Gorgia, R. Eisele, J. M. Aeschlimann, *et al.* [1985]. Plasma flupenthixol concentrations and clinical response in acute schizophrenia. *Ther Drug Monit*, 7, 411–414.)

2020 consensus paper authored jointly by the Therapeutic Drug Monitoring (TDM) task force of the German Arbeitsgemeinschaft für Neuropsychopharmakologie und Pharmakopsychiatrie (AGNP) and the American Society for Clinical Psychopharmacology (ASCP) presents flupenthixol level ranges based on the *cis* isomer [12]. There is no information on flupenthixol's metabolic pathways or drug–drug interactions, with the exception of information suggesting carbamazepine may decrease levels by 50% or more [13].

Despite being a slightly older antipsychotic, zuclopenthixol's metabolic pathways have been better characterized and were published in a 2010 paper [9]. As zuclopenthixol only consists of the active isomer of clopenthixol, there is no confusion in the literature regarding interpretation of plasma level data. This combination of a well-characterized potential for drug interactions, less confusing plasma level data, and the availability of the LAI and shorter-duration injectable zuclopenthixol acetate make zuclopenthixol preferable to flupenthixol where both products are available. There is surprisingly little Positron Emission Tomography (PET) imaging information on dopamine D_2 receptor occupancy for both antipsychotics, and the one study for flupenthixol used the summed total of *cis* and *trans* isomers, making interpretation more complicated [7]. The only PET study for zuclopenthixol does provide some insight into dosing, and informs estimates of the response threshold and point of futility [5]. Flupenthixol was assigned a Level 2 recommendation (recommended) for use of plasma level monitoring in the 2020 consensus paper authored jointly by the Therapeutic Drug Monitoring (TDM) task force of the German Arbeitsgemeinschaft für Neuropsychopharmakologie und Pharmakopsychiatrie (AGNP) and the American Society for Clinical Psychopharmacology (ASCP) [12]. The consensus paper contains no information on zuclopenthixol.

Essential Information for Oral and Long-Acting Injectable Zuclopenthixol and Flupenthixol

1 Essential Oral Zuclopenthixol Information

Despite being launched 50 years ago, there is a substantial body of data on kinetics, bioavailability and oral dose–plasma level correlations (Table 10.1). As a substrate for the polymorphic cytochrome P450 (CYP) 2D6 enzyme, the effects of genetic polymorphisms and of CYP 2D6 inhibitors have been studied [1, 9]. Zuclopenthixol levels are lowered by the inducer carbamazepine in a dose-dependent manner [9]. As with most antipsychotics, the half-life is sufficiently long to support once daily dosing, and it should always be administered at bedtime for reasons of tolerability (see Chapter 5) and to insure that levels obtained in the morning are approximately 12h from the last dose.

Table 10.1 Oral zuclopenthixol and flupenthixol kinetic facts

	Basic facts	Inhibition effects	Induction effects
Zuclopenthixol	Not approved in the US $T_{1/2}$ 29 (12–28) hours [1] Absolute oral bioavailability: 60%–80% [14] T_{max} 4 (2–12) hours [1] Metabolism: Primarily 2D6, and 3A4 [9] **Formulations:** Tablets	Exposure to the strong CYP 2D6 inhibitors fluoxetine or paroxetine increased plasma levels by 93% and 78%, respectively [9] This effect is lessened for patients on zuclopenthixol decanoate [9], but CYP 2D6 poor metabolizers may have 60% higher dose-adjusted plasma levels than extensive metabolizers [15]	Carbamazepine decreased levels by 67%, and the effect was dose-dependent [9]
Flupenthixol	Not approved in the US $T_{1/2}$ 35 (26–36) hours [16, 17] Absolute oral bioavailability: 40%–55% [17] T_{max} 4 (3–6) hours [16, 17] Metabolism: Unknown **Formulations:** Tablets*	The effects of CYP inhibitors are not known	One pharmacovigilance monitoring study noted that median plasma flupenthixol levels in carbamazepine-exposed individuals were more than 50% lower than levels in unexposed patients [13]

* The tablet form of flupenthixol is a racemic mixture of the *cis* and *trans* isomers. The depot only contains the active *cis* isomer. In patients taking the oral formulation, the *trans* isomer is present at higher serum levels in 93% of samples assayed, with 59% having a *trans/cis* ratio between 1.5 and 2.5 (range 0.77–6.0) [6]. As there is almost no information on flupenthixol drug interactions or metabolism, and laboratories may not be clear if reported flupenthixol levels are the summed total of *cis* and *trans* isomers or just the *cis* isomer, use of oral flupenthixol should be eschewed in lieu of zuclopenthixol when possible.

2 Essential Oral Flupenthixol Information

The depot formulation is an ester of *cis*-flupenthixol, but oral flupenthixol is a racemic mixture of the active *cis* and inactive *trans* isomers. The basic kinetic properties of oral flupenthixol are well known [16, 17], but there is no data on drug metabolism, and no drug–drug interaction studies, with the exception of one pharmacovigilance study noting lower mean plasma levels when used concurrently with carbamazepine [13]. The AGNP/ASCP consensus paper lists CYP 2D6 as a metabolic pathway, but it is unclear how this conclusion was reached. Many antipsychotics interact with CYP 2D6 and exert inhibitory effects on that enzyme but are metabolized by other CYP isoenzymes. Perazine is one classic example: it increases risperidone levels by inhibition of CYP 2D6 and CYP 3A4, but is primarily metabolized via CYP 1A2, CYP 2C19 and CYP 3A4 [18, 19]. Flupenthixol weakly binds to CYP 2D6, but the role played by CYP 2D6 or any enzyme in its metabolism has not been characterized [20]. As with most antipsychotics, the half-life is sufficiently long to support once daily dosing, and it should always be administered at bedtime for reasons of tolerability (see Chapter 5) and to insure that the morning trough is approximately 12h from the last dose. As there is almost no information on flupenthixol drug interactions or metabolism, and laboratories may not be clear if reported flupenthixol levels are the summed total of *cis* and *trans* isomers or just the *cis* isomer, use of oral flupenthixol should be eschewed in lieu of oral zuclopenthixol when possible.

3 Essential Long-Acting Injectable Zuclopenthixol Information

Zuclopenthixol decanoate is the long-acting injectable (LAI) formulation and should not be confused with zuclopenthixol acetate, another oil-based preparation with very short duration of action (Table 10.2). Due to the short T_{max} for zuclopenthixol decanoate, it could potentially be loaded, but there are no well-designed studies to estimate the optimal method, nor easy-to-follow oral dose conversion formulas as exist for haloperidol. The manufacturer labeling notes that the mean steady state preinjection level on zuclopenthixol decanoate 200 mg every 2 weeks is 10 ng/ml, and the mean level on 20 mg/d of oral is 13 ng/ml, suggesting that 200 mg of depot every 2 weeks is roughly equivalent to 15 mg/d of oral [1]. PET imaging studies have established that an initial target range for dopamine antagonists is 65%–80% D_2 receptor occupancy [21], but the one PET study found that a plasma zuclopenthixol level of 10 ng/ml is associated with an estimated 91% D_2 receptor occupancy, and thus may generate unwanted adverse effects [5]. As will be discussed below, a level of 2.5 ng/ml generates 71% occupancy, suggesting that initial zuclopenthixol decanoate doses of 50 mg every 2 weeks may be more appropriate [5].

4 Essential Long-Acting Flupenthixol Information

Flupenthixol decanoate is an ester of the active *cis* isomer, and is available in two concentrations (20 mg/ml, 100 mg/ml) in an oil-based vehicle (Table 10.2). The manufacturer labeling recommends a loading strategy with an initial dose of 20 mg (or 5 mg in frail, cachectic, or elderly patients), and a second dose of 20–40 mg

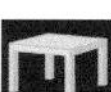

Table 10.2 Zuclopenthixol decanoate and flupenthixol decanoate essentials* [24–26, 1]

	Vehicle	Concentration	Dosage	T_{max} (days)	$T_{1/2}$ (days) multiple dosing	Able to be loaded	Maintenance dose: oral equivalence
Zuclopenthixol decanoate	Coconut oil (Viscoleo)	200 mg/ml	25–100 mg/2–4 weeks **Max:** 400 mg/2 weeks	3–7	19	Yes	See Section B, 3: "Essential Long-Acting Injectable Zuclopenthixol Information"
Flupenthixol decanoate**	Coconut oil (Viscoleo)	20 mg/ml 100 mg/ml	20–40 mg/2–4 weeks **Max:** 100 mg/2 weeks	4–7	17	Yes	See Section B, 4: "Essential Long-Acting Injectable Flupenthixol Information"

Note: There is an oil-based injectable zuclopenthixol acetate (trade name Clopixol-Acuphase®) for short-term use with very different kinetic parameters than the depot formulation. T_{max} is 24–48 hours followed by a gradual decline, with levels approximately one-third the maximum by 3 days post-injection. The average maximum serum zuclopenthixol level (C_{max}) for 100 mg zuclopenthixol acetate is 41 ng/ml, which is estimated to be associated with an extremely high level of D_2 receptor occupancy (98%) [5, 1].

* Available in Australia, New Zealand, Canada, UK

** The tablet form of flupenthixol is a racemic mixture of the *cis* and *trans* isomers, but only the *cis* isomer is active. Flupenthixol decanoate only contains the active *cis* isomer. As oral zuclopenthixol and the depot form contain only the *cis* isomer, and there is better information on drug–drug interactions, use of flupenthixol should be eschewed in lieu of zuclopenthixol when possible

(For further reading about use of LAI antipsychotics, please see the comprehensive edited book ***Antipsychotic Long-Acting Injections***, now in its 2nd edition [27])

administered 4–10 days later based on response and adverse effects [22]. Given the kinetic parameters, a week's interval is reasonable before administering the second dose, but there is no plasma level data on this strategy. No dose conversion is provided for transition between oral and depot flupenthixol in the package insert, nor plasma levels for any depot dosage [22]. Fortunately, a 2019 review provided detailed information on the correlation between depot doses and steady state trough *cis*-flupenthixol levels from five studies published between 1980 and 1993 (total n = 96) [23]. The steady state level ranged from 0.10–0.63 for each milligram of flupenthixol decanoate administered **per week**, with a mean of 0.29 [23]. A patient receiving 40 mg/2 weeks is receiving the equivalent of 20 mg/week, and thus would have an estimated preinjection trough level of 20 x 0.29 = 0.58 ng/ml. For practical purposes, the difficulty in converting from oral flupenthixol rests on whether the laboratory is reporting *cis*-flupenthixol levels, or the summed total of *cis*- and *trans*-flupenthixol. Assuming one has a steady state *cis*-flupenthixol level on oral therapy, an estimate of the depot dose can be calculated. However, given the limited information on drug–drug interactions, and the issues with laboratory assay methods for oral flupenthixol levels, use of flupenthixol should be eschewed in lieu of zuclopenthixol when possible.

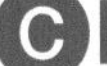

C The Therapeutic Threshold for Zuclopenthixol and Flupenthixol

1 Clinical Evidence for a Therapeutic Threshold for Zuclopenthixol

Clinical evidence, especially from fixed-dose, prospective, randomized trials, is the most important tool we have for estimation of plasma level response thresholds (see Chapter 2), but this type of data is almost nonexistent for zuclopenthixol. From a flexibly dosed open-label study of 16 adult patients with an acute exacerbation of "paranoid psychosis," plasma levels as low as 3 ng/ml appeared effective, with levels < 5 ng/ml associated with lower rates of neurological adverse effects [28]. Cross-sectional data from a group of 20 adult schizophrenia patients found that levels as low as 7 ng/ml could be effective in some patients [2]. There is one fixed-dose study of zuclopenthixol decanoate 200 mg/3 weeks conducted in 26 adult schizophrenia patients followed for 6 months [4]. Response was defined as ≥ 50% reduction in the Brief Psychiatric Rating Scale (BPRS). At study endpoint, 58% were classified as responders, with mean preinjection trough levels of 5.38 ± 2.05 ng/ml, while nonresponders had a significantly lower mean trough level of 3.78 ± 0.84 ng/ml ($p < 0.01$) [4]. The lowest plasma level in a responder was 3.17 ng/ml, while 3 nonresponders had levels under 3.18 ng/ml (2.81 –3.05 ng/ml) [4]. A gradual dose reduction study was performed in 23 adult outpatients with schizophrenia who were stabilized on zuclopenthixol decanoate 200 mg every 2 weeks, and the dose slowly reduced by 25% every 12 weeks until a predetermined level of exacerbation was reached [29]. With this study design, the mean minimum effective plasma level was 8.83 ng/ml, with a range of 2.81–28.0 ng/ml, substantially higher than estimates for the treatment of acute psychosis [29]. It should be noted that the intent to treat sample was larger, but 9 patients could not tolerate the dosing schedule, thus limiting the discovery of lower response thresholds. Based on available data, one can postulate that levels < 3.0 ng/ml are less likely to be effective, but the supporting evidence is not strong. Nonetheless, this information should inform initial dosing. The manufacturer labeling notes that the mean steady state serum level on zuclopenthixol 20 mg/d is 13 ng/ml [1]. The smallest tablet is 10 mg, so 5 mg (one half-tablet) might not be an unreasonable starting dose, especially in more antipsychotic-naïve patients, and would generate an estimated 12h trough level of 3.25 ng/ml.

2 Imaging Evidence for a Therapeutic Threshold for Zuclopenthixol

There is only PET study for zuclopenthixol which performed multiple scans in normal volunteers over a period of 31 hours after an IM injection of 12.5 mg zuclopenthixol acetate [5]. The fitted curve (Figure 10.2) allows an estimated threshold level close

Figure 10.2 Fitted D_2 occupancy curve for serum zuclopenthixol levels [5]

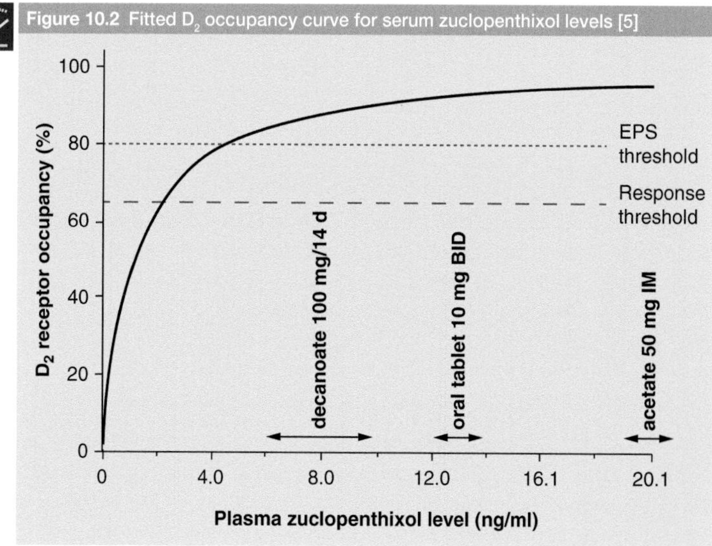

(Adapted from: S. Nyberg, L. Farde, A. Bartfai, *et al.* [1995]. Central D2 receptor occupancy and effects of zuclopenthixol acetate in humans. *Int Clin Psychopharmacol*, 10, 221–227.)

to 2.0 ng/ml to achieve 65% D_2 receptor occupancy (1.87 ng/ml) [5]. In the absence of well-designed fixed-dose trials, this calculated level should be given significant consideration. Of great concern, the manufacturer labeling notes that a 100 mg IM dose of zuclopenthixol acetate generates a mean C_{max} plasma level of 41 ng/ml [1]. This level is estimated to generate 98% D_2 occupancy, and may be intolerable to a substantial group of patients [1]. The mean steady state level of 10 ng/ml for patients on zuclopenthixol decanoate 200 mg every 2 weeks is associated with 91% D_2 occupancy, also exceeding the tolerability threshold for some individuals.

3 Clinical Evidence for a Therapeutic Threshold for Flupenthixol

There are no fixed-dose flupenthixol trials, but one study stratified responders and nonresponders in an attempt to find a therapeutic threshold [10]. This trial was a prospective open-label study of 23 adult patients with schizophrenia spectrum disorders during which oral flupenthixol was flexibly dosed based on clinical criteria, with response defined as ≥ 50% decrease in symptoms using the BPRS. Levels of both *cis* and *trans* isomers were measured together, and plasma *cis*-flupenthixol levels were defined as the summed total divided by 2. Using this estimate, the response rate for *cis*-flupenthixol levels under 2.0 ng/ml was 31%, but increased to 80% for levels > 2.0 ng/ml [10]. Subsequently, these same investigators (and others) found that the ratio of *trans* to *cis* isomers was not 1:1, but approximately 2:1 [6, 11]. Since only one-third of the summed plasma level is *cis*-flupenthixol, the new threshold estimate from this study is 1.33 ng/ml, which more closely aligns with imaging data. In a minimum effective dose study, 24 adult schizophrenia patients stabilized on flupenthixol decanoate underwent gradual dose reduction by 25% every 12 weeks until clinical exacerbation occurred by defined criteria [30]. The mean level at which exacerbation occurred was 3.39 ng/ml, substantially higher than estimates for treatment of acute psychosis. As with the zuclopenthixol reduction study, there may be aspects of study design that provide values higher than those achieved during prospective studies of acute psychosis [29].

4 Imaging Evidence for a Therapeutic Threshold for Flupenthixol

The only data correlating flupenthixol plasma levels and D_2 occupancy comes from a 2007 PET study of 13 subjects on mean oral flupenthixol doses of 5.7 ± 1.4 mg/d (Figure 10.3) [7]. Although not explicitly stated in the paper, the plasma levels reported are from the summed totals of the *cis* and the inactive *trans* isomers, so the correlations must be adjusted based on the fact that the *trans* to *cis* ratio at steady state is roughly 2:1 [6, 11]. Since one-third of the summed plasma level is

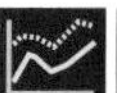

Figure 10.3 Fitted D_2 occupancy curve for the summed total of serum *cis*- and *trans*-flupenthixol levels [7]

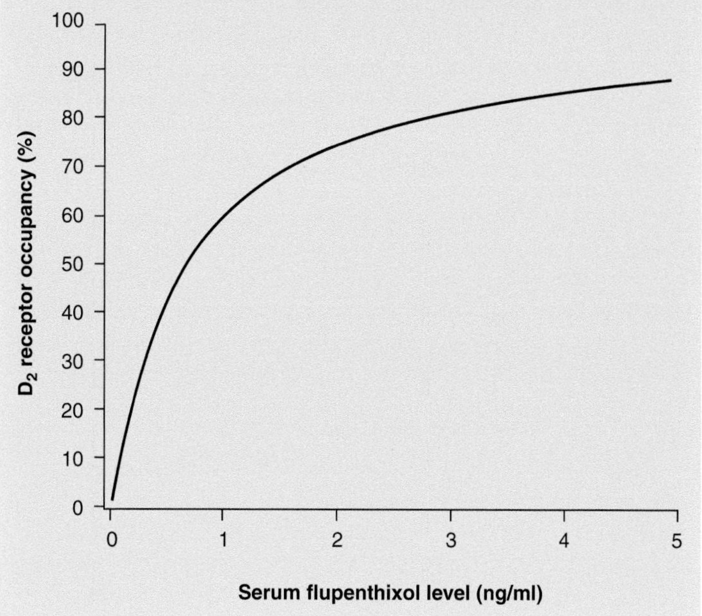

(Adapted from: M. Reimold, C. Solbach, S. Noda, *et al*. [2007]. Occupancy of dopamine D (1), D (2) and serotonin (2A) receptors in schizophrenic patients treated with flupenthixol in comparison with risperidone and haloperidol. *Psychopharmacology*, 190, 241–249.)

cis-flupenthixol, the reported EC_{50} value (0.68 ng/ml) becomes 0.227 ng/ml (0.68 ÷ 3), and the plasma level associated with 65% D_2 occupancy can be calculated as 0.43 ng/ml. The clinically calculated threshold of 1.33 ng/ml for *cis*-flupenthixol is now estimated to generate 85% D_2 occupancy. Given this small pool of data, a recent review published in 2012 chose a plasma level threshold of 0.5 ng/ml for *cis*-flupenthixol, a value that reasonably fits the newer imaging data [8]. Future PET studies using depot flupenthixol, which only contains the *cis* isomer, will be very helpful in further defining the exact relationship between the active isomer and D_2 antagonism.

The Point of Futility for Zuclopenthixol and Flupenthixol

1 Clinical Evidence for a Point of Futility for Zuclopenthixol

As with most potent D_2 antagonists, a trial of zuclopenthixol may be terminated due to neurological adverse effects, or the unpleasant, dysphoric subjective experience associated with excessive D_2 blockade ***for that patient*** (see Chapter 5 for discussion of clinical endpoints) [31]. Defining the point of futility addresses an important question for treating extremely ill schizophrenia patients, and creates an easily understood concept: further titration beyond this point is of limited value with an estimated < 5% chance of response (Chapter 2). From extremely well-studied D_2 antagonists such as haloperidol and fluphenazine, the point of futility typically appears when more than 90% of patients find treatment intolerable, and this correlates with > 90% D_2 receptor occupancy [32–34]. Sadly, published clinical studies do not provide rates of neurological adverse effects by plasma level, although one prospective study with 23 adult schizophrenia patients noted that mean plasma levels did not significantly differ in patients who did or did not require antiparkinsonian medication [10].

2 Imaging Evidence for a Point of Futility for Zuclopenthixol

Given the inadequacies of the clinical data, one has to look at the plasma level associated with > 90% D_2 receptor occupancy to estimate a point of futility. As noted above, there is only one PET study for zuclopenthixol based on multiple scans obtained in normal volunteers over a period of 31 hours after an IM injection of 12.5 mg zuclopenthixol acetate [5]. The fitted curve (Figure 10.2) allows an estimate of a threshold level to achieve 90% D_2 receptor occupancy, and this occurs at approximately 9 ng/ml. As this is one study, the level of evidence is low. It should be noted again that the mean trough level on 20 mg/d of oral zuclopenthixol is 13 ng/ml, which corresponds to 93% D_2 antagonism, suggesting this dose might be at the upper limit of tolerability in most patients [1].

3 Clinical Evidence for a Point of Futility for Flupenthixol

There is some information about the association of treatment-limiting adverse effects and plasma levels based on data from flupenthixol decanoate studies (Figure 10.4) [23]. A 2019 review noted that the relationship between doses and rates of neurological adverse effects appeared linear within the range of flupenthixol decanoate 10–40 mg every 2 weeks, but the rate on any dose did not exceed 70%. Moreover, this relationship with first-generation antipsychotics is not linear but sigmoidal, with the curve flattening appreciably at plasma levels where 70% of

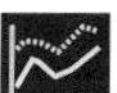

Figure 10.4 Rates of neurological adverse effects by flupenthixol decanoate dose every 2 weeks [23]

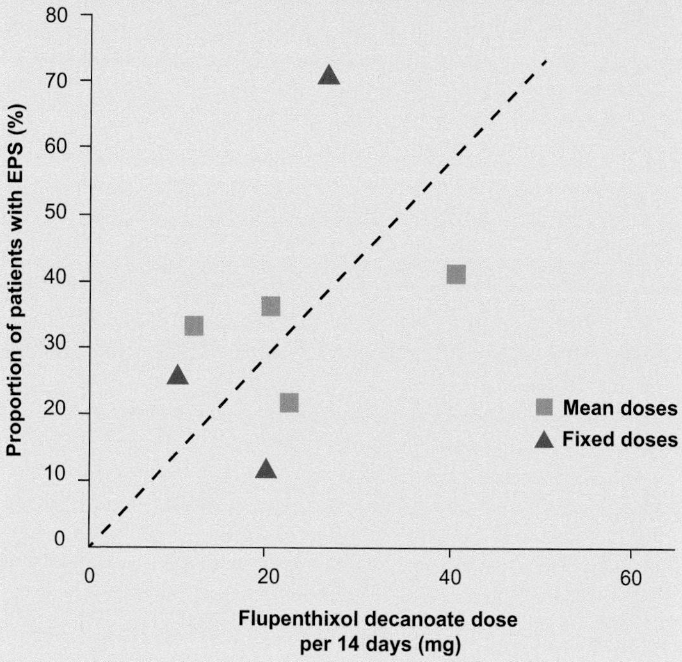

Proportion of patients with EPS (%)

0 10 20 30 40 50 60 70 80

Mean doses

Fixed doses

0 20 40 60

Flupenthixol decanoate dose per 14 days (mg)

(Adapted from: L. Bailey and D. Taylor [2019]. Estimating the optimal dose of flupenthixol decanoate in the maintenance treatment of schizophrenia – a systematic review of the literature. *Psychopharmacology (Berl)*, 236, 3081–3092.)

patients experience intolerable adverse effects [33]. Unfortunately, there is insufficient information to estimate the point at which 90% or more might experience intolerable adverse effects, to arrive at a point of futility.

4 Imaging Evidence for a Point of Futility for Flupenthixol

Clinical data indicate that the risk for neurological adverse effects increases with higher *cis*-flupenthixol plasma levels [23], but there are no PET studies to provide correlates [10]. Nonetheless, from the one PET study of oral flupenthixol previously mentioned, we can calculate a plasma level that achieves 90% D_2 occupancy as a proxy for the point of futility, and this level is 2.3 ng/ml [7]. This conclusion is derived from one study, and *cis*-flupenthixol levels are not directly reported in that trial (just the summed total of *cis* and *trans* levels), so one could reasonably consider a level up to 3.0 ng/ml, which corresponds to 93% D_2 occupancy, in those who are tolerating the medication and have ongoing positive psychotic symptoms. The upper limit of the therapeutic range in the AGNP/ASCP consensus paper is 5.0 ng/ml, and their recommended laboratory alert level is 15.0 ng/ml, which would correspond to estimated D_2 occupancies of 96% and 99%, respectively [12]. Based on the calculations presented here, those limits seem extremely high.

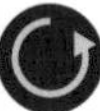

Summary Points

a Less is known about flupenthixol's metabolism and potential for drug–drug interactions, so zuclopenthixol should be used where both options are available. Zuclopenthixol is metabolized via CYP 2D6 and CYP 3A4.

b Zuclopenthixol is available in an oral and an LAI formulation (zuclopenthixol decanoate). There is an oil-based injectable zuclopenthixol acetate (trade name Clopixol-Acuphase®) for short-term use, with very different kinetic parameters from the depot formulation. Zuclopenthixol acetate should not be used in lieu of the decanoate. (Doses of zuclopenthixol acetate [Clopixol-Acuphase®] in younger or antipsychotic-naïve patients should be in the range of 12.5 mg or 25 mg, as the peak plasma level from a single 100 mg dose is 41 ng/ml, which is estimated to generate an extremely high level of D_2 receptor occupancy [98%].)

c The oral dose–plasma level correlation for oral zuclopenthixol is 0.65 (i.e. 10 mg yields a 12h trough of 6.5 ng/ml). The mean preinjection trough steady state level on zuclopenthixol decanoate 200 mg every 2 weeks is 10 ng/ml.

d There is limited data to help define the therapeutic threshold and point of futility for zuclopenthixol and flupenthixol. From the available clinical and imaging data, the therapeutic threshold for zuclopenthixol is estimated to occur at 2.0 ng/ml, and the point of futility at 9.0 ng/ml, but the degree of confidence in these values is low. Nonetheless, there is sufficient information to indicate that starting doses in younger or antipsychotic-naïve patients might be as low as 5 mg orally at bedtime, or a zuclopenthixol decanoate dose of 50 mg every 2 weeks.

References

1. **Lundbeck Canada Inc. (2016).** Clopixol, Clopixol-Acuphase, Clopixol Depot product monograph. St. Laurent, Canada.
2. **Jørgensen, A., Aaes-Jørgensen, T., Gravem, A., *et al.* (1985).** Zuclopenthixol decanoate in schizophrenia: serum levels and clinical state. *Psychopharmacology (Berl)*, 87, 364–367.
3. **Amdisen, A., Aaes-Jørgensen, T., Thomsen, N. J., *et al.* (1986).** Serum concentrations and clinical effect of zuclopenthixol in acutely disturbed, psychotic patients treated with zuclopenthixol acetate in Viscoleo. *Psychopharmacology (Berl)*, 90, 412–416.
4. **Szukalski, B., Lipska, B., Welbel, L., *et al.* (1986).** Serum levels and clinical response in long-term pharmacotherapy with zuclopenthixol decanoate. *Psychopharmacology (Berl)*, 89, 428–431.
5. **Nyberg, S., Farde, L., Bartfai, A., *et al.* (1995).** Central D2 receptor occupancy and effects of zuclopenthixol acetate in humans. *Int Clin Psychopharmacol*, 10, 221–227.
6. **Balant-Gorgia, A. E., Balant, L. P., Gex-Fabry, M., *et al.* (1987).** Stereoselective disposition of flupenthixol: influence on steady-state plasma concentrations in schizophrenic patients. *Eur J Drug Metab Pharmacokinet*, 12, 123–128.
7. **Reimold, M., Solbach, C., Noda, S., *et al.* (2007).** Occupancy of dopamine D (1), D (2) and serotonin (2A) receptors in schizophrenic patients treated with flupenthixol in comparison with risperidone and haloperidol. *Psychopharmacology*, 190, 241–249.
8. **Baumann, P., Kirchherr, H., Berney, P., *et al.* (2012).** Flupenthixol: relevance of stereoselective therapeutic drug monitoring. *Psychopharmacology (Berl)*, 221, 719–720.
9. **Davies, S. J., Westin, A. A., Castberg, I., *et al.* (2010).** Characterisation of zuclopenthixol metabolism by in vitro and therapeutic drug monitoring studies. *Acta Psychiatr Scand*, 122, 444–453.
10. **Balant-Gorgia, A. E., Eisele, R., Aeschlimann, J. M., *et al.* (1985).** Plasma flupenthixol concentrations and clinical response in acute schizophrenia. *Ther Drug Monit*, 7, 411–414.
11. **Walter, S., Bauer, S., Roots, I., *et al.* (1998).** Quantification of the antipsychotics flupenthixol and haloperidol in human serum by high-performance liquid chromatography with ultraviolet detection. *J Chromatogr B Biomed Sci Appl*, 720, 231–237.
12. **Schoretsanitis, G., Kane, J. M., Correll, C. U., *et al.* (2020).** Blood levels to optimize antipsychotic treatment in clinical practice: a joint consensus statement of the American Society of Clinical Psychopharmacology (ASCP) and the Therapeutic Drug Monitoring (TDM) Task Force of the Arbeitsgemeinschaft für Neuropsychopharmakologie und Pharmakopsychiatrie (AGNP). *J Clin Psychiatry*, 81, http://doi.org/10.4088/JCP.4019cs13169.
13. **Gex-Fabry, M., Balant-Gorgia, A. E., and Balant, L. P. (1997).** Therapeutic drug monitoring databases for postmarketing surveillance of drug–drug interactions: evaluation of a paired approach for psychotropic medication. *Ther Drug Monit*, 19, 1–10.
14. **Patteet, L., Morrens, M., Maudens, K. E., *et al.* (2012).** Therapeutic drug monitoring of common antipsychotics. *Ther Drug Monit*, 34, 629–651.
15. **Linnet, K. and Wiborg, O. (1996).** Influence of Cyp2D6 genetic polymorphism on ratios of steady-state serum concentration to dose of the neuroleptic zuclopenthixol. *Ther Drug Monit*, 18, 629–634.
16. **Balant-Gorgia, A. E. and Balant, L. (1987).** Antipsychotic drugs: clinical pharmacokinetics of potential candidates for plasma concentration monitoring. *Clin Pharmacokinet*, 13, 65–90.
17. **Lundbeck Limited (2017).** Depixol Tablets 3 mg – summary of product characteristics. St Albans, UK.
18. **Wójcikowski, J., Pichard-Garcia, L., Maurel, P., *et al.* (2004).** The metabolism of the piperazine-type phenothiazine neuroleptic perazine by the human cytochrome P-450 isoenzymes. *Eur Neuropsychopharmacol*, 14, 199–208.

19. **Paulzen, M., Haen, E., Hiemke, C., *et al.* (2017).** Cytochrome P450-mediated interaction between perazine and risperidone: implications for antipsychotic polypharmacy. *Br J Clin Pharmacol*, 83, 1668–1675.
20. **Norlén, M. and Allard, P. (1997).** [3H]GBR 12935 binding in platelets: a possible association with cytochrome P-450IID6? *Eur J Pharmacol*, 332, 227–230.
21. **Kapur, S., Zipursky, R., Roy, P., *et al.* (1997).** The relationship between D2 receptor occupancy and plasma levels on low dose oral haloperidol: a PET study. *Psychopharmacology*, 131, 148–152.
22. **Lundbeck Australia (2020).** Fluanxol Depot and Fluanxol Concentrated Depot package insert. North Ryde, NSW, Australia.
23. **Bailey, L. and Taylor, D. (2019).** Estimating the optimal dose of flupenthixol decanoate in the maintenance treatment of schizophrenia – a systematic review of the literature. *Psychopharmacology (Berl)*, 236, 3081–3092.
24. **Jann, M. W., Ereshefsky, L., and Saklad, S. R. (1985).** Clinical pharmacokinetics of the depot antipsychotics. *Clin Pharmacokinet*, 10, 315–333.
25. **Taylor, D. (2009).** Psychopharmacology and adverse effects of antipsychotic long-acting injections: a review. *Br J Psychiatry Suppl*, 52, S13–19.
26. **Lambert, T. and Taylor, D. (2016).** Pharmacology of antipsychotic long-acting injections. In P. Haddad, T. Lambert, and J. Lauriello, eds., *Antipsychotic Long-Acting Injections*, 2nd edn. New York: Oxford University Press, pp. 31–57.
27. **Haddad, P., Lambert, T., and Lauriello, J., eds. (2016).** *Antipsychotic Long-Acting Injections*, 2nd edn. New York: Oxford University Press.
28. **Bjørndal, F. and Aaes-Jørgensen, T. (1984).** Serum concentration in acute paranoid psychosis treated with cis(Z)-clopenthixol. *Nord Psykiatr Tidsskr* 38, 229–233.
29. **Solgaard, T., Kistrup, K., Aaes-Jørgensen, T., *et al.* (1994).** Zuclopenthixol decanoate in maintenance treatment of schizophrenic outpatients: minimum effective dose and corresponding serum levels. *Pharmacopsychiatry*, 27, 119–123.
30. **Kistrup, K., Gerlach, J., Aaes-Jorgensen, T., *et al.* (1991).** Perphenazine decanoate and cis(z)-flupenthixol decanoate in maintenance treatment of schizophrenic outpatients: serum levels at the minimum effective dose. *Psychopharmacology*, 105, 42–48.
31. **Viala, A., Ba, B., Durand, A., *et al.* (1988).** Comparative study of the pharmacokinetics of zuclopenthixol decanoate and fluphenazine decanoate. *Psychopharmacology (Berl)*, 94, 293–297.
32. **Van Putten, T., Marder, S. R., Mintz, J., *et al.* (1992).** Haloperidol plasma levels and clinical response: a therapeutic window relationship. *Am J Psychiatry*, 149, 500–505.
33. **Midha, K. K., Hubbard, J. W., Marder, S. R., *et al.* (1994).** Impact of clinical pharmacokinetics on neuroleptic therapy in patients with schizophrenia. *J Psychiatry Neurosci*, 19, 254–264.
34. **Regenthal, R., Kunstler, U., Junhold, U., *et al.* (1997).** Haloperidol serum concentrations and D2 dopamine receptor occupancy during low-dose treatment with haloperidol decanoate. *Int Clin Psychopharmacol*, 12, 255–261.

11 Chlorpromazine, Loxapine, Thiothixene, Trifluoperazine

QUICK CHECK

PRINCIPLES

- These antipsychotics provide an inexpensive method of delivering D_2 antagonism, with varying degrees of plasma level data to define a therapeutic threshold or point of futility. Use is limited because there are no comparable long-acting injectable versions, and due to the paucity of kinetic information on drug–drug interactions for certain agents. Other first-generation antipsychotic options should be sought for maintenance treatment.
- Chlorpromazine has poor tolerability for long-term treatment, in part due to the high risk for anticholinergic adverse effects. Moreover, this anticholinergic burden also exacerbates the cognitive dysfunction of schizophrenia.
- Chlorpromazine is occasionally used for short-term management of agitation or aggression, and has a short-acting intramuscular formulation (25 mg/ml). Intramuscular doses should be 1/3 of the comparable oral dose to account for the low bioavailability of oral chlorpromazine.

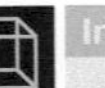

InfoBox Oral Chlorpromazine, Loxapine, Thiothixene, and Trifluoperazine Plasma Level Essentials

	Oral dose correlation (bedtime dosing, 12h trough)*	Level of evidence	Therapeutic threshold	Level of evidence	Point of futility	Level of evidence
Chlorpromazine	400 mg QHS = 22.3 (20-fold variation) [1] 400 mg QHS = 23 ng/ml [2, 3] **Multiply oral dose by 0.06**	Moderate	3.0–30.0 ng/ml [2, 4, 5]	Low	100 ng/ml [2, 4, 5]	Moderate
Loxapine	100 mg/d = 21.8 ng/ml [6] **Multiply oral dose by 0.22**	High	3.8 ng/ml [7, 8]	Moderate	18.4 ng/ml [7, 8]	Low
Thiothixene	Nonsmokers 25.0 mg/d = 1.24 ng/ml Smokers 32.4 mg = 1.33 ng/ml [9] **Nonsmoker: multiply oral dose by 0.05** **Smoker: multiply oral dose by 0.04**	High	1.0 ng/ml [10]	Low	12 ng/ml [10]	Low
Trifluoperazine	Unknown	–	1.0 ng/ml [11]	Moderate	2.3 ng/ml [11]	Low

* See Table 11.1 for effects of CYP inhibitors/inducers on this relationship

As discussed in Chapter 6, first-generation antipsychotics (FGAs) are therapeutically as effective as newer antipsychotics, and their utility derives from low cost and the availability of long-acting injectable (LAI) preparations for certain agents. While there are close to 3 dozen FGAs available worldwide, many have very limited or regional use (e.g. melperone, chlorprothixene, perazine), some are rarely used (thioridazine, pimozide) due to disproportionate effects on the rate-corrected QT interval (QTc) of the EKG, and some are so poorly characterized that plasma level data is virtually nonexistent (molindone). (For many years pimozide had a niche use for delusional parasitosis based on a small number of poorly designed studies; recent data indicate no unique efficacy benefit compared to the much safer antipsychotic risperidone, so there is no reason to use pimozide in modern psychiatric practice [35].) As discussed in Chapter 12, FGAs are not therapeutically inferior to second-generation antipsychotics (SGAs) when treating patients who do not have treatment-resistant schizophrenia, but have a higher risk of neurological adverse effects. When used in equipotent dosages, the risk for D_2-related adverse effects is roughly equal among all FGAs unless the specific molecule has an inherent mechanism (e.g. potent muscarinic antagonism for chlorpromazine) that helps to lessen this risk. The tolerability issues seen with low-potency FGAs such as chlorpromazine (sedation, anticholinergic adverse effects, orthostasis) are markedly diminished in medium- and higher-potency FGAs.

The four FGAs presented in this chapter represent a group that are generally available worldwide, but none has a comparable LAI formulation, so there is no reason to initiate these antipsychotics as maintenance treatments for schizophrenia or other serious mental illnesses. Nonetheless, there are a small number of patients who remain on oral therapy, so the kinetic information is summarized, and levels provided for the therapeutic threshold and point of futility where there is sufficient information to generate an estimate. All of these molecules are more than 45 years old, so in some instances there is virtually no imaging data, or there are no fixed-dose studies from which to estimate plasma level cutpoints. The absence of this data is a compelling reason to opt for other FGAs that are better characterized for maintenance treatment, especially when there might be an LAI option. Among these four antipsychotics, some are distinguished by unique tolerability profiles (e.g. sedation from chlorpromazine can be useful in acute situations), or unusual aspects of the molecule that have engendered debate. As will be discussed below, a mythos emerged around loxapine that it might be an SGA based on *in vitro* binding assays showing higher affinity for serotonin $5HT_{2A}$ than for dopamine D_2 receptors [36, 37]. Imaging data disproved this hypothesis in 1997 [8], but there are other interesting features of loxapine, including an inhaled aerosolized powder for acute treatment of agitation in adults with schizophrenia or bipolar I [38], and antidepressant activity from the metabolite amoxapine (see Section B) [39]. Clinicians should understand the appropriate dosing for intramuscular (IM) chlorpromazine, and realize that concepts around loxapine's unique efficacy or tolerability have been discredited. A passing familiarity is sufficient for the two other FGAs mentioned in this chapter so that one can effectively manage existing patients, or convert those patients to other FGAs when the older drug is removed from the market.

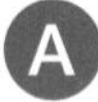

A Chlorpromazine

1 Oral Pharmacokinetic Information

The discovery of chlorpromazine's antipsychotic properties was of historical importance in the history of psychopharmacology [40]. Arvid Carlsson's Nobel Prize-winning insight that both chlorpromazine and haloperidol induced parkinsonism via nigrostriatal dopamine blockade was one of the foundational paradigms for the nascent field of biological psychiatry [41]. While of great historical importance, chlorpromazine has no role as maintenance treatment for serious mental illness due to its high affinity for and antagonism at muscarinic receptors, histamine H_1 and alpha$_1$-adrenergic receptors [20]. The dose-dependent risk for anticholinergic adverse effects, sedation, and orthostasis make this an unappealing choice for anything other than short-term management of agitated or extremely psychotic inpatients until other medications become effective. (Chlorpromazine is available as a rectal suppository for nausea, but phenothiazines with lower D_2 and alpha$_1$-adrenergic affinity are preferred, such as prochlorperazine.) Chlorpromazine is one of the few antipsychotics where knowledge of oral bioavailability is critical to deciding on the appropriate IM dose. As noted in Table 11.1, the mean oral bioavailability for a 100 mg dose is 18.4%, with a maximum of 34.2% [14]. Chlorpromazine IM dosages must therefore be no more than one-third (33%) of the comparable oral dose. Failure to follow this dose reduction formula for IM dosing can result in profound sedation and orthostasis if the oral dose in milligrams is given by injection, with falls or syncope a possible result. Like most phenothiazines, chlorpromazine is metabolized via cytochrome P450 (CYP) 1A2 and 2D6, with the latter playing a more prominent role [19]. An active metabolite 7-OH chlorpromazine is present at levels 34 ± 4.3% of the parent compound, with one study indicating a relative antidopaminergic binding affinity 60% of that seen with chlorpromazine [42, 43]. Due to genetic variations in CYP 2D6 and CYP 1A2 activity, and the effects of smoking on CYP 1A2 activity, chlorpromazine concentration–dose relationships in fixed-dose studies vary over a

Table 11.1 Oral kinetic facts for chlorpromazine, loxapine, thiothixene, and trifluoperazine

	Basic facts	Inhibition effects	Induction effects
Chlorpromazine	US FDA approval: Nov. 20, 1957 $T_{1/2}$ 11.05–15 h (range 8–33 h) [12, 13, 14, 15–18, 19] $T_{1/2}$ 11.1 ± 4.33 h (10 mg) IV Absolute oral bioavailability: [14, 20] **Mean (SD) Max** 25 mg 8.07% (3.52) 14.7% 100 mg 18.4% (8.11) 34.2% T_{max} 1.4–2.0 hours Metabolism: CYP 2D6 and to a lesser extent CYP 1A2 convert chlorpromazine to an active metabolite 7-OH chlorpromazine (CPZ). 7-OH CPZ is present at levels 34 ± 4.3% of the parent compound [16] **Formulations:** Tablets, oral solution or syrup (also acute intramuscular)[a]	Strong CYP 1A2 and CYP 2D6 inhibitors will increase exposure as much as 38% and 70% respectively [12, 13, 15–18, 19]	Carbamazepine lowers plasma levels on average 61% (range 28%–84%) [21] Phenobarbital lowers plasma levels 36%–60% [22, 23] Cigarette or cannabis smoking increases clearance 38%–50%
Loxapine	US FDA approval: Feb. 25, 1975 $T_{1/2}$ 4 h (oral) $T_{1/2}$ 7.61 h (inhaled) [24][b] NB: metabolites have longer half-lives Absolute oral bioavailability: 33% [25] T_{max} 1–3 hours (oral) T_{max} 1.13 minutes (inhaled) Metabolism: Substrate of CYP 1A2, CYP 2D6, and CYP 3A4 [26]. 7-OH loxapine is formed by CYP 2D6 and 3A4 [24], and has 4.6 times higher D_2 affinity than loxapine [27, 26]. Plasma 7-OH loxapine levels are 33%–65% that of loxapine [6, 8, 25]. 8-OH loxapine is formed via CYP 1A2 but is inactive [28, 29] **Formulations:** Capsules, Inhaled (10 mg only)	Effects of inhibitors not well documented, but the availability of multiple P450 pathways suggests that the effects might not be clinically relevant [24]. However, the absence of drug interaction information suggests that addition of, or discontinuation of, strong CYP 2D6 or 3A4 inhibitors necessitates a repeat plasma level to document the new steady state	No impact of smoking [26]. Effects of CYP 3A4 inducers not well documented, but the availability of multiple P450 pathways suggests that the effects might not be clinically relevant [24]. However, the absence of drug interaction information suggests that addition of, or discontinuation of, strong CYP 3A4 inducers necessitates a repeat plasma level to document the new steady state

	Basic facts	Inhibition effects	Induction effects
Thiothixene	US FDA approval: July 24, 1967 $T_{1/2}$ 16.4 h Absolute oral bioavailability: Unknown T_{max} 1–3 hours [30] Metabolism: Substrate of CYP 1A2, CYP 3A4, and possibly 2C19 [9, 31] **Formulations:** Capsules	Strong 2D6 inhibitors do not increase thiothixene levels [31]. No data on use with strong CYP 1A2 inhibitors, but cimetidine, a weak inhibitor of CYP 1A2 and CYP 3A4, was associated with > 3-fold increase in plasma levels [9]. Monitoring of plasma levels suggested when used with inhibitors of CYP or 3A4, and possibly also 2C19 (omeprazole, esomeprazole)	Strong inducers lower plasma levels over 70%. Suggest monitoring of plasma levels when strong inducers (e.g. phenytoin, carbamazepine, rifampin) are used for more than 14 days. Smokers require 45% higher dosages to achieve comparable plasma levels to nonsmokers
Trifluoperazine	US FDA approval: Apr. 16, 1959 $T_{1/2}$ 12.5–15.7 h (oral) [32, 33] Absolute oral bioavailability: Unknown T_{max} 2.8 ± 0.5 hours [32] Metabolism: Poorly characterized, but CYP 2D6 implicated [33, 34] Formulations: Tablets	Limited data, but one case report of severe neurological side effects upon addition of paroxetine, a strong CYP 2D6 inhibitor. Use dose reduction and plasma levels to guide treatment when moderate or strong CYP 2D6 inhibitors added [33, 34]	Limited data. Use plasma levels to guide treatment when strong inducers added (carbamazepine, phenytoin, phenobarbital). No impact of smoking [33, 34]

[a] As oral chlorpromazine has very low bioavailability, dosages of the acute intramuscular formulation (25 mg/ml) must be 1/3 of the usual oral dose.

[b] Due to the risk of bronchospasm and its potential for respiratory distress and respiratory arrest, inhaled loxapine is only available at healthcare facilities that have enrolled in the mandated risk-mitigation program [24].

20-fold range [1, 2]. Figure 11.1 shows the scatterplot from a fixed-dose study of 225 mg BID reflecting the wide range of steady state values [2]. Figure 11.2 is one of several fixed-dose studies that provided data on steady state levels from weeks 2 (and later) of chlorpromazine treatment, and the conversion factor in the InfoBox

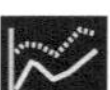

Figure 11.1 Chlorpromazine 12h trough plasma levels during a fixed-dose study (225 mg BID) [2] (divide pmol/ml by 3.14 to get ng/ml)

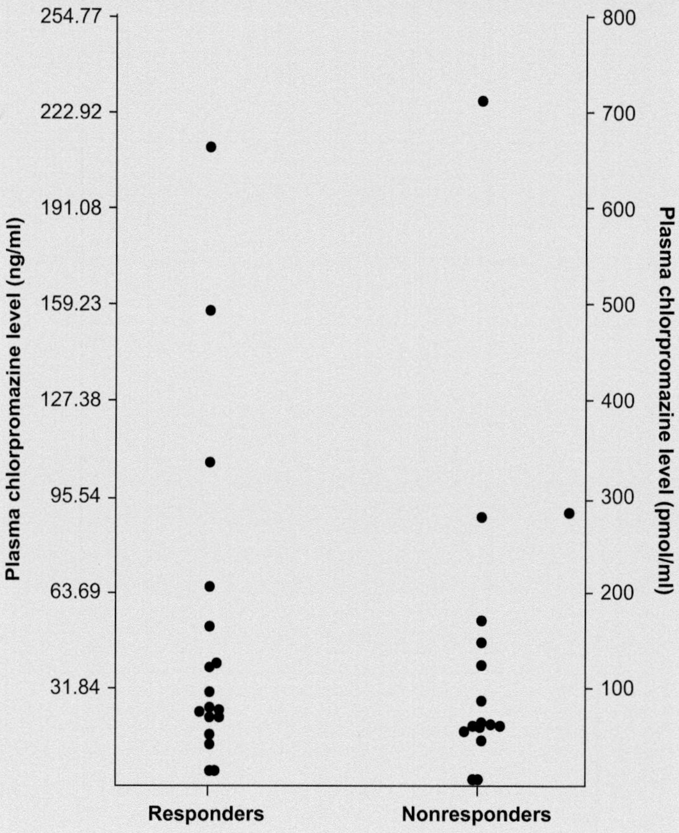

(Adapted from: T. Van Putten, P. R. May, and D. J. Jenden [1981]. Does a plasma level of chlorpromazine help? *Psychol Med*, 11, 729–734.)

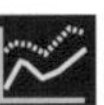

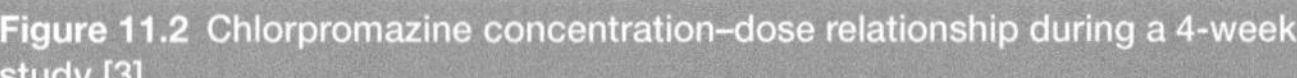

Figure 11.2 Chlorpromazine concentration–dose relationship during a 4-week study [3]

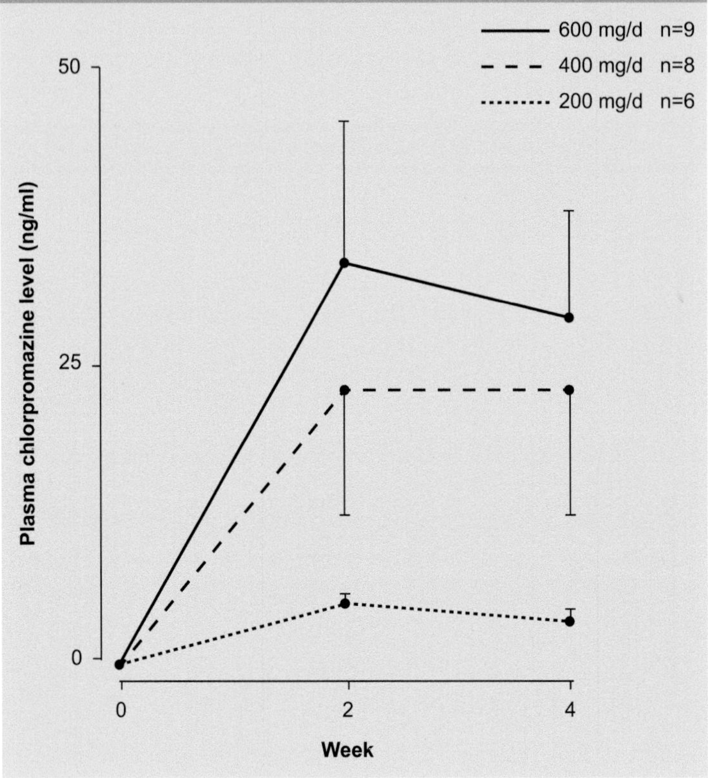

(Adapted from: B. Wode-Helgodt and G. Alfredsson [1981]. Concentrations of chlorpromazine and two of its active metabolites in plasma and cerebrospinal fluid of psychotic patients treated with fixed drug doses. *Psychopharmacology (Berl)*, 73, 55–62.)

presents a mean value from that trial and other fixed-dose studies [2, 3, 1]. However, given the enormous variability in plasma levels for any given dose, a single plasma level may be difficult to interpret – a repeat level on the same dose will generally be needed before conclusions can be drawn about adherence or kinetic issues (see Chapter 4). Chlorpromazine was assigned a Level 2 recommendation (recommended) for use of plasma level monitoring in the 2020 consensus paper authored jointly by the Therapeutic Drug Monitoring (TDM) task force of the German Arbeitsgemeinschaft für Neuropsychopharmakologie und Pharmakopsychiatrie (AGNP) and the American Society for Clinical Psychopharmacology (ASCP) [44].

2 Therapeutic Threshold and Point of Futility

The early literature on chlorpromazine plasma levels from the late 1960s through 1978 had multiple methodological issues in study design and for the laboratory assays [45], including difficulty in distinguishing the parent compound from its numerous metabolites [46]; these studies resulted in recommended plasma level ranges that subsequent fixed-dose studies found to be toxic [47–49, 22]. Papers published from 1978 onwards were largely in agreement that plasma chlorpromazine levels > 100 ng/ml are generally intolerable, and often result in lack of improvement, dysphoria, or symptomatic worsening as patients are subjected to excessively high levels of D_2 antagonism [50, 1–3]. Unfortunately, authors of these older papers continued to publish articles through the mid-1980s indicating that trough plasma levels up to 300–350 ng/ml may be part of the therapeutic range [51, 52]. The persistence of this older data in the peer-reviewed literature could be one reason why the AGNP/ASCP 2020 consensus paper suggests an upper limit for the therapeutic reference range at 300 ng/ml [44]. To help put this value into context, Figures 11.2 and 11.3 present plasma level data for chlorpromazine 600 mg/d (in divided doses) indicating that 12h trough values are roughly in the range of 25–35 ng/ml [3]. Using the defined daily dose conversion (see Chapter 6), chlorpromazine 600 mg/d is equal to 16 mg/d of oral haloperidol [53]. Thus, achieving a chlorpromazine plasma level of 300 ng/ml would require the patient to be exposed to a haloperidol equivalent of more than 100 mg/d. In a fixed-dose study of 48 subjects published in 1981, the highest level recorded was 340 ng/ml, and this individual appeared grossly overmedicated [2]. The AGNP/ASCP paper also sets a laboratory alert level at 600 ng/ml – whether such a level generated from modern laboratory assays is even survivable is unclear.

That most of the early plasma level literature is unusable creates enormous difficulties in defining the therapeutic threshold and point of futility for chlorpromazine [46]. To some extent, this is an academic problem since there is no compelling reason to use chlorpromazine as a maintenance treatment for schizophrenia due to its poor tolerability and the availability of numerous alternatives. In particular, high muscarinic affinity and related central nervous system anticholinergic burden is associated with an adverse impact on cognitive function [54, 55]. With those caveats in mind, the few fixed-dose studies published from 1978 to 1981 with newer laboratory assays

Figure 11.3 Changes in plasma chlorpromazine levels over 24 hours in patients on 200 mg thrice daily [3]

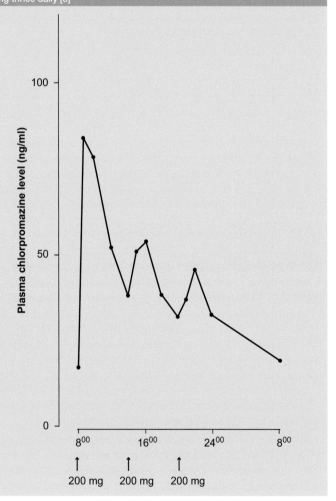

(Adapted from: B. Wode-Helgodt and G. Alfredsson [1981]. Concentrations of chlorpromazine and two of its active metabolites in plasma and cerebrospinal fluid of psychotic patients treated with fixed drug doses. *Psychopharmacology (Berl)*, 73, 55–62.)

provide a range of plasma levels from which to infer a therapeutic response threshold ranging from 3 to 40 ng/ml [50, 2, 3]. A fixed-dose trial of 400 mg/d appeared in 1984 but only provided linear correlations with changes in psychiatric symptoms, and did not report an analysis of responders versus nonresponders [1]. The extremes of this range seem implausible, as those plasma levels would be associated with daily chlorpromazine dosages of 50 mg and 600 mg, and equivalent haloperidol dosages of 1.33 mg and 16 mg [53]. As a mental exercise, one could use the haloperidol equivalent dose (and level) to estimate a chlorpromazine response threshold. The response threshold for haloperidol is 2 ng/ml (see Chapter 7), which corresponds to an oral haloperidol dose of 2.56 mg, and a chlorpromazine dose of 96.15 mg (i.e. the haloperidol dose multiplied by 37.5; see Table 6.1). Rounding off this value to 100 mg of chlorpromazine, the estimated plasma level for chlorpromazine response is 6.0 ng/ml. This is conjectural, and, as noted previously, chlorpromazine has no role as maintenance treatment, so an evidence-based value for its response threshold will likely never be known due to the absence of interest in clinical studies with this antipsychotic. When the clinical data is limited, Positron Emission Tomography (PET) imaging results can be helpful to identify a plasma level associated with 65% striatal D_2 receptor occupancy, the imaging-based threshold for response to D_2 antagonist antipsychotics [56]. While there are multiple animal PET imaging studies with chlorpromazine, the absence of human data makes it difficult to estimate a plasma level correlate of 65% D_2 receptor occupancy [57, 58].

There is more support for a point of futility based on later fixed-dose studies, with cutpoints suggested on the basis of extremely poor tolerability at higher levels [59]. The analysis of one large fixed-dose study (n = 48) provides the best defensible estimate for a point of futility, as the authors report on the plasma level ranges for responders with or without adverse effects, and the clinical outcome of nonresponders whose plasma levels were increased [2]. The upper plasma level at which response occurred without adverse effects was 72 ng/ml, and the three responders with adverse effects had plasma levels of 105 ng/ml, 158 ng/ml, and 207 ng/ml [2]. The highest level recorded among all subjects was 340 ng/ml; this individual was a nonresponder and appeared overmedicated. The patient with a plasma level of 105 ng/ml met response criteria but still manifested significant residual symptomatology; when his dose was increased, he became markedly worse. While blinded to plasma level results during the trial, the authors argue the best course of action for that patient would have been dose reduction to a level < 100 ng/ml if the level had been known, given the evidence he was very close to the point of intolerability with a level of 105 ng/ml. A similar pattern of intolerability for levels > 100 ng/ml was seen from outcomes of the 11 nonresponders who were eligible for dose increases based on the absence of adverse effects. Of these 11 patients, six achieved plasma levels > 95 ng/ml – none improved, and four of six became worse with bizarre, agitated, and hostile behaviors reported in three of this group [2]. This study thus showed that only two of 48 (4.2%) might respond to and tolerate chlorpromazine plasma levels exceeding 100 ng/ml, and the one responding patient with a level of 105 ng/ml was likely overmedicated. This value of 4.2% satisfies the basic criterion for a point of futility, since the expectation of response to plasma chlorpromazine levels > 100 ng/ml is < 5%. As discussed previously, the AGNP/ASCP upper end of the therapeutic range is listed as 300 ng/ml, but this is inconsistent with results employing modern laboratory methods [44].

B Loxapine

1 Oral Pharmacokinetic Information

Loxapine is interesting since it represents how disproven ideas gain traction and persist despite significant evidence to the contrary. Early analyses of clozapine's receptor affinities postulated that the high ratio of $5HT_{2A}$ to D_2 affinities was one possible explanation for its effectiveness, and this model was exploited to create a series of SGAs [8]. While no subsequent SGA matched clozapine's efficacy in resistant schizophrenia, the combination of potent $5HT_{2A}$ antagonism and lesser D_2 affinity helped to lessen the rates of neurological adverse effects from D_2 blockade, and SGAs (with the exception of the three partial agonist antipsychotics) all have $5HT_{2A}/D_2$ ratios that exceed 1.0 [20]. Using PET imaging, this *in vitro* difference translates to near saturation of the $5HT_{2A}$ receptor at lower dosages, and significant differences between $5HT_{2A}$ and D_2 occupancy in the usual clinical dosage range [8]. Risperidone is an SGA with high D_2 affinity, but $5HT_{2A}$ receptor occupancy exceeds D_2 occupancy by 15%–20% until risperidone is pushed to plasma levels that exceed 80% D_2 occupancy, at which point neurological adverse effects become more apparent [8]. In the absence of PET data on loxapine, investigators initially latched onto the *in vitro* finding that its $5HT_{2A}/D_2$ ratio was > 1.0, with values of 2.6–6.8 reported in papers published from 1989 to 1996, and thereby claimed that loxapine is an atypical antipsychotic [60, 61, 36]. There were two substantial flaws in this argument: (a) Loxapine's clinical activity relates not only to its binding affinity but also to that of the active metabolite 7-OH loxapine. Research dating back to the late 1970s noted that 7-OH loxapine is present at levels 33%–65% of the parent compound [6, 25], and with 4.6 times greater potency at D_2 receptors [27]; (b) All evidence from clinical trials is consistent with the profile of an FGA, with no efficacy or tolerability advantages over other antipsychotics

[62, 63]. A 1997 PET study conclusively put to rest any arguments that loxapine has a CNS profile comparable to SGAs by demonstrating that $5HT_{2A}$ occupancy did not exceed D_2 occupancy at any dose (Figure 11.4) [8]. This human imaging result is partly related to the significant D_2 antagonism from 7-OH loxapine, and the fact that the *in vitro* $5HT_{2A}$ affinity did not translate to the 80%–100% receptor occupancy seen with SGAs at low dosages [8]. Sadly, the unsupported hypothesis of loxapine's atypicality occasionally is seen in current literature. A 2018 paper reported results from PET autoradiographic imaging of brain slices incubated with loxapine suggesting an 'atypical' antipsychotic profile, but the authors did note that the absence of 7-OH loxapine and its significant D_2 blocking effects is a limitation in interpreting the study results [64]. The most recent comprehensive review of loxapine published in 2015 underscores that it appears no different from other FGAs [63]. There is, however, one interesting aspect of loxapine's metabolism – namely, that another active metabolite, amoxapine, has antidepressant properties [65, 66]. Amoxapine is formed by

Figure 11.4 Fitted D_2 and $5HT_2$ occupancy curves based on daily loxapine dose (mg) [8]

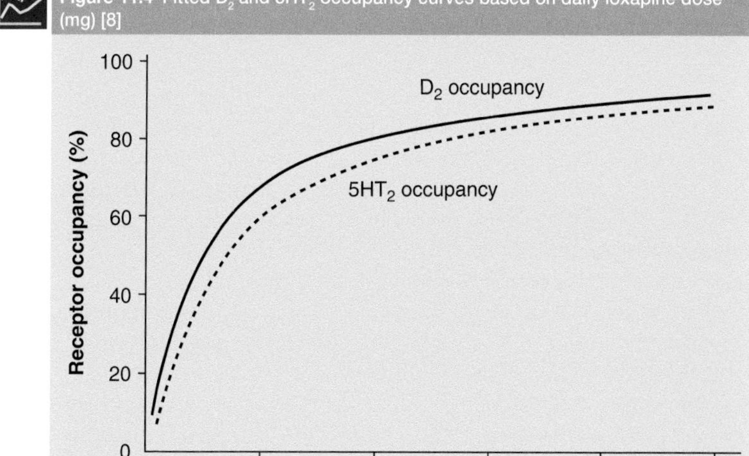

(Adapted from: S. Kapur, R. Zipursky, G. Remington, *et al.* [1997]. PET evidence that loxapine is an equipotent blocker of 5-HT2 and D2 receptors: implications for the therapeutics of schizophrenia. *Am J Psychiatry*, 154, 1525–1529.)

N-demethylation of loxapine and is present at levels approximately 24% of loxapine itself [6]. Amoxapine has moderate affinity for the norepinephrine transporter (Ki 16 nM) and serotonin transporter (Ki 56 nM), and possesses an *in vitro* $5HT_{2A}$–D_2 ratio close to 40, with a Ki of 0.50 nM at $5HT_{2A}$ and 20 nM at D_2 [20]. It was marketed as an antidepressant, and the combination of high $5HT_{2A}$ and low D_2 affinity consistent with an SGA-like picture was confirmed in PET studies [67]; however, amoxapine possessed sufficient D_2 antagonism to induce akathisia or parkinsonism in some patients [68, 69]. Amoxapine also shared some unfortunate features with tricyclic antidepressants, including anticholinergic effects and fatal cardiotoxicity in overdose, and consequently is not used in modern psychiatric practice [70, 71]. An inhaled form of loxapine was approved in the US in 2012 (and in 2013 in the European Union), which administers a 10 mg dose using a proprietary heated enclosed device [24]. In the clinical trials, the only adverse effects occurring at rates ≥ 2% and more than placebo were dysgeusia (loxapine 14% versus placebo 5%), and sedation (loxapine 14% versus placebo 5%), despite a T_{max} of 1.13 minutes and maximum loxapine levels of 257 ± 219 ng/ml [24]. The inhaled system induced bronchospasm in 0.8% (compared with 0% for placebo), and is therefore only administered at healthcare facilities that have enrolled in the mandated risk-mitigation program, severely restricting more widespread use [24].

Loxapine was one of the last FGAs to be developed (US approval 1975) and is less well studied than other FGAs. Information is lacking on drug–drug interactions, and there is a paucity of clinical data from which to estimate a response threshold and point of futility. Those issues, combined with the absence of any efficacy advantage and the lack of an LAI formulation, should dissuade clinicians from routine use as maintenance therapy for schizophrenia. Tracking adherence requires knowledge of the concentration–dose relationship, and fortunately this information does exist. Studies from the late 1970s suggested that the 12h trough plasma level was 0.12–0.15 times the oral dose [72], but that data was superseded by a 1991 study using higher-quality laboratory methods. The 1991 analysis utilized 31 specimens from 17 patients, including repeat specimens from the same individuals on different dosages, and found a conversion factor of 0.22 [6]. That value of 0.22 is supported by plasma level data obtained during a 1997 PET study that found a conversion factor of 0.24 [8]. Although loxapine's metabolic pathways were extensively characterized in 2011 [26], the absence of clinically relevant drug interaction studies makes interpretation of levels in patients on CYP inhibitors or inducers challenging. Loxapine was assigned a Level 3 recommendation (useful) for use of plasma level monitoring in the 2020 AGNP/ASCP consensus paper [44].

2 Therapeutic Threshold and Point of Futility

As with many FGAs, early studies used doses that are now recognized as too high, based on PET D_2 occupancy data, and the plasma level data that was amassed was not systematically evaluated and classified for responders and nonresponders [73, 72, 8]. The US product label continues to recommend dosages in the range of 60–100 mg/d, with a maximum of 250 mg/d [74], although subsequent studies indicate that many respond to doses under 50 mg/d [37]. In the absence of relevant plasma level data, inferences on the response threshold must be drawn from PET imaging studies to calculate the plasma level associated with 65% striatal D_2 occupancy. Two PET studies investigating loxapine were published by the same group in 1996 and 1997, and generated occupancy curves tied to dose, with the 1997 paper providing a conversion factor to plasma levels [7, 8]. The two reported mean doses that resulted in 50% D_2 occupancy were very similar (8.9 mg, 9.6 mg) and, from their average value, one arrives at a plasma level of 2.04 ng/ml for the EC_{50} [7, 8]. From this EC_{50}, the plasma level correlate of 65% D_2 antagonism is 3.79 ng/ml, which corresponds to an oral loxapine dose of 17.2 mg, very consistent with the graphical depiction by dose in Figure 11.4. This threshold value is close to the lower therapeutic range value of 5 ng/ml presented in the AGNP/ASCP consensus paper, although their methodology is not made explicit [44].

Estimating a point of futility from loxapine clinical data is not possible, but for most D_2 antagonist antipsychotics this corresponds to over 90% D_2 receptor occupancy in imaging studies. Using the EC_{50} of 2.04 ng/ml, a plasma level of 18.4 ng/ml is expected to achieve 90% D_2 occupancy, and this corresponds to an oral dose of 83.5 mg. As discussed in Chapter 5, a subset of schizophrenia patients can tolerate heroic doses of antipsychotics without D_2-related neurological adverse effects, but the manufacturer's recommended maximum dose of 250 mg/d is equivalent to a trough plasma level of 55.0 ng/ml and 96% D_2 receptor occupancy [74]. The estimate of 18.4 ng/ml to yield 90% D_2 occupancy is better supported by modern data, and close to the AGNP/ASCP laboratory alert level of 20 ng/ml [44].

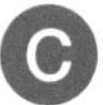

Thiothixene

1 Oral Pharmacokinetic Information

Thiothixene (also known as tiotixene) is another FGA that is used occasionally, but with no unique or special properties to advocate for its use, especially given the limited plasma level data and the absence of an LAI formulation. As with chlorpromazine, there were significant methodological issues in measuring thiothixene levels, so data prior to 1984 are considered suspect, as are some studies published through 1987 using radioreceptor assays that likely included metabolites [75–81]. A study in 1984 was among the first to use gas chromatography [10], and the subsequent use of high-performance thin layer chromatography (HPLC) greatly improved the accuracy and limits of detection for thiothixene [80, 81]. There is limited plasma level data after 1988, with the exception of a therapeutic drug monitoring study published in 1991 using HPLC, in which levels in a group of 59 psychiatric inpatients were classified by smoking status and use of CYP inhibitors or inducers [9]. The authors provided concentration–dose relationships for the 49% of patients not receiving CYP inhibitors or inducers, and this information is the source of the conversion factors in the InfoBox. The metabolic pathway for thiothixene has never been clarified, but inferences can be drawn from the impact of smoking in the 1991 paper, and from a 1997 study documenting lack of kinetic effects with paroxetine [9, 31]. Thiothixene was not mentioned in the 2020 AGNP/ASCP consensus paper [44].

2 Therapeutic Threshold and Point of Futility

As was common at that time, several thiothixene studies pursued extremely high dosages to determine the limits of response and tolerability, with daily doses up to 400 mg used in some trials of treatment-resistant patients [79, 82]. A 1984 trial is the only source of information from which to estimate a response threshold due to its randomized, fixed-dose design, and also the use of gas chromatography for plasma level analysis [10]. In that trial, 19 adult schizophrenia patients were randomly assigned to thiothixene 16 mg/d, 30 mg/d, or 60 mg/d, with percent change in symptoms at day 14 correlated with steady state 12h trough plasma levels (Figure 11.5) [10]. Symptom improvement of at least 40% was seen in 3 of 9 patients with day 14 plasma levels in the range of 0.45 to 1.0 ng/ml; in 3 of 5 patients with levels of 1.0 to 2.0 ng/ml; and in 4 of 4 patients with levels 2.5 to 10.5 ng/ml. One patient with a level of 15 ng/ml after 2 weeks became worse, leading the authors to suggest an upper limit of 12 ng/ml. The investigators suggested a response threshold of 2 ng/ml, but a responder analysis indicates that 73% of subjects with levels ≥ 1.0 ng/ml were responders, compared to 25% of those with day 14 levels < 1.0 ng/ml. From this sparse evidence, a response threshold of 1.0 ng/ml is suggested, with a point of futility of 12.0 ng/ml. The absence of any PET imaging data further weakens these conclusions, and the lack of data emphasizes that thiothixene is not an optimal choice to commence schizophrenia treatment when other, better-studied FGAs are available. For patients who are on thiothixene monotherapy for schizophrenia, consider switching to another FGA, especially one with more complete information on drug

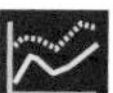

Figure 11.5 Correlation between plasma thiothixene levels at day 14 and change in schizophrenia symptoms [10]

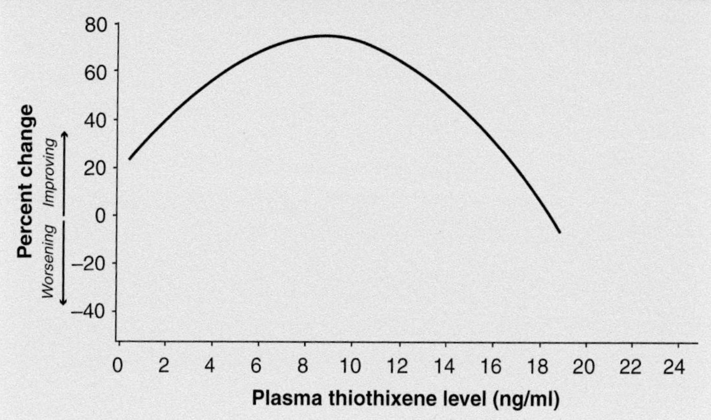

(Adapted from: M. L. Mavroidis, D. R. Kanter, J. Hirschowitz, *et al.* [1984]. Clinical relevance of thiothixene plasma levels. *J Clin Psychopharmacol*, 4, 155–157.)

metabolism and drug–drug interactions, ideally an FGA with an LAI option. Part of the concern with older FGAs is that manufacturers may abruptly stop producing the medication due to its limited market, so more widely used FGAs are always better choices.

D Trifluoperazine

1 Oral Pharmacokinetic Information

Trifluoperazine is a phenothiazine synthesized in the 1950s as an alternative to the more sedating chlorpromazine. Unlike fluphenazine, a long-acting injectable version of trifluoperazine was never developed, and in many countries the only form is an oral tablet, with liquid preparations and short-acting injectables no longer available. As with thiothixene, many basic parameters for trifluoperazine have not been defined, including absolute oral bioavailability, oral concentration–dose relationships, the specific contribution of CYP isoenzymes to phase 1 metabolism, and the potential kinetic effects of CYP inhibitors and inducers. As discussed in Chapter 5, trifluoperazine is historically important for defining concepts about antipsychotic trial adequacy based on the results of a trifluoperazine titration study by Professor George

Simpson [83]. The primary outcome of that trial was to delineate the dosage range that achieved a predefined level of neurological adverse effects (e.g. parkinsonism, akathisia, dystonia) with ongoing weekly trifluoperazine titration [83]. The study was eventually terminated as one subject had reached 480 mg/d of trifluoperazine (equivalent to 192 mg/d of haloperidol), yet had one of the lowest neurological adverse effect ratings. That trial clearly indicated the existence of a subgroup for whom D_2-related adverse effects may not limit ongoing antipsychotic titration, and justified setting an upper limit or point of futility for plasma antipsychotic levels to prevent ongoing titration when the chance of response was close to zero. Trifluoperazine was not mentioned in the 2020 AGNP/ASCP consensus paper [44].

2 Therapeutic Threshold and Point of Futility

As with other FGAs, sensitive assay techniques were not developed until the 1980s [84], so there is no prior usable information from which to correlate response and plasma trifluoperazine levels. There is also no D_2 occupancy imaging data for trifluoperazine. Fortunately, a fixed-dose study of 5 mg BID was published in 1989 in 36 adult schizophrenia patients with an acute exacerbation of their illness [11]. The investigators purposely chose a relatively modest trifluoperazine dose with the explicit intent of defining a therapeutic threshold. Subjects were started on trifluoperazine after a mean washout of 17.9 ± 7 days, with 12h trough plasma levels obtained on days 11 and 15. Response was defined as > 25% improvement on BPRS at 2 weeks, or > 50% improvement on the Global Assessment Scale (GAS). Based on the scatterplot (Figure 11.6), subjects were classified in 3 plasma level groups: low ≤ 1.0 ng/ml; medium > 1.0 and ≤ 2.3 ng/ml; and high > 2.3 ng/ml. BPRS response rates were clearly tied to endpoint plasma levels: 0/19 subjects responded with levels ≤ 1 ng/ml, 9/12 (75%) responded with levels > 1.0–2.3 ng/ml, and 0/5 responded at levels > 2.3 ng/ml. A nearly identical pattern was seen using the higher threshold of > 50% improvement in GAS: 1/19 subjects responded with levels ≤ 1 ng/ml, 5/12 (41.7%) responded with levels > 1.0–2.3 ng/ml, and 0/5 responded at levels > 2.3 ng/ml [11]. This represents the only interpretable data from which to infer a response threshold, but the finding of 0% response on day 15 is consistent with our modern understanding that less than minimal response after 2 weeks of a given antipsychotic dose (and plasma level) indicates high likelihood of nonresponse at later time points (see Chapter 5) [85]. For this reason, the response threshold of 1.0 ng/ml appears reasonably well supported. One can base a point of futility on the finding that levels > 2.3 ng/ml were associated with 0% chance of response, but this conclusion seems less compelling given the small sample size for the cohort. Nonetheless, this is the

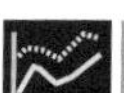

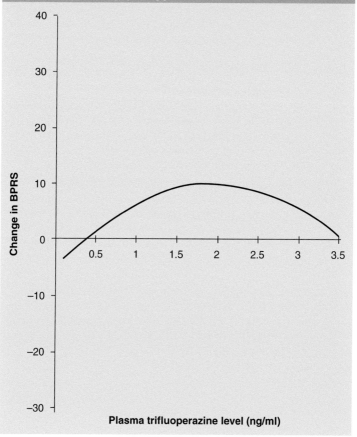

Figure 11.6 Correlation between plasma trifluoperazine levels at day 15 and change in schizophrenia symptoms [1]

(Adapted from: P. G. Janicak, J. I. Javaid, R. P. Sharma, *et al*. [1989]. Trifluoperazine plasma levels and clinical response. *J Clin Psychopharmacol*, 9, 340–346.)

only data set which addresses that issue, so for now that must suffice. As discussed previously with thiothixene, the absence of trifluoperazine imaging data further weakens these conclusions, and suggests that trifluoperazine is not an optimal choice to commence schizophrenia treatment when other, better-studied FGAs are available.

For patients on trifluoperazine monotherapy for schizophrenia, consider switching to another FGA, especially one with better information on drug metabolism and drug–drug interactions, and ideally an FGA with an LAI formulation. Manufacturers may abruptly stop producing the older FGAs such as trifluoperazine due to its limited market, so more widely used FGAs are always better choices.

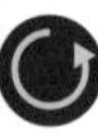

Summary Points

a All first-generation antipsychotics (FGAs) have the same mechanism of action, dopamine D_2 antagonism, and are equally effective. Clinicians typically gravitate towards those FGAs which have more robust kinetic and plasma level information, and also have long-acting injectable (LAI) options. The four antipsychotics covered in this chapter should not be used for maintenance treatment of schizophrenia due to the paucity of plasma level data, or the lack of an LAI formulation.

b For patients on existing maintenance treatment with any of these four antipsychotics, strong consideration should be given to switching to another FGA, especially for little-used antipsychotics (e.g. thiothixene, trifluoperazine) that are in peril of having production discontinued due to the limited market. Other FGAs should be sought for patients on chlorpromazine as the anticholinergic burden associated with this molecule exacerbates the cognitive dysfunction of schizophrenia.

c Chlorpromazine is used at times for management of inpatient aggression or agitation, with a short-acting intramuscular preparation available if needed (25 mg/ml). Intramuscular chlorpromazine doses must be no more than 1/3 of the comparable oral dose to account for the low oral bioavailability of chlorpromazine.

References

1. **Alfredsson, G., Bjerkenstedt, L., Edman, G., *et al.* (1984).** Relationships between drug concentrations in serum and CSF, clinical effects and monoaminergic variables in schizophrenic patients treated with sulpiride or chlorpromazine. *Acta Psychiatr Scand Suppl*, 311, 49–74.
2. **Van Putten, T., May, P. R., and Jenden, D. J. (1981).** Does a plasma level of chlorpromazine help? *Psychol Med*, 11, 729–734.
3. **Wode-Helgodt, B. and Alfredsson, G. (1981).** Concentrations of chlorpromazine and two of its active metabolites in plasma and cerebrospinal fluid of psychotic patients treated with fixed drug doses. *Psychopharmacology (Berl)*, 73, 55–62.
4. **Dahl, S. G. (1986).** Plasma level monitoring of antipsychotic drugs: clinical utility. *Clin Pharmacokinet*, 11, 36–61.
5. **Van Putten, T., Marder, S. R., Wirshing, W. C., *et al.* (1991).** Neuroleptic plasma levels. *Schizophr Bull*, 17, 197–216.
6. **Cheung, S. W., Tang, S. W., and Remington, G. (1991).** Simultaneous quantitation of loxapine, amoxapine and their 7- and 8-hydroxy metabolites in plasma by high-performance liquid chromatography. *J Chromatogr*, 564, 213–221.
7. **Kapur, S., Zipursky, R. B., Jones, C., *et al.* (1996).** The D2 receptor occupancy profile of loxapine determined using PET. *Neuropsychopharmacology*, 15, 562–566.
8. **Kapur, S., Zipursky, R., Remington, G., *et al.* (1997).** PET evidence that loxapine is an equipotent blocker of 5-HT2 and D2 receptors: implications for the therapeutics of schizophrenia. *Am J Psychiatry*, 154, 1525–1529.
9. **Ereshefsky, L., Saklad, S. R., Watanabe, M. D., *et al.* (1991).** Thiothixene pharmacokinetic interactions: a study of hepatic enzyme inducers, clearance inhibitors, and demographic variables. *J Clin Psychopharmacol*, 11, 296–301.
10. **Mavroidis, M. L., Kanter, D. R., Hirschowitz, J., *et al.* (1984).** Clinical relevance of thiothixene plasma levels. *J Clin Psychopharmacol*, 4, 155–157.
11. **Janicak, P. G., Javaid, J. I., Sharma, R. P., *et al.* (1989).** Trifluoperazine plasma levels and clinical response. *J Clin Psychopharmacol*, 9, 340–346.
12. **Otagiri, M., Maruyama, T., Imai, T., *et al.* (1987).** A comparative study of the interaction of warfarin with human alpha 1-acid glycoprotein and human albumin. *J Pharm Pharmacol*, 39, 416–420.
13. **Castaneda-Hernandez, G., Bravo, G., and Godfraind, T. (1991).** Chlorpromazine treatment increases circulating digoxin like immunoreactivity in the rat. *Proc West Pharmacol Soc*, 34, 501–503.
14. **Yeung, P. K., Hubbard, J. W., Korchinski, E. D., *et al.* (1993).** Pharmacokinetics of chlorpromazine and key metabolites. *Eur J Clin Pharmacol*, 45, 563–569.
15. **Chetty, M., Miller, R., and Moodley, S. V. (1994).** Smoking and body weight influence the clearance of chlorpromazine. *Eur J Clin Pharmacol*, 46, 523–526.
16. **Yoshii, K., Kobayashi, K., Tsumuji, M., *et al.* (2000).** Identification of human cytochrome P450 isoforms involved in the 7-hydroxylation of chlorpromazine by human liver microsomes. *Life Sci*, 67, 175–184.
17. **Sunwoo, Y., Ryu, J., Jung, C., *et al.* (2004).** Disposition of chlorpromazine in Korean healthy subjects with CYP2D6*10B mutation. *Clin Pharmacol Ther*, 75, P90–P90.
18. **Gardiner, S. J. and Begg, E. J. (2006).** Pharmacogenetics, drug-metabolizing enzymes, and clinical practice. *Pharmacol Rev*, 58, 521–590.
19. **Wojcikowski, J., Boksa, J., and Daniel, W. A. (2010).** Main contribution of the cytochrome P450 isoenzyme 1A2 (CYP1A2) to N-demethylation and 5-sulfoxidation of the phenothiazine neuroleptic chlorpromazine in human liver: a comparison with other phenothiazines. *Biochem Pharmacol*, 80, 1252–1259.

20. **Meyer, J. M. (2018).** Pharmacotherapy of psychosis and mania. In L. L. Brunton, R. Hilal-Dandan and B. C. Knollmann, eds., *Goodman & Gilman's The Pharmacological Basis of Therapeutics*, 13th edn. Chicago, IL: McGraw-Hill, pp. 279–302.
21. **Raitasuo, V., Lehtovaara, R., and Huttunen, M. O. (1994).** Effect of switching carbamazepine to oxcarbazepine on the plasma levels of neuroleptics: a case report. *Psychopharmacology (Berl)*, 116, 115–116.
22. **Curry, S. H., Davis, J. M., Janowsky, D. S., *et al.* (1970).** Factors affecting chlorpromazine plasma levels in psychiatric patients. *Arch Gen Psychiatry*, 22, 209–215.
23. **Loga, S., Curry, S., and Lader, M. (1975).** Interactions of orphenadrine and phenobarbitone with chlorpromazine: plasma concentrations and effects in man. *Br J Clin Pharmacol*, 2, 197–208.
24. **Galen US Inc. (2019).** Adasuve package insert. Souderton, PA 18964.
25. **Alexza Pharmaceuticals Inc. (2011).** Adasuve (loxapine) inhalation powder NDA 022549 – Psychopharmacologic Drug Advisory Committee briefing document, 12 December 2011. Food and Drug Administration.
26. **Luo, J. P., Vashishtha, S. C., Hawes, E. M., *et al.* (2011).** In vitro identification of the human cytochrome p450 enzymes involved in the oxidative metabolism of loxapine. *Biopharm Drug Dispos*, 32, 398–407.
27. **Coupet, J. and Rauh, C. E. (1979).** 3H-Spiroperidol binding to dopamine receptors in rat striatal membranes: influence of loxapine and its hydroxylated metabolites. *Eur J Pharmacol*, 55, 215–218.
28. **Midha, K. K., Hubbard, J. W., McKay, G., *et al.* (1993).** The role of metabolites in a bioequivalence study I: loxapine, 7-hydroxyloxapine and 8-hydroxyloxapine. *Int J Clin Pharmacol Ther Toxicol*, 31, 177–183.
29. **Wong, Y. C., Wo, S. K., and Zuo, Z. (2012).** Investigation of the disposition of loxapine, amoxapine and their hydroxylated metabolites in different brain regions, CSF and plasma of rat by LC-MS/MS. *J Pharm Biomed Anal*, 58, 83–93.
30. **Hobbs, D. C., Welch, W. M., Short, M. J., *et al.* (1974).** Pharmacokinetics of thiothixene in man. *Clin Pharmacol Ther*, 16, 473–478.
31. **Guthrie, S. K., Hariharan, M., Kumar, A. A., *et al.* (1997).** The effect of paroxetine on thiothixene pharmacokinetics. *J Clin Pharm Ther*, 22, 221–226.
32. **Midha, K. K., Korchinski, E. D., Verbeeck, R. K., *et al.* (1983).** Kinetics of oral trifluoperazine disposition in man. *Br J Clin Pharmacol*, 15, 380–382.
33. **Midha, K. K., Hawes, E. M., Hubbard, J. W., *et al.* (1988).** A pharmacokinetic study of trifluoperazine in two ethnic populations. *Psychopharmacology (Berl)*, 95, 333–338.
34. **Nicholson, S. D. (1992).** Extra pyramidal side effects associated with paroxetine. *West Engl Med J*, 107, 90–91.
35. **McPhie, M. L. and Kirchhof, M. G. (2020).** A systematic review of antipsychotic agents for primary delusional infestation. *J Dermatolog Treat*, 1–13.
36. **Singh, A. N., Barlas, C., Singh, S., *et al.* (1996).** A neurochemical basis for the antipsychotic activity of loxapine: interactions with dopamine D1, D2, D4 and serotonin 5-HT2 receptor subtypes. *J Psychiatry Neurosci*, 21, 29–35.
37. **Ereshefsky, L. (1999).** Pharmacologic and pharmacokinetic considerations in choosing an antipsychotic. *J Clin Psychiatry*, 60 Suppl 10, 20–30.
38. **Spyker, D. A., Riesenberg, R. A., and Cassella, J. V. (2015).** Multiple dose pharmacokinetics of inhaled loxapine in subjects on chronic, stable antipsychotic regimens. *J Clin Pharmacol*, 55, 985–994.
39. **Midha, K. K., Hubbard, J. W., McKay, G., *et al.* (1999).** The role of metabolites in a bioequivalence study II: amoxapine, 7-hydroxyamoxapine, and 8-hydroxyamoxapine. *Int J Clin Pharmacol Ther*, 37, 428–438.
40. **Lopez-Munoz, F., Alamo, C., Cuenca, E., *et al.* (2005).** History of the discovery and clinical introduction of chlorpromazine. *Ann Clin Psychiatry*, 17, 113–135.
41. **Baumeister, A. A. (2013).** The chlorpromazine enigma. *J Hist Neurosci*, 22, 14–29.

42. **Sakalis, G., Chan, T. L., Gershon, S., *et al.* (1973).** The possible role of metabolites in therapeutic response to chlorpromazine treatment. *Psychopharmacologia*, 32, 279–284.
43. **Dahl, S. G. and Hall, H. (1981).** Binding affinity of levomepromazine and two of its major metabolites of central dopamine and alpha-adrenergic receptors in the rat. *Psychopharmacology (Berl)*, 74, 101–104.
44. **Schoretsanitis, G., Kane, J. M., Correll, C. U., *et al.* (2020).** Blood levels to optimize antipsychotic treatment in clinical practice: a joint consensus statement of the American Society of Clinical Psychopharmacology (ASCP) and the Therapeutic Drug Monitoring (TDM) Task Force of the Arbeitsgemeinschaft für Neuropsychopharmakologie und Pharmakopsychiatrie (AGNP). *J Clin Psychiatry*, 81, https://doi:.org/10.4088/JCP.4019cs13169.
45. **Rivera-Calimlim, L. (1982).** Problems in therapeutic blood monitoring of chlorpromazine. *Ther Drug Monit*, 4, 41–49.
46. **May, P. R. and Van Putten, T. (1978).** Plasma levels of chlorpromazine in schizophrenia: a critical review of the literature. *Arch Gen Psychiatry*, 35, 1081–1087.
47. **Curry, S. H. (1968).** The determination and possible significance of plasma levels of chlorpromazine in psychiatric patients. *Agressologie*, 9, 115–121.
48. **Curry, S. H. and Marshall, J. H. (1968).** Plasma levels of chlorpromazine and some of its relatively non-polar metabolites in psychiatric patients. *Life Sci*, 7, 9–17.
49. **Sakalis, G., Curry, S. H., Mould, G. P., *et al.* (1972).** Physiologic and clinical effects of chlorpromazine and their relationship to plasma level. *Clin Pharmacol Ther*, 13, 931–946.
50. **Wode-Helgodt, B., Borg, S., Fyrö, B., *et al.* (1978).** Clinical effects and drug concentrations in plasma and cerebrospinal fluid in psychotic patients treated with fixed doses of chlorpromazine. *Acta Psychiatr Scand*, 58, 149–173.
51. **Rivera-Calimlim, L. and Hershey, L. (1984).** Neuroleptic concentrations and clinical response. *Annu Rev Pharmacol Toxicol*, 24, 361–386.
52. **Curry, S. H. (1985).** The strategy and value of neuroleptic drug monitoring. *J Clin Psychopharmacol*, 5, 263–271.
53. **Leucht, S., Samara, M., Heres, S., *et al.* (2016).** Dose equivalents for antipsychotic drugs: the DDD method. *Schizophr Bull*, 42 Suppl 1, S90–94.
54. **Ang, M. S., Abdul Rashid, N. A., Lam, M., *et al.* (2017).** The impact of medication anticholinergic burden on cognitive performance in people with schizophrenia. *J Clin Psychopharmacol*, 37, 651–656.
55. **Eum, S., Hill, S. K., Rubin, L. H., *et al.* (2017).** Cognitive burden of anticholinergic medications in psychotic disorders. *Schizophr Res*, 190, 129–135.
56. **Kapur, S., Zipursky, R., Jones, C., *et al.* (2000).** Relationship between dopamine D(2) occupancy, clinical response, and side effects: a double-blind PET study of first-episode schizophrenia. *Am J Psychiatry*, 157, 514–520.
57. **Kusumi, I., Takahashi, Y., Suzuki, K., *et al.* (2000).** Differential effects of subchronic treatments with atypical antipsychotic drugs on dopamine D2 and serotonin 5-HT2A receptors in the rat brain. *J Neural Transm (Vienna)*, 107, 295–302.
58. **Barth, V. N., Chernet, E., Martin, L. J., *et al.* (2006).** Comparison of rat dopamine D2 receptor occupancy for a series of antipsychotic drugs measured using radiolabeled or nonlabeled raclopride tracer. *Life Sci*, 78, 3007–3012.
59. **Midha, K. K., Hubbard, J. W., Marder, S. R., *et al.* (1994).** Impact of clinical pharmacokinetics on neuroleptic therapy in patients with schizophrenia. *J Psychiatry Neurosci*, 19, 254–264.
60. **Meltzer, H. Y., Matsubara, S., and Lee, J. C. (1989).** The ratios of serotonin2 and dopamine2 affinities differentiate atypical and typical antipsychotic drugs. *Psychopharmacol Bull*, 25, 390–392.
61. **Leysen, J. E., Janssen, P. M., Schotte, A., *et al.* (1993).** Interaction of antipsychotic drugs with neurotransmitter receptor sites in vitro and in vivo in relation to pharmacological and clinical effects: role of 5HT2 receptors. *Psychopharmacology (Berl)*, 112, S40–54.
62. **Chakrabarti, A., Bagnall, A., Chue, P., *et al.* (2007).** Loxapine for schizophrenia. *Cochrane Database Syst Rev*, 2007, CD001943.

63. **Popovic, D., Nuss, P., and Vieta, E. (2015).** Revisiting loxapine: a systematic review. *Ann Gen Psychiatry*, 14, 15.
64. **Ferreri, F., Drapier, D., Baloche, E., *et al.* (2018).** The in vitro actions of loxapine on dopaminergic and serotonergic receptors. Time to consider atypical classification of this antipsychotic drug? *Int J Neuropsychopharmacol*, 21, 355–360.
65. **Sa, D. S., Kapur, S., and Lang, A. E. (2001).** Amoxapine shows an antipsychotic effect but worsens motor function in patients with Parkinson's disease and psychosis. *Clin Neuropharmacol*, 24, 242–244.
66. **Apiquian, R., Fresan, A., Ulloa, R. E., *et al.* (2005).** Amoxapine as an atypical antipsychotic: a comparative study vs risperidone. *Neuropsychopharmacology*, 30, 2236–2244.
67. **Kapur, S., Cho, R., Jones, C., *et al.* (1999).** Is amoxapine an atypical antipsychotic? Positron-emission tomography investigation of its dopamine2 and serotonin2 occupancy. *Biol Psychiatry*, 45, 1217–1220.
68. **Sunderland, T., Orsulak, P. J., and Cohen, B. M. (1983).** Amoxapine and neuroleptic side effects: a case report. *Am J Psychiatry*, 140, 1233–1235.
69. **Gaffney, G. R. and Tune, L. E. (1985).** Serum neuroleptic levels and extrapyramidal side effects in patients treated with amoxapine. *J Clin Psychiatry*, 46, 428–429.
70. **Buckley, N. A. and McManus, P. R. (1998).** Can the fatal toxicity of antidepressant drugs be predicted with pharmacological and toxicological data? *Drug Saf*, 18, 369–381.
71. **Uno, J., Obara, K., Suzuki, H., *et al.* (2017).** Inhibitory effects of antidepressants on acetylcholine-induced contractions in isolated guinea pig urinary bladder smooth muscle. *Pharmacology*, 99, 89–98.
72. **Simpson, G. M., Cooper, T. B., Lee, J. H., *et al.* (1978).** Clinical and plasma level characteristics of intramuscular and oral loxapine. *Psychopharmacology (Berl)*, 56, 225–232.
73. **Clark, M. L., Paredes, A., Costiloe, J. P., *et al.* (1977).** Evaluation of two dose levels of loxapine succinate in chronic schizophrenia. *Dis Nerv Syst*, 38, 7–10.
74. **Actavis Pharma Inc. (2016).** Loxapine package insert. Parsippany, NJ 07054.
75. **Bergling, R., Mjorndal, T., Oreland, L., *et al.* (1975).** Plasma levels and clinical effects of thioridazine and thiothixene. *J Clin Pharmacol*, 15, 178–186.
76. **Reifler, B. V., Ward, N., Davis, C. M., *et al.* (1981).** Thiothixene plasma levels and clinical response in acute schizophrenia. *J Clin Psychiatry*, 42, 207–211.
77. **Yesavage, J. A., Becker, J., Werner, P. D., *et al.* (1982).** Serum level monitoring of thiothixene in schizophrenia: acute single-dose levels at fixed doses. *Am J Psychiatry*, 139, 174–178.
78. **Yesavage, J. A., Holman, C. A., Cohn, R., *et al.* (1983).** Correlation of initial thiothixene serum levels and clinical response: comparison of fluorometric, gas chromatographic, and RBC assays. *Arch Gen Psychiatry*, 40, 301–304.
79. **Hollister, L. E., Lombrozo, L., and Huang, C. C. (1987).** Plasma concentrations of thiothixene and clinical response in treatment-resistant schizophrenics. *Int Clin Psychopharmacol*, 2, 77–82.
80. **Davis, C. M. and Harrington, C. A. (1988).** Quantitation of thiothixene in plasma by high-performance thin-layer chromatography and fluorometric detection. *Ther Drug Monit*, 10, 215–223.
81. **Dilger, C., Salama, Z., and Jaeger, H. (1988).** Improved high-performance liquid chromatographic method for the determination of tiotixene in human serum. *Arzneimittelforschung*, 38, 1522–1525.
82. **Huang, C. C., Gerhardstein, R. P., Kim, D. Y., *et al.* (1987).** Treatment-resistant schizophrenia: controlled study of moderate- and high-dose thiothixene. *Int Clin Psychopharmacol*, 2, 69–75.
83. **Simpson, G. M. and Kunz-Bartholini, E. (1968).** Relationship of individual tolerance, behavior and phenothiazine produced extrapyramidal system disturbance. *Dis Nerv System*, 29, 269–274.
84. **Midha, K. K., Hubbard, J. W., Cooper, J. K., *et al.* (1981).** Radioimmunoassay for trifluoperazine in human plasma. *Br J Clin Pharmacol*, 12, 189–193.
85. **Samara, M. T., Leucht, C., Leeflang, M. M., *et al.* (2015).** Early improvement as a predictor of later response to antipsychotics in schizophrenia: a diagnostic test review. *Am J Psychiatry*, 172, 617–629.

12 Important Concepts about Second-Generation Antipsychotics

QUICK CHECK

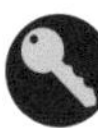

PRINCIPLES

- Most second-generation antipsychotics (SGAs) rely on D_2 receptor antagonism as the mechanism of action (MOA), but neurological tolerability is improved compared to first-generation antipsychotics by serotonin $5HT_{2A}$ antagonism
- For some SGAs, the point of futility is not defined by neurological adverse effects but by other tolerability concerns (e.g. orthostasis, sedation), or, for partial agonist antipsychotics, when 100% D_2 receptor occupancy is achieved
- SGAs approved more than 10 years ago have extensive plasma level data, and several have long-acting injectable (LAI) preparations
- Certain SGA LAIs can be loaded, and this shortens the time to reach therapeutic plasma levels, and the time to steady state

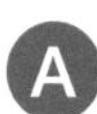

Why Use a Second-Generation Antipsychotic?

As described in Chapter 6, antipsychotics have limited efficacy differences for adult schizophrenia patients who are not treatment resistant, but marked differences in tolerability [1, 2]. The trend toward use of second-generation antipsychotics (SGAs) relates to lower risk for neurological adverse effects (e.g. parkinsonism, dystonia, akathisia) compared to first-generation antipsychotics (FGAs) [1]. For most SGAs, the primary therapeutic mechanism is identical to that for FGAs, dopamine D_2 receptor antagonism, but the neurological tolerability profile of SGAs is improved by the property of serotonin $5HT_{2A}$ antagonism. In the nigrostriatal pathway, $5HT_{2A}$ antagonism interferes with serotonin-mediated limits on presynaptic dopamine release. By allowing more dopamine release from the presynaptic neuron, $5HT_{2A}$ antagonism can mitigate the effects of postsynaptic D_2 receptor blockade [3]. This insight led to the synthesis of numerous serotonin–dopamine antagonist SGAs [3], and to the use of mirtazapine, an antidepressant with moderate $5HT_{2A}$ affinity, for antipsychotic-induced akathisia [4]. The tolerability trade-off for certain SGAs has been increased risk of metabolic adverse effects, particularly for older compounds such as clozapine, olanzapine, quetiapine, sertindole, risperidone, and its metabolite paliperidone [2]. Many of the serotonin–dopamine antagonist SGAs were created in the hope of harnessing clozapine's unique efficacy profile in treatment-resistant schizophrenia, but results have been disappointing in that regard. In treatment-resistant patients, the response rate to most antipsychotics remains under 5%, for amisulpride and olanzapine under 10%, but for clozapine it is 40%–60% [5, 6]. Nonresistant schizophrenia patients can often be transitioned from one SGA to another for tolerability reasons (e.g. hyperprolactinemia, weight gain), assuming that equivalent dosages are used (Table 12.1). Concerns about QT prolongation among SGAs are confined to sertindole [7]. Now that cardiology societies have discouraged use of the flawed Bazett QT correction formula, the spurious association between clozapine use and QTc prolongation is understood to be a function of its high tachycardia prevalence and the distorted results obtained when using the Bazett formula with heart rates > 72 beats per minute [8–10]. The 2020 joint consensus paper from the Therapeutic Drug Monitoring (TDM) task force of the German Arbeitsgemeinschaft für Neuropsychopharmakologie und Pharmakopsychiatrie (AGNP) and the American Society for Clinical Psychopharmacology (ASCP) assigned a Level 1 recommendation (strongly recommended) for use of plasma level monitoring to clozapine and olanzapine [11].

What Defines the Point of Futility for Second-Generation Antipsychotics?

While FGAs share the common mechanism of action (MOA) of D_2 antagonism, SGAs are a heterogeneous group that includes agents with limited D_2 occupancy and the dopamine partial agonists [3]. Among SGAs whose principal MOA is D_2 blockade, positron imaging tomography (PET) studies indicate that the 'sweet spot' for receptor occupancy is the same as for FGAs, 65%–80%, with decreased

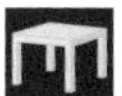

Table 12.1 Oral dose equivalency of commonly used first- and second-generation antipsychotics in acute schizophrenia [12, 13]

Medication	Oral equivalent (mg)
First generation	
Haloperidol	1.00
Fluphenazine	1.25
Trifluoperazine	2.50
Perphenazine	3.75
Thiothixene	3.75
Zuclopenthixol	3.75
Loxapine	12.5
Chlorpromazine	37.5
Second generation	
Amisulpride	82.4
Aripiprazole	1.82
Brexpiprazole	0.53
Cariprazine	1.21
Lurasidone	23.2
Risperidone	1.00
Olanzapine	2.15
Ziprasidone	29.5

Comments:

a Clozapine dose equivalencies are not provided as the primary use is for treatment-resistant schizophrenia and there are no equivalent medications [6].

b Quetiapine dose equivalents are not provided as both naturalistic and clinical trials data raise concerns about efficacy as monotherapy for schizophrenia [14, 15]. When used at doses > 400 mg/d for schizophrenia treatment, quetiapine also has substantial metabolic adverse effects [16, 17].

Note: Other antipsychotic dose equivalencies for antipsychotics not listed here can be calculated using a spreadsheet developed by Professor Stefan Leucht and colleagues [13]. The results are reported based on a variety of methods (e.g. minimum effective dose, 95% effective dose, etc.) and the spreadsheet can be downloaded from their website:

www.cfdm.de/media/doc/Antipsychotic%20dose%20conversion%20calculator.xls.

response rates below this threshold, and greater risk for neurological adverse effects above 80% [18]. Even within this group, neurological adverse effects may not always be the defining problem at higher plasma levels. For example, in a study of high-dose olanzapine, the most common adverse effect was constipation [19]. Clozapine provided the first example of an effective antipsychotic that rarely reached 60% D_2 receptor occupancy, although one cannot discount that this may contribute partly to its therapeutic effects (Figure 12.1) [6]. With this low level of D_2 antagonism, the unique efficacy profile is likely the product of multiple mechanisms possessed by clozapine and its active metabolite norclozapine, including: muscarinic M_4 cholinergic agonism, trace amine-associated receptor 1 agonism, and partial agonism at glutamatergic sites [20–24]. During clozapine titration, tolerability is typically limited by sedation, orthostasis, sialorrhea, and constipation, but not by neurological adverse effects, and the point of futility is defined primarily by cumulative adverse effect burden combined with low likelihood of response for plasma levels above 1000 ng/ml [6, 25, 11]. The early literature cited in the package insert described high rates of clozapine-related seizures at daily doses above 600 mg, but analyses of significantly larger samples call this into question, especially when patients with pre-existing seizure disorders are excluded (see Box 12.1) [26, 27]. Fear of seizure induction is no longer considered an acceptable

Figure 12.1 Fitted D_2 occupancy curve for plasma clozapine levels [21]

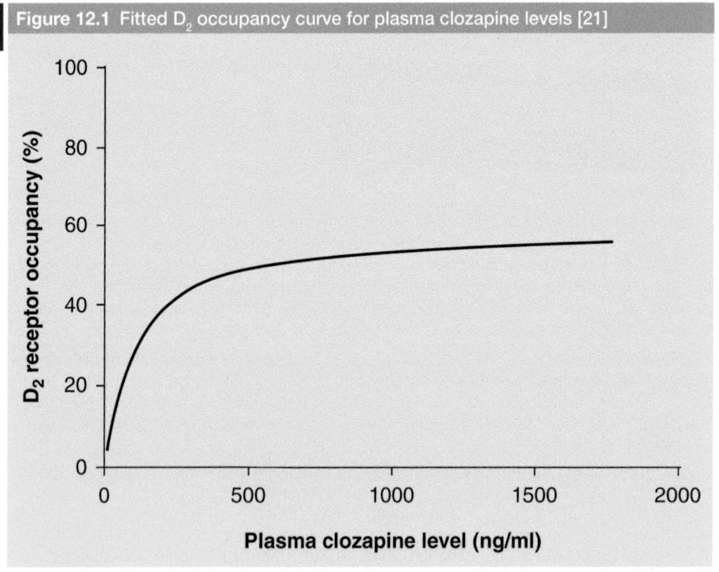

(Adapted from: H. Uchida, H. Takeuchi, A. Graff-Guerrero, *et al.* [2011]. Predicting dopamine D2 receptor occupancy from plasma levels of antipsychotic drugs: a systematic review and pooled analysis. *J Clin Psychopharmacol*, 31, 318–325.)

Box 12.1 Rates of Seizures by Dosing Groups during Early Clozapine Studies [26, 27]

	< 300 mg/d	300–599 mg/d	≥ 600 mg/d
1991 (N = 1481)	1.0%	2.7%	4.4%
1994 (N = 5629)	1.6%	0.9%	1.9%
1994 (N = 5629)*	0.9%	0.8%	1.5%

* Excluding patients with pre-existing seizure disorders

reason to forgo clozapine titration, assuming other adverse effects are managed, especially as there are no highly effective alternatives for treatment-resistant schizophrenia patients [6]. Two other SGAs possess low levels of D_2 occupancy – quetiapine and lumateperone – but ongoing titration for these medications is limited by different considerations. For quetiapine, the biggest concerns relate to sedation, its unacceptably high metabolic adverse risk profile, and poor effectiveness data when used as monotherapy for schizophrenia [14–16]. Use of quetiapine should be avoided as monotherapy for schizophrenia in lieu of other options. Lumateperone is an antipsychotic recently available in the United States with only one approved dose (42 mg); moreover, there is a signal that higher dosages (e.g. 84 mg) are not necessarily more effective for schizophrenia [28, 29].

The three partial agonists (aripiprazole, brexpiprazole and cariprazine) have high affinity for the D_2 receptor and are only effective at occupancy levels ≥ 80% (Figures 12.2 and 12.3) [3]. For aripiprazole and cariprazine, the therapeutic range of D_2 occupancy may extend to 100%. Unfortunately, the laws of mathematics and mass action preclude occupying more than 100% of available receptors; therefore, plasma antipsychotic levels associated with saturation of the D_2 receptor become the defined points of futility as further modulation of D_2-mediated neurotransmission is literally impossible [30–32]. According to PET studies, the aripiprazole dose associated with 100% D_2 occupancy is approximately 45 mg/d [31], while for cariprazine this dose is slightly above 12 mg [32]. The unique properties of partial agonist antipsychotics thus present a different set of rules for defining futility based on receptor occupancy and not tolerability, but once one grasps this concept the plasma levels which achieve 100% D_2 occupancy become hard endpoints to end further antipsychotic titration for these three antipsychotics.

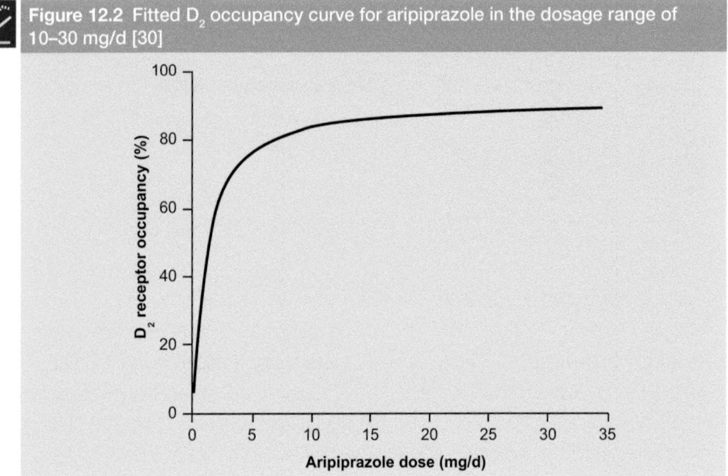

Figure 12.2 Fitted D_2 occupancy curve for aripiprazole in the dosage range of 10–30 mg/d [30]

(Adapted from: D. Mamo, A. Graff, R. Mizrahi, *et al.* [2007]. Differential effects of aripiprazole on D(2), 5-HT(2), and 5-HT(1A) receptor occupancy in patients with schizophrenia: a triple tracer PET study. *Am J Psychiatry*, 164, 1411–1417.)

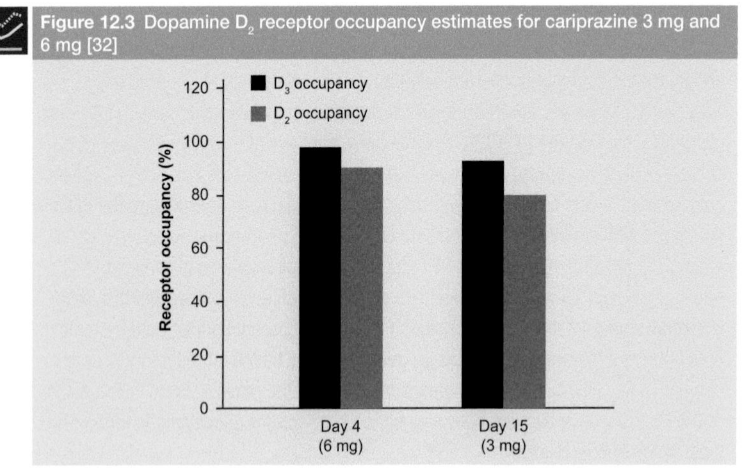

Figure 12.3 Dopamine D_2 receptor occupancy estimates for cariprazine 3 mg and 6 mg [32]

(Adapted from: R. R. Girgis, M. Slifstein, D. D'Souza, *et al.* [2016]. Preferential binding to dopamine D3 over D2 receptors by cariprazine in patients with schizophrenia using PET with the D3/D2 receptor ligand [(11)C]-(+)-PHNO. *Psychopharmacology (Berl)*, 233, 3503–3512.)

References

1. **Huhn, M., Nikolakopoulou, A., Schneider-Thoma, J., *et al.* (2019).** Comparative efficacy and tolerability of 32 oral antipsychotics for the acute treatment of adults with multi-episode schizophrenia: a systematic review and network meta-analysis. *Lancet*, 394, 939–951.
2. **Pillinger, T., McCutcheon, R. A., Vano, L., *et al.* (2020).** Comparative effects of 18 antipsychotics on metabolic function in patients with schizophrenia, predictors of metabolic dysregulation, and association with psychopathology: a systematic review and network meta-analysis. *Lancet Psychiatry*, 7, 64–77.
3. **Meyer, J. M. (2018).** Pharmacotherapy of psychosis and mania. In L. L. Brunton, R. Hilal-Dandan and B. C. Knollmann, eds., *Goodman & Gilman's The Pharmacological Basis of Therapeutics*, 13th edn. Chicago, IL: McGraw-Hill, pp. 279–302.
4. **Poyurovsky, M. and Weizman, A. (2018).** Very low-dose mirtazapine (7.5 mg) in treatment of acute antipsychotic-associated akathisia. *J Clin Psychopharmacol*, 38, 609–611.
5. **Kahn, R. S., Winter van Rossum, I., Leucht, S., *et al.* (2018).** Amisulpride and olanzapine followed by open-label treatment with clozapine in first-episode schizophrenia and schizophreniform disorder (OPTiMiSE): a three-phase switching study. *Lancet Psychiatry*, 5, 797–807.
6. **Meyer, J. M. and Stahl, S. M. (2019).** *The Clozapine Handbook*. Cambridge: Cambridge University Press.
7. **Xiong, G. L., Pinkhasov, A., Mangal, J. P., *et al.* (2020).** QTc monitoring in adults with medical and psychiatric comorbidities: expert consensus from the Association of Medicine and Psychiatry. *J Psychosom Res*, 135, 110138.
8. **Indik, J. H., Pearson, E. C., Fried, K., *et al.* (2006).** Bazett and Fridericia QT correction formulas interfere with measurement of drug-induced changes in QT interval. *Heart Rhythm*, 3, 1003–1007.
9. **Nielsen, J., Graff, C., Kanters, J. K., *et al.* (2011).** Assessing QT prolongation of antipsychotic drugs. *CNS Drugs*, 25, 473–490.
10. **Vandenberk, B., Vandael, E., Robyns, T., *et al.* (2016).** Which QT correction formulae to use for QT monitoring? *J Am Heart Assoc*, 5, e003264.
11. **Schoretsanitis, G., Kane, J. M., Correll, C. U., *et al.* (2020).** Blood levels to optimize antipsychotic treatment in clinical practice: a joint consensus statement of the American Society of Clinical Psychopharmacology (ASCP) and the Therapeutic Drug Monitoring (TDM) Task Force of the Arbeitsgemeinschaft für Neuropsychopharmakologie und Pharmakopsychiatrie (AGNP). *J Clin Psychiatry*, 81, http://doi.org/10.4088/JCP.4019cs13169.
12. **Leucht, S., Samara, M., Heres, S., *et al.* (2016).** Dose equivalents for antipsychotic drugs: the DDD method. *Schizophr Bull*, 42 Suppl 1, S90–94.
13. **Leucht, S., Crippa, A., Siafis, S., *et al.* (2020).** Dose-response meta-analysis of antipsychotic drugs for acute schizophrenia. *Am J Psychiatry*, 177, 342–353.
14. **Asmal, L., Flegar, S. J., Wang, J., *et al.* (2013).** Quetiapine versus other atypical antipsychotics for schizophrenia. *Cochrane Database Syst Rev*, CD006625.
15. **Vanasse, A., Blais, L., Courteau, J., *et al.* (2016).** Comparative effectiveness and safety of antipsychotic drugs in schizophrenia treatment: a real-world observational study. *Acta Psychiatr Scand*, 134, 374–384.
16. **Meyer, J. M., Davis, V. G., Goff, D. C., *et al.* (2008).** Change in metabolic syndrome parameters with antipsychotic treatment in the CATIE Schizophrenia Trial: prospective data from phase 1. *Schizophr Res*, 101, 273–286.
17. **Meyer, J. M. (2010).** Antipsychotics and metabolics in the post-CATIE era. *Curr Top Behav Neurosci*, 4, 23–42.

18. **Kapur, S., Zipursky, R., Jones, C., *et al.* (2000).** Relationship between dopamine D(2) occupancy, clinical response, and side effects: a double-blind PET study of first-episode schizophrenia. *Am J Psychiatry*, 157, 514–520.
19. **Kelly, D. L., Richardson, C. M., Yang, Y., *et al.* (2006).** Plasma concentrations of high-dose olanzapine in a double-blind crossover study. *Hum Psychopharmacol*, 21, 393–398.
20. **Schwieler, L., Linderholm, K. R., Nilsson-Todd, L. K., *et al.* (2008).** Clozapine interacts with the glycine site of the NMDA receptor: electrophysiological studies of dopamine neurons in the rat ventral tegmental area. *Life Sci*, 83, 170–175.
21. **Uchida, H., Takeuchi, H., Graff-Guerrero, A., *et al.* (2011).** Predicting dopamine D2 receptor occupancy from plasma levels of antipsychotic drugs: a systematic review and pooled analysis. *J Clin Psychopharmacol*, 31, 318–325.
22. **McKinzie, D. L. and Bymaster, F. P. (2012).** Muscarinic mechanisms in psychotic disorders. *Handb Exp Pharmacol*, **213**, 233–265.
23. **Pei, Y., Asif-Malik, A., and Canales, J. J. (2016).** Trace amines and the trace amine-associated receptor 1: pharmacology, neurochemistry, and clinical implications. *Front Neurosci*, 10, 148.
24. **Dedic, N., Jones, P. G., Hopkins, S. C., *et al.* (2019).** SEP-363856, a novel psychotropic agent with a unique, non-D2 receptor mechanism of action. *J Pharmacol Exp Ther*, 371, 1–14.
25. **Meyer, J. M. (2020).** Monitoring and improving antipsychotic adherence in outpatient forensic diversion programs. *CNS Spectr*, 25, 136–144.
26. **Devinsky, O., Honigfeld, G., and Patin, J. (1991).** Clozapine-related seizures. *Neurology*, 41, 369–371.
27. **Pacia, S. V. and Devinsky, O. (1994).** Clozapine-related seizures: experience with 5,629 patients. *Neurology*, 44, 2247–2249.
28. **Vyas, P., Hwang, B. J., and Brasic, J. R. (2019).** An evaluation of lumateperone tosylate for the treatment of schizophrenia. *Expert Opin Pharmacother*, 30, 1–7.
29. **Meyer, J. M. (2020).** Lumateperone for schizophrenia. *Curr Psychiatr*, 19, 33–39.
30. **Mamo, D., Graff, A., Mizrahi, R., *et al.* (2007).** Differential effects of aripiprazole on D(2), 5-HT(2), and 5-HT(1A) receptor occupancy in patients with schizophrenia: a triple tracer PET study. *Am J Psychiatry*, 164, 1411–1417.
31. **Sparshatt, A., Taylor, D., Patel, M. X., *et al.* (2010).** A systematic review of aripiprazole – dose, plasma concentration, receptor occupancy, and response: implications for therapeutic drug monitoring. *J Clin Psychiatry*, 71, 1447–1556.
32. **Girgis, R. R., Slifstein, M., D'Souza, D., *et al.* (2016).** Preferential binding to dopamine D3 over D2 receptors by cariprazine in patients with schizophrenia using PET with the D3/D2 receptor ligand [(11)C]-(+)-PHNO. *Psychopharmacology (Berl)*, 233, 3503–3512.

13 Clozapine

QUICK CHECK

PRINCIPLES

- Clozapine is the only antipsychotic that effectively treats resistant forms of schizophrenia and mania, and also is uniquely effective for schizophrenia spectrum patients with aggression, suicidality, or polydipsia.
- Due to its adverse effect profile, clozapine has a wealth of plasma level data to define concentration–dose relationships on the basis of gender and smoking status. Laboratories also routinely report norclozapine levels, allowing clinicians to calculate the metabolic ratio.
- Clozapine is metabolized primarily via CYP 1A2, but also via other CYP isoenzymes. Cigarette smoking induces CYP 1A2 expression by generating aryl hydrocarbons from the burnt plant matter. Vaping does not have the same effect on CYP 1A2 activity.
- Numerous receiver operating characteristic (ROC) curve analyses have been performed to identify the clozapine response threshold, with the consensus in the literature set at 350 ng/ml.
- Unlike most antipsychotics, clozapine is a very weak D_2 antagonist whose efficacy derives from multiple mechanisms of action. For clozapine, the point of futility is defined primarily by decreasing tolerability at plasma levels > 1000 ng/ml from sedation, orthostasis, constipation, tachycardia, and sialorrhea,

but not from D_2-related adverse effects such as parkinsonism, akathisia, or dystonia. Early concerns that clozapine doses > 600 mg/d disproportionately induce seizure activity have not been borne out by later analyses. The relationship between dose (or plasma level) and seizure induction is not straightforward, as some can develop seizures during titration at low doses.

- Pursuing trough clozapine levels up to 1000 ng/ml (assuming tolerability) should be considered in inadequate responders given the lack of effective options for treatment-resistant schizophrenia. The AGNP/ASCP consensus paper sets the laboratory alert level at 1000 ng/ml, implying that above this level the risk for adverse drug reactions is expected to increase, but that levels up to this point are acceptable if tolerated.

InfoBox Clozapine Plasma Level Essentials

Oral dose correlation (bedtime dosing, 12 h trough)	Level of evidence	Therapeutic threshold	Level of evidence	Point of futility	Level of evidence
Females: estimated dose needed to achieve the therapeutic threshold of 350 ng/ml at steady state: [1] 265 mg -> 350 ng/ml (nonsmokers) 440 mg -> 350 ng/ml (smokers) **Males: estimated dose needed to achieve the therapeutic threshold of 350 ng/ml at steady state: [1]** 325 mg -> 350 ng/ml (nonsmokers) 525 mg -> 350 ng/ml (smokers) **Female smoker: multiply oral dose by 0.80[a]** **Female nonsmoker: multiply oral dose by 1.32** **Male smoker: multiply oral dose by 0.67[b]** **Male nonsmoker: multiply oral dose by 1.08** (see Table 13.1 for effects of CYP inhibitors/inducers) (see Box 13.2 for discussion of the Metabolic Ratio)	High	350 ng/ml	High	1000 ng/ml	High

[a] This applies to a 40-year-old female, 70 kg, with a metabolic ratio (clozapine/norclozapine) = 1.32

[b] This applies to a 40-year-old male, 80 kg, with a metabolic ratio (clozapine/norclozapine) = 1.32

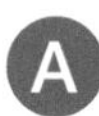

Basic Pharmacokinetic Information for Clozapine

Many clinicians not trained in the use of plasma antipsychotic levels are still familiar with the concept that levels are used commonly during clozapine treatment [2]. Clozapine occupies a special place in the management of severely mentally ill patients as it is the only effective antipsychotic for treatment-resistant schizophrenia, and for schizophrenia patients with aggression, polydipsia, or a history of suicidality [3]. Approximately one-third of schizophrenia patients are treatment resistant, but one limitation to clozapine use is prescriber fear of adverse effects, or lack of comfort with managing clozapine's spectrum of relatively unusual adverse effects [4, 5]. When treatment resistance is rigorously defined, the response rate to antipsychotics other than clozapine is < 5%, and for higher-dose olanzapine 7% [6], yet patients are often subjected to multiple trials of other antipsychotics in the hope that clozapine can be avoided. Adding to confusion in this area are numerous papers in which patients with varying degrees of treatment resistance and intolerance are grouped together, leading the unwary reader to question clozapine's benefit in treatment-resistant patients [7]. What most of these studies omit is a crucial element of the pivotal clozapine trial design created by Dr. John Kane in 1988: demonstrating in a prospective manner failure to respond to high levels of D_2 antagonism (see Box 13.1) [8]. In the 1988 pivotal trial, fewer than 2% of patients met response criteria in the prospective haloperidol arm (mean dose 61 mg/d) [8]. Unfortunately, many studies use "modified Kane criteria" and skip this step, and thus report unrealistically high response rates for antipsychotics other than clozapine. When treatment resistance is defined using all of the Kane criteria, the response rate to olanzapine at doses up to 50 mg/d ranges from 0% to 7% [6, 9, 10], but the response rate was reported as 50% in an olanzapine trial where the third criterion was completely omitted [11]. There is little question that, when all three Kane criteria are satisfied, the anticipated response rate to antipsychotics other than clozapine is extremely small, compared to rates ≥ 40% for clozapine [12, 13].

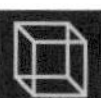

Box 13.1 Essential Components of the Kane Definition of Treatment-Resistant Schizophrenia for Patients Enrolled in the Pivotal Clozapine Trial [8]

1. At least three periods of treatment in the preceding five years with antipsychotics (from at least two different chemical classes) at dosages equivalent to or greater than 1000 mg/d of chlorpromazine for a period of six weeks, each without significant symptomatic relief.
2. No period of good functioning within the preceding five years.

3 Failure to respond to a **prospective high-dose trial** of a typical antipsychotic (haloperidol at doses up to 60 mg/d or higher administered with benztropine 6 mg/d). Response was defined as a 20% decrease in the BPRS total score, plus either a post-treatment CGI severity rating of mildly ill (≤ 3) or a post-treatment BPRS score ≤ 35.

As investigators sought to unravel the properties that underlie clozapine's efficacy, it became evident that clozapine possesses numerous and novel mechanisms of action. This realization is important not only for research into treatment-resistant schizophrenia, but also for the debate on how clozapine's kinetic profile should dictate dosing. Clozapine has a mean peripheral half-life of only 12 hours, although it is converted to the active metabolite norclozapine whose half-life is almost twice as long, and whose levels are 75% of the parent compound [14]. Although clozapine is very sedating, early titration schedules recommended twice daily dosing; however, in the 30 years since US approval on September 26, 1989, single bedtime dosing (QHS) has become the norm, with 75% of patients at two academic sites in North America having all of their clozapine dosed QHS without apparent loss of efficacy [15]. If clozapine's primary mechanism was solely dependent on dopamine D_2 antagonism QHS dosing might be concerning, since studies indicate that clozapine only transiently reaches 60% D_2 receptor occupancy (Figure 13.1) [16]. One of the early mysteries surrounding clozapine was the virtual absence of neurological adverse effects as expected from animal and human studies with first-generation antipsychotics [3]. Low level D_2 occupancy was clearly not the reason for clozapine's effectiveness, especially as efficacy concerns surround the extremely weak D_2 antagonist quetiapine based on poor outcomes documented in clinical trials and naturalistic data sets [17, 18].

Potent $5HT_{2A}$ antagonism may partly explain clozapine's sustained efficacy with QHS dosing since the time course of receptor occupancy shows sustained high-level blockade throughout the day (Figure 13.2) [16]. That $5HT_{2A}$ antagonism is a therapeutic antipsychotic mechanism has been proven with studies of pimavanserin, a medication with even higher $5HT_{2A}$ affinity than clozapine, and which is approved in the US for Parkinson's disease psychosis [19]. While that mechanism by itself may not adequately treat schizophrenia, a controlled study demonstrated that the addition of the potent $5HT_{2A}$ antagonist pimavanserin to a low level of D_2 antagonism (risperidone 2 mg/d) enhances its efficacy in schizophrenia patients [20]. When a higher level of D_2 occupancy already exists (e.g. haloperidol 2 mg/d), adjunctive pimavanserin did not improve efficacy, although it did help to mitigate the development of neurological adverse effects. Since clozapine is a weak D_2 antagonist (Ki 160 nM) [21], high

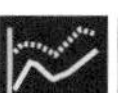

Figure 13.1 Predicted time course of D_2 occupancy with clozapine 200 mg/day (solid line), 300 mg/day (dotted line), and 400 mg/day (dashed line) [16]

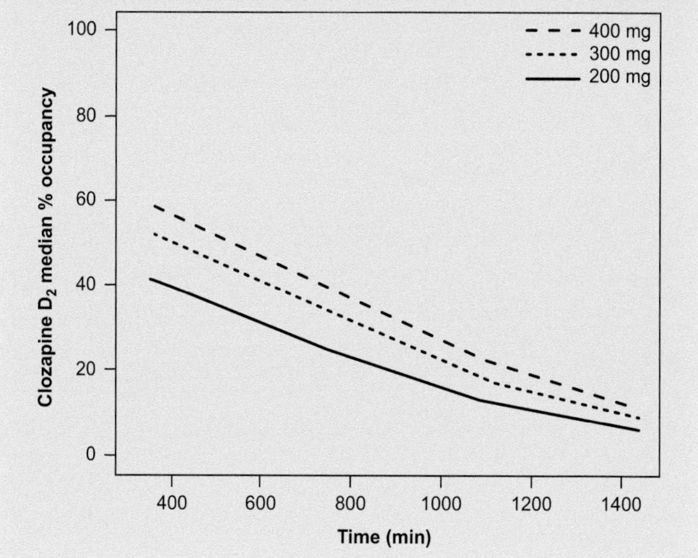

(Adapted from: C. H. Li, R. E. Stratford, Jr., N. Velez de Mendizabal, *et al.* [2014]. Prediction of brain clozapine and norclozapine concentrations in humans from a scaled pharmacokinetic model for rat brain and plasma pharmacokinetics. *J Transl Med*, 12, 203.)

affinity for the $5HT_{2A}$ receptor is certainly one of its therapeutic mechanisms, but there are others: partial agonist properties at the *N*-methyl-D-aspartate glutamate receptor glycine binding site [22]; stimulation of muscarinic M_4 receptors mediated by norclozapine [23–25]; agonism of the intracellular trace amine associated receptor type 1 (TAAR1) [26–28]. The extent of these contributions and the time course of central nervous system activity at these sites are unknown, but it is reasonable to speculate they contribute sufficiently for once daily dosing to be successful in the majority of patients, despite clozapine's short peripheral half-life.

Clozapine has a complex metabolic pathway primarily mediated by cytochrome P450 (CYP) 1A2, but which involves multiple other CYP isoenzymes (Table 13.1). Given the important role of CYP 1A2, smoking cigarettes (or cannabis leaf) reduces clozapine levels 40%–50% via induction of CYP 1A2 expression by aryl hydrocarbons

Figure 13.2 Predicted time course of $5HT_{2A}$ occupancy with clozapine 200 mg/day (solid line), 300 mg/day (dotted line), and 400 mg/day (dashed line) [16]

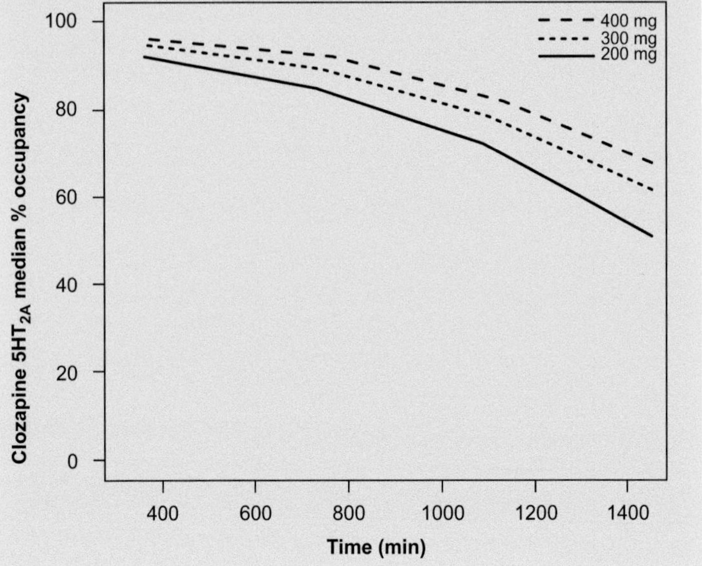

(Adapted from: C. H. Li, R. E. Stratford, Jr., N. Velez de Mendizabal, *et al.* [2014]. Prediction of brain clozapine and norclozapine concentrations in humans from a scaled pharmacokinetic model for rat brain and plasma pharmacokinetics. *J Transl Med*, 12, 203.)

from the burnt plant matter [29]. Vaping, which involves inhalation of a heated water-based solution, does not burn any organic matter, and does not induce CYP 1A2 [30]. As CYP 1A2 activity is lower in females than males, the concentration–dose relationship equations must be modified for both smoking behavior and for gender [1]. As is true for risperidone, one unique benefit of clozapine plasma level monitoring is the routine reporting of levels for its metabolite by most commercial laboratories. Using the norclozapine level, clinicians can calculate the ratio of trough clozapine–norclozapine levels, also known as the metabolic ratio (MR). As noted in Box 13.2, the largest studies have found a mean population MR of 1.32 [1], but other values are reported in meta-analyses of different data sets (e.g. 1.73) [31]. The MR is genetically determined, so any alterations in MR reflect changes to smoking behavior, changes in medications that alter clozapine metabolism (e.g. starting or stopping), or erratic timing of the dose with respect to the 12h trough so that more or less clozapine has been metabolized when the level is drawn. As discussed in Chapters 1 and 4, a drop in the MR coinciding with a decrease in the clozapine level means the patient either has poor adherence or has started smoking. If smoking is the culprit, the MR will remain below the prior baseline on subsequent levels, but the level will not decrease further and will remain within 30% of the new baseline. However, poor adherence usually surfaces as large jumps in the plasma clozapine level (i.e. > 50%) between determinations. Clozapine is also susceptible to other drug–drug interactions, and this complexity underscores the need for plasma level monitoring. Clozapine was assigned a Level 1 recommendation (strongly recommended) for use of plasma level monitoring in the 2020 consensus paper authored jointly by the Therapeutic Drug Monitoring

Table 13.1 Clozapine kinetic facts [14, 36, 3]

Basic facts	Inhibition effects	Induction effects
US FDA approval: Sept. 30, 1989 Absolute oral bioavailability: 60% $T_{1/2}$ 12 (4–66) hours $T_{1/2}$ 22.5 hours (norclozapine)* T_{max} 2.5 hours Metabolism: The mean contributions of CYPs 1A2, 2C19, 3A4, 2C9, and 2D6 are 30%, 24%, 22%, 12%, and 6%, respectively. In some studies, CYP 1A2 is responsible for 40%–55% of clozapine biotransformation. CYP 1A2 is the most important form at low concentrations, which is in agreement with clinical findings **Formulations:** Tablets, oral dissolving tablet (ODT); oral suspension (50 mg/ml); intramuscular (25 mg/ml) ***(in some countries)***	Fluvoxamine, a strong CYP 1A2 inhibitor, increases plasma levels 5–10-fold. Strong CYP 2D6 or CYP 3A4 inhibitors increase trough plasma levels approximately two-fold	Carbamazepine, phenytoin, phenobarbital, rifampin, and omeprazole decrease clozapine trough levels by up to 50%. Smoking as few as 7–12 cigarettes/day is sufficient to induce CYP 1A2 fully, with a net increase of 1.66-fold in enzyme activity. The clozapine concentration–dose ratio is approximately 50% lower in smokers (see below) Upon smoking cessation, CYP 1A2 activity declines with a half-life of 38.6 hours (range 27.4–54.4 hours). CYP 1A2 activity will therefore return to baseline after 5 half-lives, or 8 days on average. Loss of smoking-related 1A2 induction results in ≥ 50% increase in plasma levels

* In the largest data set available, the steady state ratio of clozapine to norclozapine in nonsmokers is 1.32 [1]. Other studies report different values (e.g. 1.73) [31], but the important concept is that this is genetically determined and only modified by exposure to medications or other chemicals (e.g. cigarette smoke) that alter cytochrome P450 activity, or by erratic timing of the clozapine dose with respect to plasma level determinations. (See Box 13.2 for a discussion of the metabolic ratio, and Chapters 1 and 4 for how timing of blood draws may alter the metabolic ratio.)

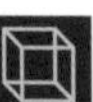

Box 13.2 Guidelines for Interpreting the Metabolic Ratio (MR) [3]

1. MR = 1.32: The expected mean value for nonsmokers who are CYP 1A2 extensive metabolizers according to large studies, but a range of values are reported in the literature [31].
2. MR ≪ 1.32: Trough values of 1.00 or less reflect exposure to an inducer (e.g. smoking, carbamazepine, omeprazole, phenytoin), or CYP 1A2 ultrarapid metabolizer status.
3. MR ≫ 1.32: Trough values greater than 2.00 reflect exposure to inhibitors of the main CYP enzymes involved in clozapine metabolism – 1A2, 2C19, 2D6, or 3A4 – or poor metabolizer status, especially at CYP 1A2 or CYP 2D6. As clozapine is principally metabolized via CYP 1A2, strong CYP 2D6 or CYP 3A4 inhibitors will typically increase clozapine levels by 40%–100%, generating MR values in the range of 1.80–2.60. Conversely, strong CYP 1A2 inhibitors (e.g. fluvoxamine, ciprofloxacin) may increase clozapine levels up to ten-fold, with resulting MR values of 3.00 or greater. CYP poor metabolizers will typically have MR values comparable to those seen with use of strong 2D6 or 3A4 inhibitors.
4. MR ≥ 3.0 during serious infectious illness: A marked increase in MR from baseline in the context of serious bacterial or viral infections may occur (e.g. severe enough to necessitate hospitalization), with MR values on average around 3.0 (range 1.4–8.6). This change in clozapine metabolism reflects an inhibitory effect of inflammatory cytokines on CYP 1A2 activity [33–35].

(TDM) task force of the German Arbeitsgemeinschaft für Neuropsychopharmakologie und Pharmakopsychiatrie (AGNP) and the American Society for Clinical Psychopharmacology (ASCP) [32].

B The Therapeutic Threshold for Clozapine

1 Clinical Evidence

Management of clozapine's adverse effects is something that any capable clinician can master, and developing this expertise not only is a source of professional pride to many providers, but also permits a larger pool of patients to have a successful clozapine trial. Clozapine response and levels have been extensively studied, with multiple investigators generating receiver operating characteristic (ROC) curves. Clinical evidence, especially from fixed-dose, prospective, randomized trials, is the most important tool we have for estimation of plasma level response thresholds (see Chapter 2), but the need for extended titration to effective doses (and plasma levels) renders this more difficult for clozapine. Clozapine was the first antipsychotic with a published ROC analysis, and a seminal 1991 article outlined the considerations in using what was then a novel analytic method for psychiatry [37]. The 1991 paper by Dr. Paul Perry from the College of Pharmacy, University of Iowa, discussed the balance between maximizing sensitivity (the probability of response in subjects who have high clozapine plasma concentrations) and minimizing specificity (the probability of no response to clozapine at low clozapine plasma levels). Perry commented that because false positives represent nonresponders to clozapine, **sensitivity is of greater importance**. The plasma level data Perry analyzed came from a fixed-dose trial in treatment-resistant patients titrated to a clozapine dose of 400 mg/d over 8–24 days [37]. Of the 29 patients who completed the study, 82.6% reached 400 mg/d; one received 450 mg/d; and five ended up on lower dosages due to tolerability issues (n = 3 on 300 mg/d, and one each on 250 mg/d and 350 mg/d). Response was defined as ≥ 20% improvement in the Brief Psychiatric Rating Scale (BPRS) total score from baseline to the end of week 4, and a final BPRS score < 35. From the endpoint plasma levels and symptom ratings, a clozapine level ≥ 350 ng/ml correctly predicted response in 63.6% of responders (i.e. sensitivity), and a level < 350 ng/ml predicted nonresponse in 77.8% of nonresponders (i.e. specificity) [37].

A subsequent 1995 study calculated the clozapine response threshold from an ROC analysis of 45 subjects, utilizing a slightly different study design that explored higher dosages and plasma levels than the 1991 protocol: treatment-resistant adult patients were titrated to 500 mg/d by day 14, the dose was held fixed at least through day 21, and subsequent doses were adjusted as clinically indicated up to a maximum of 900 mg/d [13]. Response was defined as ≥ 20% improvement in the BPRS total score from baseline to week 6, and either an endpoint clinical global impression (CGI) severity scale rating of mildly ill (score of 3 or below) or a BPRS ≤ 35. At week 6, the mean daily clozapine dose was 623.2 mg ± 203.5 mg, and the mean plasma clozapine level was 571.6 ± 441.8 ng/ml. The week 6 response rate was 40.5%. As shown in Table 13.2 and Figure 13.3, several cutpoints were statistically significant, but the trough clozapine level of 350 ng/ml best satisfied the criterion noted by Perry by maximizing sensitivity [13].

While 350 ng/ml has become the most widely supported response threshold, other values as high as 550 ng/ml are reported based on ROC and other discriminant function analyses [12, 38]. For example, one fixed-dose, 4-week trial titrated 58 subjects to 400 mg/d, and found that a plasma level of 420 ng/ml optimally distinguished responders from nonresponders: only 8% with levels < 420 ng/ml responded, compared with 60% responders with levels > 420 ng/ml [12]. Response criteria were identical to those used in the 1995 trial. When plasma levels were increased above 420 ng/ml in nonresponders with levels under 420 ng/ml, using

Figure 13.3 Receiver operating characteristic (ROC) curve from 1995 data on the proportion of clozapine responders and nonresponders for plasma clozapine levels in 50 ng/ml increments plotted from the data in Table 13.2 [13]

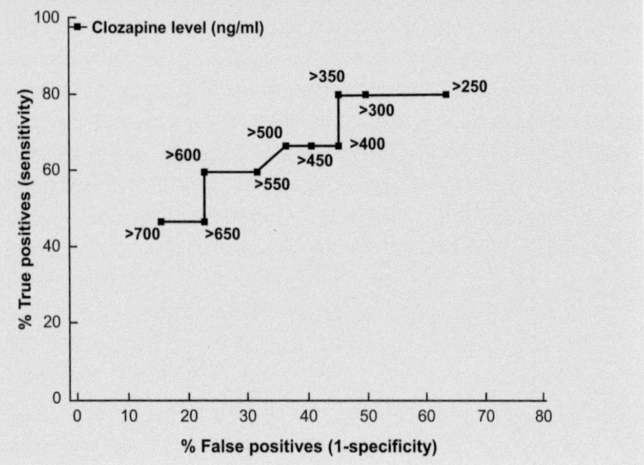

(Adapted from: M. H. Kronig, R. A. Munne, S. Szymanski, *et al.* [1995]. Plasma clozapine levels and clinical response for treatment-refractory schizophrenic patients. *Am J Psychiatry*, 152, 179–182.)

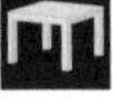

Table 13.2 Responders (sensitivity) and nonresponders (1-specificity) for plasma clozapine levels in 50 ng/ml increments [13]

Blood level (ng/ml)	% Responders (sensitivity)	% Nonresponders (1-specificity)	*p*
250	80.0	63.6	0.28
300	80.0	50.0	0.06
350	80.0	45.5	**<0.04**
400	66.7	45.5	0.20
450	66.7	40.9	0.12
500	66.7	36.4	0.07
550	60.0	31.8	0.09
600	60.0	22.7	**<0.03**
650	46.7	22.7	0.12
700	46.7	13.6	**<0.03**

a double-blind random assignment procedure, the response rate was 73% if week 12 levels were > 420 ng/ml, compared with a response rate of 29% when week 12 levels were < 420 ng/ml [12]. Other studies and analyses using the combined total of clozapine and norclozapine levels, or clozapine–norclozapine ratios, have not proven superior for optimizing clozapine response than the 12h trough clozapine level.

As with all estimates of response threshold, the clozapine plasma level of 350 ng/ml is an initial target in nonresponders. Chapter 5 presents an extensive discussion of the 2-week rule which states that less than minimal response to a given dose (and level) after 2 weeks indicates a low probability of eventual response. Given the extended titration often needed to achieve clozapine response, questions were raised whether clozapine is an exception to this 2-week rule. Fortunately, we have an explicit answer to this question from a study of 50 treatment-resistant schizophrenia inpatients treated with clozapine for at least 12 months (regardless of response status) using a standardized dose escalation protocol [39]. By study end, 34 subjects (68%) met response criteria, and it took an average of 60 ± 87 days for responders to reach the clozapine dose where response was achieved. Importantly, once a patient reached the dose where response occurred, the average time to response was **17 ± 14 days** (range = 2–56 days). All 34 subjects who did respond met the response criteria within 8 weeks of the clozapine dose escalation – no late response was found in the remaining 16 subjects despite a mean follow-up period of 75 ± 50 weeks [39]. That response was seen in an average of 2.5 weeks when titrated to the point where the patient would respond is consistent with the 2-week rule. Adding one standard deviation (14 days) to this value captures 68.3% of subjects and increases the time frame to wait for response to 31 days. This extension of the 2-week rule to 1 month allows identification of the majority of clozapine responders, bearing in mind that this rule should only be applied once patients have exceeded the response threshold of 350 ng/ml. Under no circumstances should patients be left on a given dose and plasma level for > 8 weeks hoping for 'late response' as was touted in the early clozapine literature [39].

2 Imaging Evidence

For antipsychotics that work via D_2 antagonism, effective antipsychotic response is associated with striatal receptor occupancy of 65% [40]. Clozapine quickly became the exception to this dictum as early single-photon emission computerized tomography (SPECT) and Positron Emission Tomography (PET) studies quickly noted that the majority of clozapine patients had ≤ 50% D_2 receptor occupancy [41–43]. A graphical representation of this relationship depicts the individual data points from

Figure 13.4 Fitted D_2 occupancy curve for plasma clozapine levels [44]

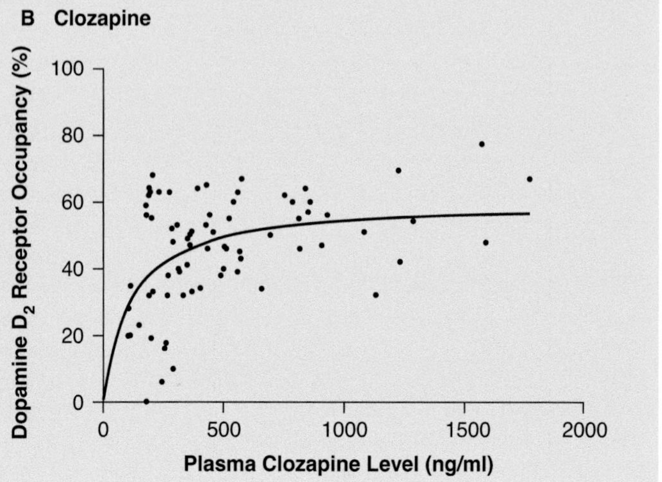

(Adapted from: H. Uchida, H. Takeuchi, A. Graff-Guerrero, *et al.* [2011]. Predicting dopamine D2 receptor occupancy from plasma levels of antipsychotic drugs: a systematic review and pooled analysis. *J Clin Psychopharmacol*, 31, 318–325.)

all available imaging studies through 2011 (Figure 13.4) [44]. Even for patients at the extreme upper end of the response curve (1000 ng/ml), mean D_2 receptor occupancy is significantly below 60%. Neuroimaging clearly differentiated clozapine from earlier antipsychotics, but has not shed any additional insights into the necessary plasma level for clozapine response beyond that achieved from clinical analyses.

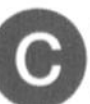

C The Point of Futility for Clozapine

1 Clinical Evidence

As with all antipsychotics, tolerability decreases at higher plasma levels, but for clozapine the limiting adverse effects are not related to D_2 antagonism. Orthostasis, sialorrhea, tachycardia, constipation, and sedation comprise the most common issues, with no evidence that higher plasma levels are related to risk for severe neutropenia [45]. (See paragraph below about seizure risk.) An extensive review of the literature correlating clozapine response, plasma levels, and tolerability concerns was published in 2013, with the explicit goal of identifying an upper limit for clozapine response from 70 relevant papers [45]. The authors noted the near absence of studies intended to find an upper limit for either clinical response or safety. The two papers which specifically mentioned a safety-related threshold provided values of 1000 and 1300 ng/ml, and one paper mentioned a 'supratherapeutic' range > 750 ng/ml. In parsing through data from ten studies examining the relationship between clinical response and clozapine levels, it became apparent that no prospective studies had examined levels above 450 ng/ml, although two retrospective analyses identified 600 ng/ml and 838 ng/ml as upper thresholds beyond which clinical response falls off [46, 47]. The 2020 AGNP/ASCP consensus paper set the laboratory alert level at 1000 ng/ml, implying that above this level the risk for adverse drug reactions is expected to increase and require patient reassessment for tolerability, but that lower levels are acceptable if tolerated [32].

Earlier versions of the AGNP recommendations also mention 1000 ng/ml as the laboratory alert level [47], and this has been suggested as the point of futility [48]. The logic underlying the choice of 1000 ng/ml as the point of futility rests on several arguments: (1) while the data are sparse for response rates in the region of 838–1000 ng/ml, there is no obvious safety concern to limit pursuing a clozapine level up to 1000 ng/ml, assuming tolerability; (2) given the absence of viable options to clozapine, patients should be provided every opportunity to respond to clozapine [48, 3].

While early clozapine literature focused heavily on dose-dependent seizure rates, the bigger source of morbidity (and, rarely, mortality) is from constipation and ileus, a risk which is doubled by concurrent anticholinergic burden from other medications [49]. Although papers commenting on this risk and the need for aggressive constipation treatment have appeared for over a decade [49, 50], it was not until January 2020 that the US FDA strengthened the package label to warn clinicians about the potentially serious consequences of inadequately treated constipation, or adding systemically active anticholinergic medications to clozapine therapy [51]. Constipation management is addressed in most patients starting from the first day of clozapine treatment, but it deserves greater attention at higher plasma levels due to the anticholinergic burden. In nonsmokers it is estimated that every 50 mg of clozapine is the equivalent of 1 mg benztropine; thus, a patient on 600 mg/d clozapine is receiving the equivalent of 12 mg/d benztropine [52, 3].

Unfortunately, the comprehensive 2013 review did not mention ileus, and concluded: "There is a lack of consistent evidence linking plasma [clozapine] levels to any serious side effects" [45]. Even more unfortunate was the fact that an earlier portion of the paper referred to outdated information on a dose-dependent association with seizures: "Also of significant concern, though, is risk of seizures, which increases in a dose-dependent fashion: <300 mg/day = 1%; 300–600 mg/day = 2.7%, and >600 mg/day = 4.4% (Devinsky et al. 1991)." Sadly, many sources, including the package labeling, continue to refer to the 1991 data (n = 1481) [53], despite the fact that a 1994 study with a sample size 4 times larger (n = 5629) found significantly lower seizure rates, and a risk difference of only 0.3% between low dose (< 300 mg/d) and high dose exposure (≥ 600 mg/d) (Table 13.3) [54]. Not only do the 1994 data (and subsequent smaller reviews) question any dose relationship [55], the 1994 publication also makes two important points: (1) patients without prior seizure history have a risk **across all doses of only 3.2%**; (2) 600 mg/d does not present a threshold for markedly increased risk that requires enhanced monitoring. The overall low rate found in the analysis of 5629 patients also undermines any recommendation that individuals exceeding 600 mg/d should receive prophylaxis with divalproex [54, 3]. Not only will anticonvulsant therapy be unnecessary in over 96% of clozapine-treated patients, the use of divalproex is itself associated with neutropenia risk [56, 57]. A case-control analysis found that the concurrent use of valproate with clozapine more than doubled neutropenia risk (odds ratio 2.28; p = 0.006) [57]. Given the extremely low incidence of seizures across all clozapine dosages, fear of seizure induction is not an evidence-based reason to deprive patients of a clozapine trial with levels up to 1000 ng/ml (if tolerated), especially considering there are no comparably effective options for treatment-resistant schizophrenia and other conditions that preferentially respond to clozapine [3]. When clinicians pursue high clozapine levels in search of efficacy in nonresponders, the entire range of common adverse effects may need to be addressed (e.g. orthostasis, sialorrhea, sedation, constipation, tachycardia). While there is no perfect study to provide an answer, the accumulated information points to 1000 ng/ml as a reasonably supported point of futility for clozapine treatment of resistant schizophrenia, beyond which the expectation of response is likely < 5%.

Table 13.3 Rates of seizures by dosing groups during early clozapine studies [53, 54]

	< 300 mg/d	300–599 mg/d	≥ 600 mg/d
1991 (n = 1481)	1.0%	2.7%	4.4%
1994 (n = 5629)	1.6%	0.9%	1.9%
1994 (n = 5629)*	0.9%	0.8%	1.5%

* Excluding patients with prior seizure history

2 Imaging Evidence

As discussed previously, imaging evidence from D_2 occupancy studies has been less relevant than the clinical data in defining areas of clozapine response. While the plot in Figure 13.4 clearly depicts that some humans seemingly tolerate plasma levels > 1000 ng/ml, we have no data to indicate that these patients had greater psychiatric benefit than at 1000 ng/ml, or that any added benefit was specifically related to increased striatal D_2 occupancy [44]. Important to the discussion about a point of futility, clozapine's dose-limiting adverse effects are not tied to D_2-related neurological symptoms (e.g. parkinsonism, akathisia, dystonia), so imaging data is not helpful in this context. Given clozapine's multiple postulated mechanisms of action, it may not be possible for any study of a specific receptor to answer this question. As with derivations of the therapeutic threshold, the clinical data is the best source we have to estimate the point of futility for clozapine treatment.

Summary Points

a Clozapine is the only antipsychotic with compelling efficacy data in treatment-resistant schizophrenia, and in schizophrenia spectrum patients with psychogenic polydipsia, suicidality, or aggression that does not respond to other antipsychotics.

b Clozapine concentration–dose relationships are markedly influenced by gender and smoking status. Using the appropriate conversion formula, one can better estimate the dose needed to achieve the therapeutic threshold of 350 ng/ml.

c The point of futility is less well defined, but 1000 ng/ml is cited in many sources as a plausible upper limit beyond which likelihood of response is minimal. The primary safety concern at higher plasma levels is constipation and ileus, and not seizure risk. Clinicians who pursue higher clozapine levels in search of efficacy in nonresponders should be adept at managing constipation and other adverse effects that may limit titration.

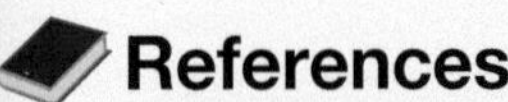

References

1. **Rostami-Hodjegan, A., Amin, A. M., Spencer, E. P., *et al.* (2004).** Influence of dose, cigarette smoking, age, sex, and metabolic activity on plasma clozapine concentrations: a predictive model and nomograms to aid clozapine dose adjustment and to assess compliance in individual patients. *J Clin Psychopharmacol*, 24, 70–78.
2. **Best-Shaw, L., Gudbrandsen, M., Nagar, J., *et al.* (2014).** Psychiatrists' perspectives on antipsychotic dose and the role of plasma concentration therapeutic drug monitoring. *Ther Drug Monit*, 36, 486–493.
3. **Meyer, J. M. and Stahl, S. M. (2019).** *The Clozapine Handbook*. Cambridge: Cambridge University Press.
4. **Cohen, D. (2014).** Prescribers fear as a major side-effect of clozapine. *Acta Psychiatr Scand*, 130, 154–155.
5. **Gee, S., Vergunst, F., Howes, O., *et al.* (2014).** Practitioner attitudes to clozapine initiation. *Acta Psychiatr Scand*, 130, 16–24.
6. **Conley, R. R., Tamminga, C. A., Bartko, J. J., *et al.* (1998).** Olanzapine compared with chlorpromazine in treatment-resistant schizophrenia. *Am J Psychiatry*, 155, 914–920.
7. **Samara, M. T., Dold, M., Gianatsi, M., *et al.* (2016).** Efficacy, acceptability, and tolerability of antipsychotics in treatment-resistant schizophrenia: a network meta-analysis. *JAMA Psychiatry*, 73, 199–210.
8. **Kane, J., Honigfeld, G., Singer, J., *et al.* (1988).** Clozapine for the treatment-resistant schizophrenic: a double-blind comparison with chlorpromazine. *Arch Gen Psychiatry*, 45, 789–796.
9. **Conley, R. R., Tamminga, C. A., Kelly, D. L., *et al.* (1999).** Treatment-resistant schizophrenic patients respond to clozapine after olanzapine non-response. *Biol Psychiatry*, 46, 73–77.
10. **Conley, R. R., Kelly, D. L., Richardson, C. M., *et al.* (2003).** The efficacy of high-dose olanzapine versus clozapine in treatment-resistant schizophrenia: a double-blind crossover study. *J Clin Psychopharmacol*, 23, 668–671.
11. **Meltzer, H. Y., Bobo, W. V., Roy, A., *et al.* (2008).** A randomized, double-blind comparison of clozapine and high-dose olanzapine in treatment-resistant patients with schizophrenia. *J Clin Psychiatry*, 69, 274–285.
12. **Potkin, S. G., Bera, R., Gulasekaram, B., *et al.* (1994).** Plasma clozapine concentrations predict clinical response in treatment-resistant schizophrenia. *J Clin Psychiatry*, 55 Suppl B, 133–136.
13. **Kronig, M. H., Munne, R. A., Szymanski, S., *et al.* (1995).** Plasma clozapine levels and clinical response for treatment-refractory schizophrenic patients. *Am J Psychiatry*, 152, 179–182.
14. **Renwick, A. C., Renwick, A. G., Flanagan, R. J., *et al.* (2000).** Monitoring of clozapine and norclozapine plasma concentration–time curves in acute overdose. *J Toxicol Clin Toxicol*, 38, 325–328.
15. **Takeuchi, H., Powell, V., Geisler, S., *et al.* (2016).** Clozapine administration in clinical practice: once daily versus divided dosing. *Acta Psychiatr Scand*, 134, 234–240.
16. **Li, C. H., Stratford, R. E., Jr., Velez de Mendizabal, N., *et al.* (2014).** Prediction of brain clozapine and norclozapine concentrations in humans from a scaled pharmacokinetic model for rat brain and plasma pharmacokinetics. *J Transl Med*, 12, 203.
17. **Asmal, L., Flegar, S. J., Wang, J., *et al.* (2013).** Quetiapine versus other atypical antipsychotics for schizophrenia. *Cochrane Database Syst Rev*, CD006625.
18. **Vanasse, A., Blais, L., Courteau, J., *et al.* (2016).** Comparative effectiveness and safety of antipsychotic drugs in schizophrenia treatment: a real-world observational study. *Acta Psychiatr Scand*, 134, 374–384.
19. **Stahl, S. M. (2016).** Mechanism of action of pimavanserin in Parkinson's disease psychosis: targeting serotonin 5HT2A and 5HT2C receptors. *CNS Spectr*, 21, 271–275.

20. **Meltzer, H. Y., Elkis, H., Vanover, K., *et al.* (2012).** Pimavanserin, a selective serotonin (5-HT)2A-inverse agonist, enhances the efficacy and safety of risperidone, 2mg/day, but does not enhance efficacy of haloperidol, 2mg/day: comparison with reference dose risperidone, 6mg/day. *Schizophr Res*, 141, 144–152.
21. **Meyer, J. M. (2018).** Pharmacotherapy of psychosis and mania. In L. L. Brunton, R. Hilal-Dandan and B. C. Knollmann, eds., *Goodman & Gilman's The Pharmacological Basis of Therapeutics*, 13th edn. Chicago, IL: McGraw-Hill, pp. 279–302.
22. **Schwieler, L., Linderholm, K. R., Nilsson-Todd, L. K., *et al.* (2008).** Clozapine interacts with the glycine site of the NMDA receptor: electrophysiological studies of dopamine neurons in the rat ventral tegmental area. *Life Sci*, 83, 170–175.
23. **Sur, C., Mallorga, P. J., Wittmann, M., *et al.* (2003).** N-desmethylclozapine, an allosteric agonist at muscarinic 1 receptor, potentiates N-methyl-D-aspartate receptor activity. *Proceedings of the National Academy of Sciences of the United States of America*, 100, 13674–13679.
24. **Barak, S. and Weiner, I. (2011).** The M_1/M_4 preferring agonist xanomeline reverses amphetamine-, MK801- and scopolamine-induced abnormalities of latent inhibition: putative efficacy against positive, negative and cognitive symptoms in schizophrenia. *Int J Neuropsychopharmacol*, 14, 1233–1246.
25. **McKinzie, D. L. and Bymaster, F. P. (2012).** Muscarinic mechanisms in psychotic disorders. *Handb Exp Pharmacol*, 233–265.
26. **Karmacharya, R., Lynn, S. K., Demarco, S., *et al.* (2011).** Behavioral effects of clozapine: involvement of trace amine pathways in *C. elegans* and *M. musculus*. *Brain Res*, 1393, 91–99.
27. **Pei, Y., Asif-Malik, A., and Canales, J. J. (2016).** Trace amines and the trace amine-associated receptor 1: pharmacology, neurochemistry, and clinical implications. *Front Neurosci*, 10, 148.
28. **Dedic, N., Jones, P. G., Hopkins, S. C., *et al.* (2019).** SEP-363856, a novel psychotropic agent with a unique, non-D2 receptor mechanism of action. *J Pharmacol Exp Ther*, 371, 1–14.
29. **Haslemo, T., Eikeseth, P. H., Tanum, L., *et al.* (2006).** The effect of variable cigarette consumption on the interaction with clozapine and olanzapine. *Eur J Clin Pharmacol*, 62, 1049–1053.
30. **Khorassani, F., Kaufman, M., and Lopez, L. V. (2018).** Supratherapeutic serum clozapine concentration after transition from traditional to electronic cigarettes. *J Clin Psychopharmacol*, 38, 391–392.
31. **Schoretsanitis, G., Kane, J. M., Ruan, C. J., *et al.* (2019).** A comprehensive review of the clinical utility of and a combined analysis of the clozapine/norclozapine ratio in therapeutic drug monitoring for adult patients. *Expert Rev Clin Pharmacol*, 12, 603–621.
32. **Schoretsanitis, G., Kane, J. M., Correll, C. U., *et al.* (2020).** Blood levels to optimize antipsychotic treatment in clinical practice: a joint consensus statement of the American Society of Clinical Psychopharmacology (ASCP) and the Therapeutic Drug Monitoring (TDM) Task Force of the Arbeitsgemeinschaft für Neuropsychopharmakologie und Pharmakopsychiatrie (AGNP). *J Clin Psychiatry*, 81, https://doi.org/10.4088/JCP.4019cs13169.
33. **Leung, J. G., Nelson, S., Takala, C. R., *et al.* (2014).** Infection and inflammation leading to clozapine toxicity and intensive care: a case series. *Ann Pharmacother*, 48, 801–805.
34. **Clark, S. R., Warren, N. S., Kim, G., *et al.* (2018).** Elevated clozapine levels associated with infection: a systematic review. *Schizophr Res*, 192, 50–56.
35. **Siskind, D., Honer, W. G., Clark, S., *et al.* (2020).** Consensus statement on the use of clozapine during the COVID-19 pandemic. *J Psychiatry Neurosci*, 45, 2.
36. **Meyer, J. M., Proctor, G., Cummings, M., *et al.* (2017).** Ciprofloxacin and clozapine – a potentially fatal but underappreciated interaction. *Case Rep Psychiatry*, 5606098, 1–7.
37. **Perry, P. J., Miller, D. D., Arndt, S. V., *et al.* (1991).** Clozapine and norclozapine plasma concentrations and clinical response of treatment-refractory schizophrenic patients. *Am J Psychiatry*, 148, 231–235.

38. **Llorca, P. M., Lancon, C., Disdier, B., *et al.* (2002).** Effectiveness of clozapine in neuroleptic-resistant schizophrenia: clinical response and plasma concentrations. *J Psychiatry Neurosci*, 27, 30–37.

39. **Conley, R. R., Carpenter, W. T., Jr., and Tamminga, C. A. (1997).** Time to clozapine response in a standardized trial. *Am J Psychiatry*, 154, 1243–1247.

40. **Kapur, S., Zipursky, R., Jones, C., *et al.* (2000).** Relationship between dopamine D(2) occupancy, clinical response, and side effects: a double-blind PET study of first-episode schizophrenia. *Am J Psychiatry*, 157, 514–520.

41. **Farde, L., Wiesel, F. A., Halldin, C., *et al.* (1988).** Central D2-dopamine receptor occupancy in schizophrenic patients treated with antipsychotic drugs. *Arch Gen Psychiatry*, 45, 71–76.

42. **Farde, L., Wiesel, F. A., Nordstrom, A. L., *et al.* (1989).** D1- and D2-dopamine receptor occupancy during treatment with conventional and atypical neuroleptics. *Psychopharmacology*, 99 S28–31.

43. **Wiesel, F. A., Farde, L., Nordstrom, A. L., *et al.* (1990).** Central D1- and D2-receptor occupancy during antipsychotic drug treatment. *Prog Neuropsychopharmacol Biol Psychiatry*, 14, 759–767.

44. **Uchida, H., Takeuchi, H., Graff-Guerrero, A., *et al.* (2011).** Predicting dopamine D2 receptor occupancy from plasma levels of antipsychotic drugs: a systematic review and pooled analysis. *J Clin Psychopharmacol*, 31, 318–325.

45. **Remington, G., Agid, O., Foussias, G., *et al.* (2013).** Clozapine and therapeutic drug monitoring: is there sufficient evidence for an upper threshold? *Psychopharmacology (Berl)*, 225, 505–518.

46. **Paz, E., Bouzas, L., Hermida, J., *et al.* (2008).** Evaluation of three dosing models for the prediction of steady-state trough clozapine concentrations. *Clin Biochem*, 41, 603–606.

47. **Hiemke, C., Baumann, P., Bergemann, N., *et al.* (2011).** AGNP consensus guidelines for therapeutic drug monitoring in psychiatry: update 2011. *Pharmacopsychiatry*, 44, 195–235.

48. **Meyer, J. M. (2014).** A rational approach to employing high plasma levels of antipsychotics for violence associated with schizophrenia: case vignettes. *CNS Spectr*, 19, 432–438.

49. **Nielsen, J. and Meyer, J. M. (2012).** Risk factors for ileus in patients with schizophrenia. *Schizophr Bull*, 38, 592–598.

50. **Meyer, J. M. and Cummings, M. A. (2014).** Lubiprostone for treatment-resistant constipation associated with clozapine use. *Acta Psychiatr Scand*, 130, 71–72.

51. **Food and Drug Administration (2020).** FDA strengthens warning that untreated constipation caused by schizophrenia medicine clozapine (Clozaril) can lead to serious bowel problems. Risk increased at higher doses or when taken with other constipating medicines. *FDA Drug Safety Communication* (January 28, 2020).

52. **de Leon, J. (2005).** Benztropine equivalents for antimuscarinic medication. *Am J Psychiatry*, 162, 627.

53. **Devinsky, O., Honigfeld, G. and Patin, J. (1991).** Clozapine-related seizures. *Neurology*, 41, 369–371.

54. **Pacia, S. V. and Devinsky, O. (1994).** Clozapine-related seizures: experience with 5,629 patients. *Neurology*, 44, 2247–2249.

55. **Williams, A. M. and Park, S. H. (2015).** Seizure associated with clozapine: incidence, etiology, and management. *CNS Drugs*, 29, 101–111.

56. **Acharya, S. and Bussel, J. B. (2000).** Hematologic toxicity of sodium valproate. *J Pediatr Hematol Oncol*, 22, 62–65.

57. **Malik, S., Lally, J., Ajnakina, O., *et al.* (2018).** Sodium valproate and clozapine induced neutropenia: a case control study using register data. *Schizophr Res*, 195, 267–273.

14 Risperidone Oral and Long-Acting Injectable; Paliperidone Oral and Long-Acting Injectable

QUICK CHECK

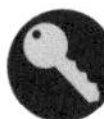

PRINCIPLES

- Risperidone and its active metabolite 9-OH risperidone (also known as paliperidone) are the most widely used second-generation antipsychotics worldwide. They provide an inexpensive method of delivering D_2 antagonism, with a well-developed literature on plasma levels to define a therapeutic threshold and estimate a point of futility.
- Laboratories routinely report 9-OH risperidone (paliperidone) levels when a risperidone level is ordered, allowing clinicians to calculate the metabolic ratio (MR). In CYP 2D6 extensive metabolizers, the ratio of risperidone to its metabolite is 0.2 on average (range 0.1–0.3).
- There are multiple long-acting injectable (LAI) preparations of risperidone and paliperidone with differing delivery systems and kinetics. Clinicians must be familiar with the kinetic properties of each LAI formulation they use, and the expected plasma levels of various dosages.

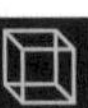

InfoBox Oral Risperidone and Paliperidone Plasma Level Essentials

	Oral dose correlation (bedtime dosing, 12h trough)	Level of evidence	Therapeutic threshold	Level of evidence	Point of futility	Level of evidence
Risperidone	10 mg = 70.0 ng/ml* **Multiply oral dose by 7.0 [1]** (see Table 14.1 for effects of CYP inhibitors/ inducers on this relationship)	High	15 ng/ml [2, 3, 4, 5, 6]	High	112 ng/ml [7, 2, 8, 9]	High
Paliperidone (9-OH risperidone)	10 mg = 40.9 ng/ml **Multiply oral dose by 4.09**** [10] (see Table 14.1 for effects of CYP inhibitors/ inducers on this relationship)	High	20 ng/ml [10]	High	90 ng/ml [11]	Moderate

* This value represents the active moiety, which is the sum of risperidone and 9-OH risperidone (paliperidone) levels. The mean steady state ratio of risperidone to 9-OH risperidone **(the metabolic ratio)** is 0.2 (range 0.1–0.3), or 1:5 [1]. The metabolic ratio (MR) is genetically determined and only modified by exposure to cytochrome P450 (CYP) inhibitors, CYP, or p-glycoprotein inducers. In those with CYP functional polymorphisms that influence risperidone metabolism, the MR may be higher (CYP 2D6 poor metabolizers), or lower (CYP 2D6 ultrarapid metabolizers), but this should not change during the course of treatment. Erratic timing of oral risperidone dosing with respect to the plasma level determination and nonadherence both alter the MR as more or less risperidone is metabolized.

From the mean ratio of 1:5 (i.e. 0.2) for risperidone and its metabolite, at steady state 1/6 of the active moiety will be risperidone, and 5/6 will be 9-OH risperidone. Below is an example:

Patient on 6 mg QHS of oral risperidone at steady state. The expected 12h trough plasma levels are as follows:

Risperidone level: 7 ng/ml
9–OH risperidone: 35 ng/ml
} Risperidone: 9–OH risperidone ratio is 0.2 (i.e. 1:5)

Active moiety level: 42 ng/ml. Total is 7.0 times the oral dose.

** Based on administration of oral paliperidone extended-release tablets. Studies find a range of 2.74–6.89, with the exception of outlying values from two Korean trials (2.57, 2.65) [10].

A Basic Pharmacokinetic Information for Oral and Long-Acting Injectable Risperidone and Paliperidone

Zotepine was approved in Japan in 1982, and is the first antipsychotic modeled on clozapine with relatively high serotonin $5HT_{2A}$ affinity, lower dopamine D_2 affinity, and a corresponding Positron Emission Tomography (PET) imaging profile that demonstrates wide separation between the $5HT_{2A}$ and D_2 occupancy curves in a manner unlike first-generation antipsychotics (FGAs) such as loxapine (see Chapter 11) [12–14]. Zotepine was never approved in the United States (US), Canada, the United Kingdom, Australia, or most European countries, leaving risperidone (US approval December 29, 1993) as the first commercially successful second-generation antipsychotic [15]. Risperidone and its active metabolite 9-OH risperidone (also known as paliperidone) are widely used due to the generally favorable tolerability profile and the presence of multiple long-acting injectable (LAI) formulations with a variety of technologies: impregnated microspheres, slowly dissolving esters, and a subcutaneously injected gel matrix [16–18]. Significant $5HT_{2A}$ antagonism lessens the risk of neurological adverse effects from D_2 antagonism compared to FGAs, and early PET studies employing risperidone were crucial in defining the optimal range of D_2 receptor occupancy for dopamine antagonist antipsychotics at 65%–80% [15, 19]. However, compared to FGAs, risperidone and paliperidone exert a disproportionate effect on serum prolactin levels relative to their D_2 affinity, and are the agents at highest risk of clinically significant hyperprolactinemia (Figure 14.1) [20]. This property often limits the use of risperidone or paliperidone, especially in first-episode schizophrenia patients who are sensitive to all forms of adverse effects related to D_2 antagonism. In a sample of 228 first-episode patients, sexual side effects were among the three biggest predictors of drug discontinuation [21]. The basis for this disproportionate impact on prolactin secretion relates to affinities for the p-glycoprotein (PGP) efflux transporter that are greater than every other antipsychotic [22–24]. Like all antipsychotics, risperidone and paliperidone are lipophilic molecules that diffuse into endothelial cells at the blood–brain barrier (BBB), but are actively transported back at high rates into the capillary lumen by PGP, creating extensive local recirculation before getting past the basal lamina and into the central nervous system (CNS) (Figure 14.2). The anterior pituitary is subjected to these locally high levels at the BBB resulting in an exaggerated effect on prolactin secretion beyond what one might expect for the D_2 affinity [25]. The same phenomenon also applies to amisulpride, resulting in a propensity to induce hyperprolactinemia close to that for risperidone/paliperidone (Figure 14.1)

Figure 14.1 Mean difference (MD) from placebo in serum prolactin levels during oral antipsychotic treatment for schizophrenia. Risperidone (RIS) and paliperidone (PAL) have the greatest effect [20]

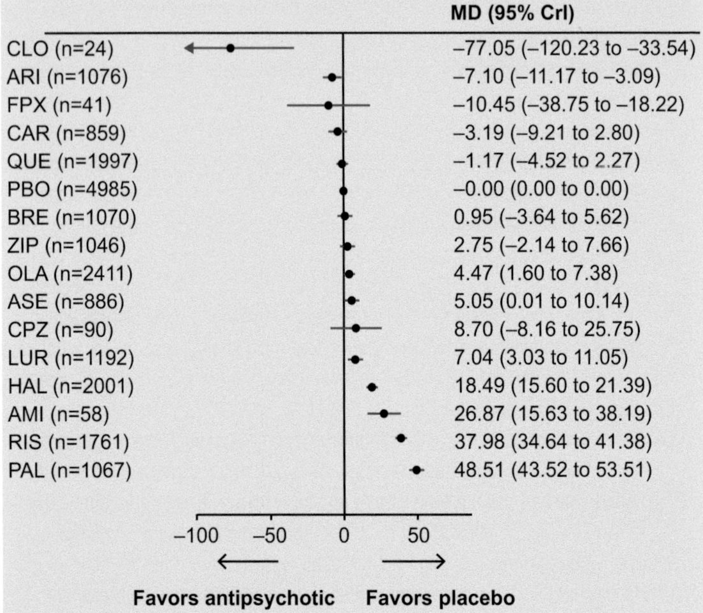

CLO - Clozapine; ARI - Aripiprazole; FPX - Flupenthixol; CAR - Cariprazine; QUE - Quetiapine; PBO - Placebo; BRE - Brexpiprazole; ZIP - Ziprasidone; OLA - Olanzapine; ASE - Asenapine; CPZ - Chlorpromazine; LUR - Lurasidone; HAL - Haloperidol; AMI - Amisulpride; RIS - Risperidone; PAL - Paliperidone

(Adapted from: M. Huhn, A. Nikolakopoulou, J. Schneider-Thoma, *et al.* [2019]. Comparative efficacy and tolerability of 32 oral antipsychotics for the acute treatment of adults with multi-episode schizophrenia: a systematic review and network meta-analysis. *Lancet*, 394, 939–951.)

[26]. Risperidone and paliperidone were assigned a Level 2 recommendation (recommended) for use of plasma level monitoring in the 2020 consensus paper authored jointly by the Therapeutic Drug Monitoring (TDM) task force of the German Arbeitsgemeinschaft für Neuropsychopharmakologie und Pharmakopsychiatrie (AGNP) and the American Society for Clinical Psychopharmacology (ASCP) [6].

Figure 14.2 Behavior of risperidone and paliperidone at the blood–brain barrier (BBB) [29]

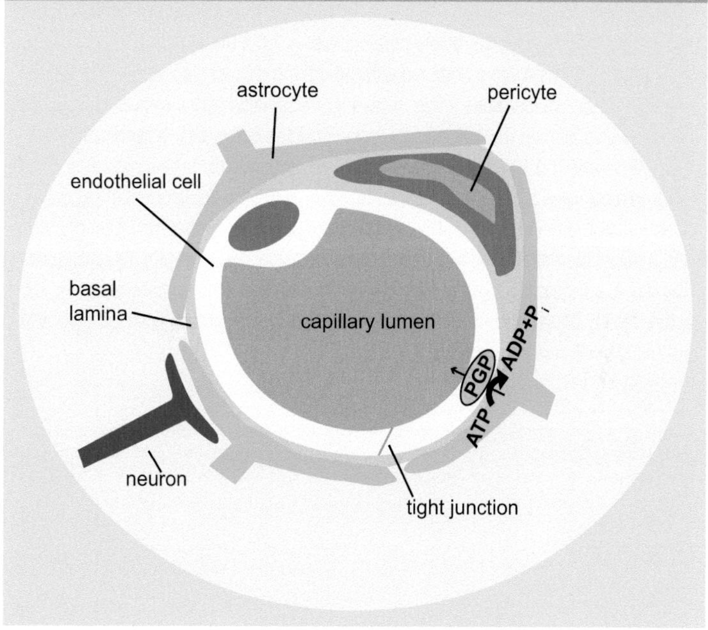

(Adapted from: F. E. O'Brien, T. G. Dinan, B. T. Griffin, *et al.* [2012]. Interactions between antidepressants and P-glycoprotein at the blood-brain barrier: clinical significance of in vitro and in vivo findings. *Br J Pharmacol*, 165, 289–312.)

B Essential Information for Oral and Long-Acting Injectable Risperidone and Paliperidone

1 Essential Oral Risperidone Information

Risperidone is metabolized primarily via cytochrome P450 (CYP) 2D6 to an active metabolite 9-OH risperidone (i.e. paliperidone) which has similar pharmacodynamic properties but a longer half-life. Due to the longer half-life of paliperidone, the steady state metabolic ratio (MR) of risperidone to paliperidone in CYP 2D6 extensive metabolizers is approximately 1:5 (i.e. 0.2, range 0.1–0.3) [1]. Since both molecules possess nearly equivalent antipsychotic activity, plasma levels are expressed as the

active moiety, which represents the sum of risperidone and paliperidone levels. As noted in the InfoBox and illustrated in Figure 14.3, there is an easily remembered mathematical relationship between the oral risperidone dose and the active moiety level: the 12h trough active moiety plasma level = 7.0 x the oral dose [1]. This easily remembered relationship, combined with the fact that most laboratories report both risperidone and paliperidone levels, provides the clinician with information about drug metabolism based on the MR. A lower than expected active moiety level combined with MR values < 0.1 can only imply one of two possibilities: (a) the patient is an ultrarapid metabolizer due to genetics (e.g. CYP 2D6 gene duplication) or exposure to an inducer (e.g. carbamazepine); or (b) the patient has missed the latest oral dose and most of the risperidone has been converted to paliperidone [30]. As discussed in Chapter 4, a repeat level will greatly clarify the situation. In an adherent patient, the active moiety plasma level will fluctuate < 30% between plasma level determinations but the MR will remain unchanged.

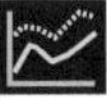

Figure 14.3 Relationship between the steady state risperidone active moiety level (risperidone + 9-OH risperidone levels) and oral risperidone dose [31]

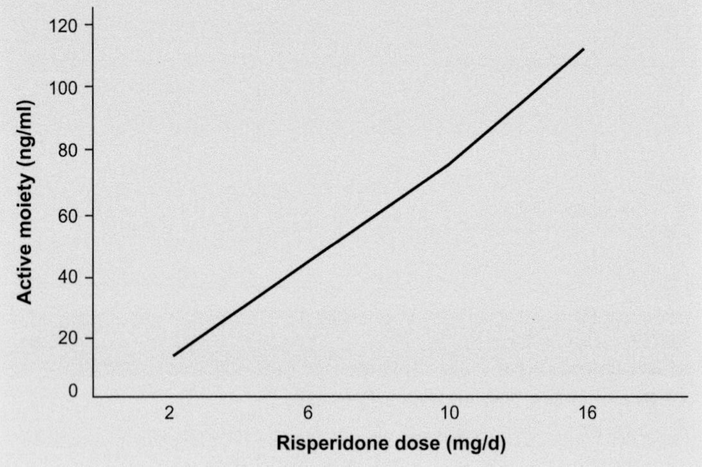

(Adapted from: J. de Leon, N. B. Sandson, and K. L. Cozza [2008]. A preliminary attempt to personalize risperidone dosing using drug–drug interactions and genetics, Part II. *Psychosomatics*, 48, 347–361.)

2 Essential Oral Paliperidone Information

There is no practical reason to use oral paliperidone, as 83% of the active moiety in patients receiving risperidone is the metabolite [1]. Paliperidone does have higher affinity for alpha$_1$-adrenergic receptors than risperidone, and orthostasis was an issue with immediate-release oral forms. Later studies used a proprietary extended-release osmotic pump, and some form of sustained-release mechanism exists in all approved generic versions of oral paliperidone [1]. Paliperidone is largely excreted unchanged, leading some clinicians to mistakenly believe it should be preferentially used in any patient with a liver function test abnormality. As discussed extensively in Chapter 3, this erroneous belief relates to the vague wording around hepatic dysfunction in older package labeling, and a fundamental misunderstanding regarding which types of liver function test abnormalities are associated with decreased drug metabolism. Modern antipsychotic labeling provides a precise definition for hepatic dysfunction using Child–Pugh criteria, the staging of which is calculated using total bilirubin, serum albumin, and the International Normalized Ratio (INR), along with two clinical features (hepatic encephalopathy, ascites) [32]. It is worth noting that the oral paliperidone package insert indicates it has not been studied in patients with severe hepatic impairment (Child–Pugh C) [27]. Oral paliperidone has much lower bioavailability than risperidone, so doses 2–2.5 times greater are needed to achieve comparable plasma levels and antipsychotic effect (Table 14.1) [33]. There is no compelling reason

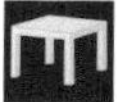

Table 14.1 Oral risperidone and paliperidone kinetic facts [27, 28]

	Basic facts	Inhibition effects	Induction effects
Risperidone	US FDA approval: Dec. 29, 1993 $T_{1/2}$ **Risperidone:** 3 hours, and 20 hours in CYP 2D6 poor metabolizers (PM) **9-OH risperidone:** 21 hours, and 30 hours in CYP 2D6 PM Absolute oral bioavailability: 70% T_{max} 1 and 3 hours for risperidone and 9-OH risperidone, respectively. In CYP 2D6 PM, T_{max} for 9-OH risperidone is 17 hours. Metabolism: CYP 2D6 **Formulations:** Tablets, oral dissolving tablets, liquid	2D6 converts risperidone to active metabolite 9-OH risperidone Strong CYP 2D6 inhibitors increase exposure to the active moiety (i.e. the AUC) by 1.5-fold (range 1.3–1.8) Strong CYP 3A4 inhibitors have no significant impact on active moiety levels	Carbamazepine decreases exposure to the active moiety (i.e. the AUC) by 49%

	Basic facts	Inhibition effects	Induction effects
Paliperidone (9-OH risperidone)	US FDA approval: Dec. 19, 2006 $T_{1/2}$ 23 hours [27] Absolute oral bioavailability: 28% [27] T_{max} 24 hours (extended-release oral tablet) Metabolism: 59% excreted unchanged, 32% appears as metabolites (primarily phase 2). 80% of elimination is renal, related to active excretion by the efflux transporter p-glycoprotein (PGP) **Formulations:** Extended-release oral tablet	No significant impact of CYP inhibitors At steady state (5 days), divalproex extended release 1000 mg once daily increased the AUC of paliperidone 12 mg by 50%	Carbamazepine use decreased steady state AUC by 37%

to use oral paliperidone before starting LAI paliperidone as the conversion to its LAI formulation can be easily achieved from oral risperidone using guidance provided in the manufacturer labeling and from the patient's active moiety plasma levels.

3 Essential Long-Acting Injectable Risperidone Information

Risperidone has two LAI formulations using very different technologies and with markedly different kinetic parameters. Risperidone microspheres was the first LAI second-generation antipsychotic available, approved in the US on October 29, 2003, and was also the first water-based LAI antipsychotic [34]. Risperidone embedded microspheres are composed of organic molecules often used in dissolving sutures (poly D, L-lactide-co-glycolide), and the powder is suspended in 2 ml sterile water for injection [34]. The doses studied in the pivotal trials were 25 mg, 50 mg, and 75 mg every 2 weeks, but the initial approved dosage range was 25–50 mg, with the 12.5 mg dose added later [35]. Dosages as high as 100 mg every 2 weeks have been studied (Table 14.3), but the cost of treatment for dosages above 50 mg is prohibitive, as 2 injections will be required every 2 weeks instead of one. Patients who require more D_2 antagonism despite maximal doses of risperidone microspheres (i.e. 50 mg/2 weeks) are candidates for an FGA LAI. Clinicians should obtain a trough active moiety level at steady state 3h–72h prior to the next injection to assess to what extent treatment failure may be related to kinetic factors (e.g. lower than expected plasma levels).

While this product represented a technological advance over oil-based FGA LAI formulations, the slow dissolution of the microspheres yielded several unfortunate kinetic properties: (a) the long T_{max} prevented any form of loading or initiation, so prolonged oral coverage is required at the outset of treatment (e.g. 3–4 weeks); (b) the long T_{max} meant that the effect of any dosage changes or missed doses was not seen for several weeks; and (c) the relatively short window of drug delivery to systemic circulation necessitated injections every 2 weeks (Figure 14.4) [36]. Another practical issue is the requirement that the kits remain refrigerated, creating storage issues for many clinics. Paliperidone palmitate was developed to overcome all of these issues with an equivalent monthly cost and a 3-month formulation, so the use of risperidone microspheres has essentially been abandoned. While the data in Table 14.3 provides the expected active moiety plasma levels for various risperidone microsphere dosages, there are large standard deviations around each mean level; any clinician who wishes to convert to paliperidone palmitate should obtain a trough active moiety level at steady state 3h–72h prior to the next risperidone microsphere injection, and not rely exclusively on the recommended conversion formulas in the paliperidone palmitate package insert [35, 37, 38]. From the active moiety level on risperidone microspheres, one can estimate the optimal monthly paliperidone palmitate dose using the formula in Table 14.4: the steady state trough paliperidone plasma level **= 0.1645 x monthly paliperidone palmitate dose** [39]. For example, 234 mg/month of paliperidone palmitate should yield a mean steady state level of 234 x 0.1645 = 38.5 ng/ml. Outside the US, dosages are based on the equivalent amount of paliperidone, not the total molecular mass of paliperidone palmitate. Thus, 156 mg of paliperidone palmitate = 100 mg paliperidone equivalent. The conversion ratio for doses outside the US now becomes **0.2566.** For 150 mg/month of paliperidone equivalent (which equals 234 mg of paliperidone palmitate), the mean steady state level is 150 x 0.2566 = 38.5 ng/ml.

Since risperidone is susceptible to the impact of CYP 2D6 inhibitors, lower dosages may be needed if concomitant use is contemplated with strong CYP 2D6 inhibitors for > 14 days (e.g. bupropion, fluoxetine, paroxetine). Conversely, dosages may need to be increased if a strong CYP 2D6 inhibitor is discontinued in a patient on established risperidone microsphere therapy [40]. The disposition of its metabolite paliperidone is influenced by use of strong CYP 3A4/PGP inducers (e.g. carbamazepine, phenytoin, phenobarbital), so the same concerns apply for concomitant use or subsequent discontinuation of an inducer. The easiest method of managing ongoing use or changes in exposure to strong CYP 2D6 inhibitors or strong CYP 3A4/PGP inducers is use of plasma active moiety levels, bearing in mind that fluoxetine's active metabolite norfluoxetine is also a strong CYP 2D6 inhibitor with a half-life of 7–14 days. The full kinetic impact of adding or stopping fluoxetine may not be realized for the five half-lives required for norfluoxetine to reach steady state, or 1–2 months.

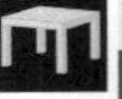

Table 14.2 Long-acting injectable risperidone and paliperidone essentials

	Vehicle	Concentration	Dosage	T_{max} (days)	$T_{1/2}$ (days) multiple dosing	Able to be loaded	Maintenance dose: oral equivalence
Risperidone microspheres	Water	All doses (12.5 mg, 25 mg, 37.5 mg, 50 mg) are reconstituted in 2 ml	12.5–50 mg/2 weeks **Max:** 50 mg/2 weeks	21	[a]	No	See Table 14.3
Risperidone subcutaneous	Water	90 mg: 0.6 ml 120 mg: 0.8 ml	90–120 mg/4 weeks **Max:** 120 mg/4 weeks	7–8 days	9–11 days	Not needed	See Figure 14.5
Paliperidone palmitate monthly[b]	Water	156 mg/ml (PP) (100 mg/ml paliperidone)	39–234 mg/4 weeks (25–150 mg/4 weeks) **Max:** 234 mg/4 weeks (150 mg/4 weeks)	13 days	25–49 days	Yes	See Table 14.4
Paliperidone palmitate 3-Month[b,c]	Water	312 mg/ml (PP) 200 mg/ml (paliperidone)	273–819 mg/12 weeks (175–525 mg/12 weeks) **Max:** 819 mg/12 weeks (525 mg/12 weeks)	84–95 days (deltoid) 118–139 days (gluteal)	30–33 days	No	[c]

PP = paliperidone palmitate

[a] Steady state plasma levels after 5 biweekly injections are maintained for 4–5 weeks, but decrease rapidly at that point with a mean half-life of 4–6 days [41].

[b] The dosages provided reflect the US label for the molecular weight of paliperidone palmitate. Outside the US, the paliperidone equivalent doses are in multiples of 25 mg, based on the conversion that 39 mg of paliperidone palmitate equals the equivalent of 25 mg paliperidone.

[c] Only for those on paliperidone palmitate monthly for at least 4 months. Cannot be converted from oral medication. The conversion from the stable dose of monthly paliperidone palmitate (PP) is below (the 39 mg PP dose was not studied). The 3-month formulation is delivered in lieu of the usual monthly dose once the patient has been on PP monthly for at least 4 months [42]:

Monthly PP dose	Monthly paliperidone equivalent	3-month PP dose	3-month paliperidone equivalent
78 mg	50 mg	273 mg	175 mg
117 mg	75 mg	410 mg	175 mg
156 mg	100 mg	546 mg	350 mg
234 mg	150 mg	819 mg	525 mg

(For further reading about use of LAI antipsychotics, please see the comprehensive edited book ***Antipsychotic Long-Acting Injections,*** now in its 2nd edition [43].)

Table 14.3 Risperidone microspheres biweekly dose and active moiety (± SD) plasma levels (ng/ml)

Dose	12-week study [37]	52-week study [35]	26-week study [38]	Daily oral risperidone equivalence
25 mg	18.7 ± 9.23	18.1 ± 16.1	–	2.63 mg
50 mg	35.5 ± 18.7	32.2 ± 18.0	29.6 ± 15.8	4.63 mg
75 mg	44.7 ± 20.6	47.4 ± 27.6	–	6.58 mg
100 mg	–	–	62.4 ± 38.0	8.91 mg

Figure 14.4 Model of active moiety levels (risperidone + 9-OH risperidone) showing the total (dark line) and the contribution of individual injections for risperidone microspheres 25 mg IM every 2 weeks, with no bridging oral therapy [36]

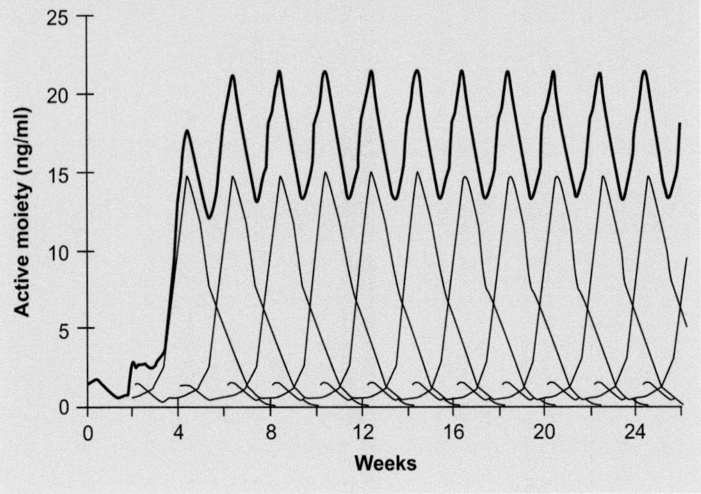

(Adapted from: W. H. Wilson [2004]. A visual guide to expected blood levels of long-acting injectable risperidone in clinical practice. *J Psychiatr Pract*, 10, 393–401.)

The most innovative departure from intramuscular LAI antipsychotic therapy was realized by the development of a monthly subcutaneous risperidone injectable, approved in the US on July 27, 2018 [44, 45]. The technology involved uses a biodegradable injectable polymer designed to deliver prolonged medication exposure after subcutaneous injection. This drug delivery system suspends and dissolves the medication of interest (in this case, risperidone) in a poly D, L-lactide-coglycolide gel and its biocompatible carrier using injection volumes < 1 ml for the currently approved dosages [46]. The viscous liquid undergoes a phase transition upon contact with tissue fluids after subcutaneous injection, resulting in an implant that releases risperidone in a controlled manner as it is resorbed. Importantly, the kinetic parameters are such that effective drug levels are seen within the first week without the need for oral coverage, and the injections are monthly [18, 47]. The kinetics for risperidone subcutaneous are thus markedly different than those for risperidone microspheres. After a single subcutaneous injection, there are two absorption peaks: the initial lower peak occurs with a T_{max} of 4–6 hours due to release of risperidone during the implant formation process; a second higher peak occurs after 10–14 days, associated with slow release from the subcutaneous depot (Figure 14.5) [18, 48, 49]. The median active moiety T_{max} of the 2nd peak ranges from 7 to 11 days, very similar to that for many other

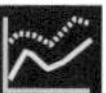

Figure 14.5 Risperidone and 9-OH risperidone levels following subcutaneous risperidone injections on day 1 and day 29 [45]

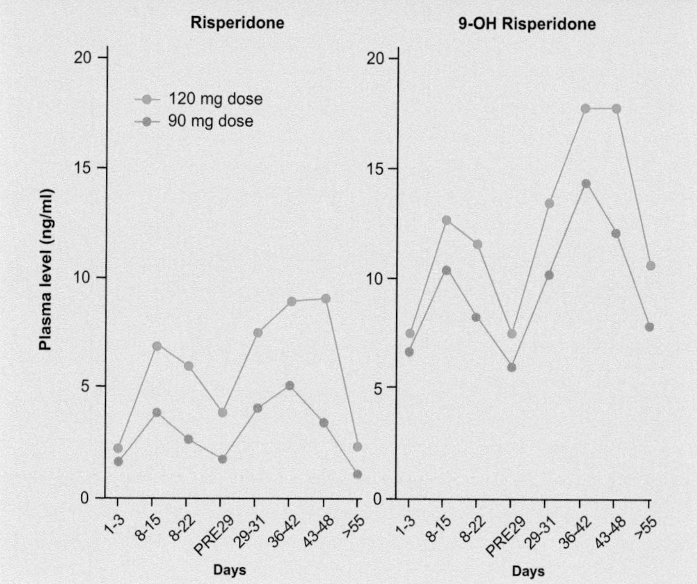

(Adapted from: V. Ivaturi, M. Gopalakrishnan, J. V. S. Gobburu, *et al.* [2017]. Exposure-response analysis after subcutaneous administration of RBP-7000, a once-a-month long-acting Atrigel formulation of risperidone. *Br J Clin Pharmacol*, 83, 1476–1498.)

14

LAI antipsychotics. Based on population pharmacokinetic modeling, the 90 mg and 120 mg subcutaneous doses are estimated to provide drug exposure equivalent to 3 mg/d and 4 mg/d of oral risperidone, respectively [18, 48, 49]. The cost of treatment for dosages above 120 mg is prohibitive as two injections will be required every 4 weeks, instead of one; however, the manufacturer is pursuing studies of a 180 mg risperidone subcutaneous injection, equivalent to 6 mg/d of oral risperidone.

While it has obvious kinetic advantages over the microsphere formulation, the gel is administered as an abdominal subcutaneous injection which poses some unique issues. One issue is the need for the patient to lie flat to gauge the proper depth and site of the abdominal injection. This requires both privacy and an exam table or other acceptable alternative. The other issue is that the firmed gel implant will be felt as a lump for several weeks which slowly decreases in size over time. It is important that the patient be educated that this is normal, and is also instructed not to rub or massage the injection site and to be aware of the placement of any belts or clothing waistbands [36]. In a manner identical to that with risperidone microspheres, the impact of strong CYP 2D6 inhibitors and strong CYP 3A4/PGP inducers, and effects of the addition or discontinuation of those agents, must be taken into account [50]. In particular, the labeling notes that strong CYP 3A4/PGP inducers may lower plasma active moiety levels to the extent that supplemental oral risperidone is required [50]. The effects of discontinuing strong CYP 2D6 inhibitors have not been studied so monitoring of active moiety plasma levels before and after will guide the need for dosing adjustments. The same rule applies for discontinuation of strong CYP 3A4/PGP inducers. As noted above, the full kinetic impact of adding or stopping fluoxetine may not be realized for the five half-lives required for norfluoxetine to reach steady state, or 1–2 months.

4 Essential Long-Acting Injectable Paliperidone Information

Paliperidone palmitate is an ester of risperidone's active metabolite delivered in a water-based intramuscular injection, and approved in the US on July 31, 2009 [51]. Paliperidone palmitate does not require refrigeration, is administered initially as a monthly injection, has a large range of dosages, and has a T_{max} of 13 days, permitting the use of a loading regimen to initiate therapy. The paliperidone palmitate standard loading regimen involves injections of 234 mg and 156 mg (equal to 150 mg and 100 mg of paliperidone equivalent) administered in the deltoid muscle (not the gluteus) one week apart; the deltoid site is utilized as it is more vascular with maximal plasma levels 28% higher than with gluteal injections (Table 14.4, Figure 14.6) [51]. This higher level of paliperidone exposure is important ***only*** during the early weeks

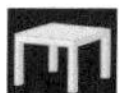

Table 14.4 Paliperidone palmitate monthly dose and plasma (ng/ml) in a 13-week trial [52]

PP dose (paliperidone equivalent)	Days	N	Mean	SD	Median	25th percentile	75th percentile	Daily oral risperidone equivalence at steady state[a]
39 mg (25 mg)	92	78	10.2	8.5	8.9	5.7	11.1	0.92 mg (~ 1 mg)
156 mg (100 mg)	92	84	21.0	13.0	18.6	10.8	25.5	3.67 mg (~ 4 mg)
234 mg (150 mg)	92	88	28.4	14.9	27.0	16.1	35.1	5.51 mg (~ 6 mg)

PP = paliperidone palmitate

[a] **Steady state plasma level estimate:** from three long-term studies (n = 69) the steady state trough paliperidone plasma level **= 0.1645 x monthly paliperidone palmitate dose** [39]. (The conversion ratio for doses outside the US now is **0.2566.** For 150 mg/month of paliperidone equivalent [which equals 234 mg of paliperidone palmitate], the mean steady state level is 150 x 0.2566 = 38.5 ng/ml.)

Example:

A patient on a monthly paliperidone palmitate dose of 156 mg would be expected to have a steady state level of 156 x 0.1645 = 25.66 ng/ml.

Using the conversion formula from the risperidone active moiety, 25.66/7.0 = 3.67 mg/d oral risperidone (approximately 4 mg/d).

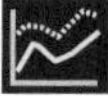

Figure 14.6 Paliperidone palmitate kinetics following initiation with deltoid injections of 234 mg (150 mg paliperidone equivalent) on day 1, and 156 mg (100 mg paliperidone equivalent) on day 8 [17]

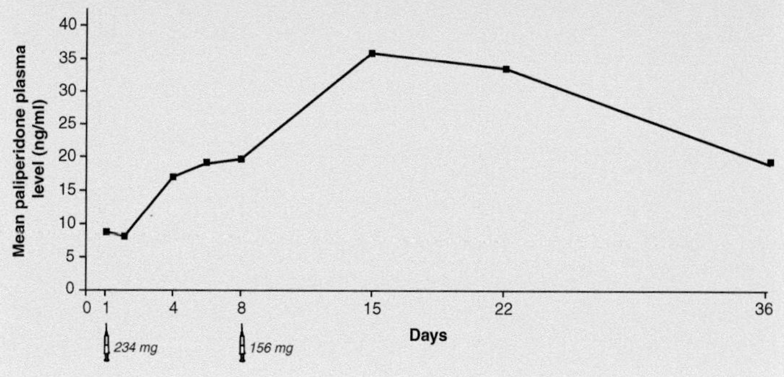

(Adapted from: M. N. Samtani, A. Vermeulen, and K. Stuyckens [2009]. Population pharmacokinetics of intramuscular paliperidone palmitate in patients with schizophrenia: a novel once-monthly, long-acting formulation of an atypical antipsychotic. *Clin Pharmacokinet*, 48, 585–600.)

14

of therapy to obviate the need for oral coverage. Subsequent injections can use the gluteal site if preferred, since the difference in exposure becomes less discernible over time. As the metabolite of risperidone, paliperidone is not influenced by CYP 2D6 factors, but is affected by exposure to strong CYP 3A4/PGP inducers. If the latter are needed for > 14 days, supplemental oral risperidone may be required since renal paliperidone excretion is increased by 35% [51]. Conversely, downwards dosage adjustment of paliperidone palmitate may be needed in a patient on established concomitant therapy with a strong CYP 3A4/PGP inducer that is subsequently discontinued. As always, these situations are best managed by use of plasma antipsychotic levels before and after the change in inducer exposure.

To extend coverage, a larger-particle sized formulation of paliperidone palmitate was created to permit a 3-month injection cycle, and was approved in the US on May 18, 2015. As noted in Table 14.2, the T_{max} is 3 months or longer, and therefore the 3-month injection is only suitable for those patients who have been on the monthly formulation of paliperidone palmitate for at least 4 months, and are therefore at steady state (Figure 14.7) [42]. The half-life of monthly paliperidone palmitate is sufficiently long that it provides antipsychotic coverage during the early weeks of the

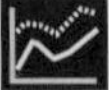

Figure 14.7 Plasma paliperidone levels following 4 months of paliperidone palmitate treatment 234 mg (150 mg paliperidone equivalent) transitioning to 819 mg (525 mg paliperidone equivalent) of the 3-month formulation on week 17

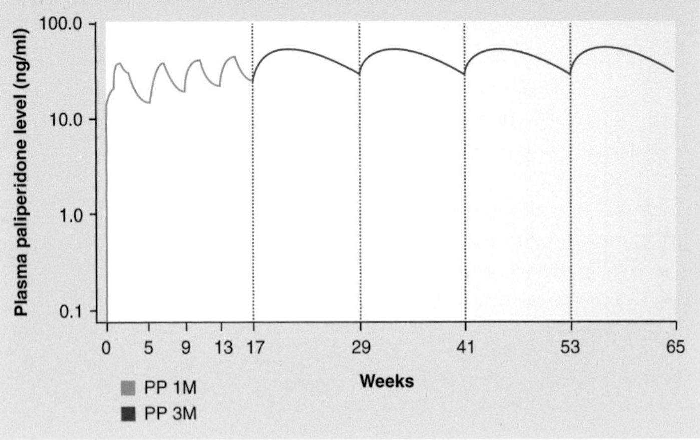

(Janssen Pharmaceutica, data on file.)

3-month injection cycle. Patients are given the 3-month formulation in lieu of the next 1-month paliperidone palmitate dose using the conversion chart (Table 14.2) [42]. Since paliperidone is the active ingredient, the 3-month formulation is susceptible to the same effects of strong CYP 3A4/PGP inducers as the 1-month preparation, and the same considerations apply during concurrent use, or after discontinuation of the inducer [42].

The Therapeutic Threshold for Risperidone and Paliperidone

1 Clinical Evidence for a Therapeutic Threshold for Risperidone

Clinical evidence, especially from fixed-dose, prospective, randomized trials, is the most important tool we have for estimation of plasma level response thresholds (see Chapter 2). By 1995, two large fixed-dose studies had been performed (total n = 1573), although this data was never analyzed mathematically using receiver operating characteristic (ROC) curves as discussed in Chapter 2 [53–55]. Nonetheless, Dr. Niina Ezewuzie (Clinical Pharmacist, Maudsley Hospital, London) and Dr. David Taylor (Chief Pharmacist, Maudsley Hospital, London) provided a review of these fixed-dose trials which graphically depicts a cutpoint for response between 3 and 4 mg/d of oral risperidone, based on a response definition of 20% symptom reduction (Figure 14.8) [7]. It should be noted that 3 mg was not an assigned dose in any of these studies: one trial (with data published separately for Canadian and US cohorts) employed arms of 2 mg, 6 mg, 10 mg, or 16 mg per day [53, 54], and one study used daily doses of 1 mg, 4 mg, 8 mg, 12 mg, or 16 mg [55]. The absence of information at 3 mg does limit the ability to detect a signal for response in this region; moreover, all of these studies were performed in chronic schizophrenia patients, so their conclusion that 2 mg is not as effective as higher dosages may not apply to the treatment of first-episode (FE) schizophrenia. Evidence for the latter assertion comes from results of an 8-week, randomized, double-blind, fixed-dose study of risperidone 2 mg/d versus 4 mg/d in 49 FE patients [56]. In that trial, the two doses proved equally effective on measures of psychiatric response, but the 2 mg/d dose group experienced significantly fewer neurological adverse effects at 8 weeks. No significant correlations to the plasma active moiety level were found for changes in psychopathology or fine motor function in this FE study.

In 2014, Stefan Leucht, a Professor of Psychiatry at Technische Universität in Munich, performed an updated analysis of 12 fixed-dose risperidone trials to determine a minimum effective dose [4]. This comprehensive examination of the clinical trials data expanded the pool of studies using the 4 mg/d dose, but not for lower dosages. The primary criterion to define a minimum effective dose was that

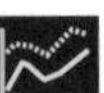

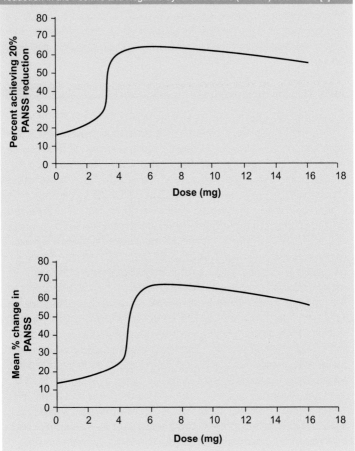

Figure 14.8 Analysis of fixed-dose risperidone studies by responders, or by reduction in the Positive and Negative Syndrome Scale (PANSS) total score [7]

(Adapted from: N. Ezewuzie and D. Taylor [2006]. Establishing a dose-response relationship for oral risperidone in relapsed schizophrenia. *J Psychopharmacol*, 20, 86–90.)

the dose was statistically significantly superior to placebo in one double-blind, randomized controlled trial (RCT), with a sensitivity analysis requiring positive results from a second RCT. Since certain lower dosages may have been studied in smaller samples, the authors meta-analyzed the results of low doses when available [4]. Their conclusions were very similar to the earlier analysis by Ezewuzie and Taylor: 4 mg/d meets the criteria for the minimum effective dose, using the sensitivity analysis that demands separation from placebo in two RCTs; the 2 mg/d dose only separated in the Canadian arm of the pivotal trial, but not the US arm, so it qualified as the minimum effective dose based on the less stringent definition of separation from placebo in one RCT [4]. A 2009 Cochrane analysis examining risperidone dosing for schizophrenia also stated bluntly in their summary conclusions: "Ultra low dose (< 2 mg/day) seemed useless" [57].

Unfortunately, there is a paucity of plasma level data from which to draw definitive conclusions, leaving one to infer the plasma level response threshold from the doses. Using the conversion that the active moiety plasma level is 7.0 times the oral dose, one arrives at a range of 14.0–28.0 ng/ml as a threshold for response to risperidone. This corresponds to the conclusions in the AGNP/ASCP consensus paper that sets a lower bound of the active moiety therapeutic range at 20 ng/ml, although their rationale for choosing that value is not explicitly delineated [6]. It is worth noting that a plasma active moiety level of 20 ng/ml corresponds almost exactly to 3 mg of oral risperidone.

2 Imaging Evidence for a Therapeutic Threshold for Risperidone

There are numerous risperidone PET imaging studies to identify the plasma level achieving 65% striatal D_2 occupancy, the level of D_2 blockade that corresponds to the response threshold for dopamine antagonist antipsychotics [58]. Figure 14.9 presents a representative picture of these results, indicating that 65% D_2 occupancy appears to occur at an active moiety level between 20 and 30 ng/ml [2]. From the imaging data, one can better estimate the plasma level associated with 65% D_2 occupancy using the calculated concentration that results in 50% receptor occupancy (the EC_{50}) [3]. The EC_{50} values from earlier studies ranged from 9.9 ng/ml to 11.06 ng/ml, with a mean value of 10.48 ng/ml [59, 41, 2, 8]. From those studies, the active moiety plasma level needed to achieve 65% D_2 occupancy is 19.5 ng/ml, equivalent to 2.8 mg/d oral risperidone. Complicating this picture is a 2011 paper which pooled the available data for risperidone-treated subjects with schizophrenia spectrum disorders in an attempt to more accurately characterize the EC_{50}, and by extension the response threshold

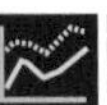

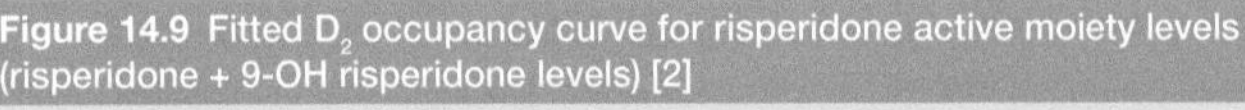

Figure 14.9 Fitted D_2 occupancy curve for risperidone active moiety levels (risperidone + 9-OH risperidone levels) [2]

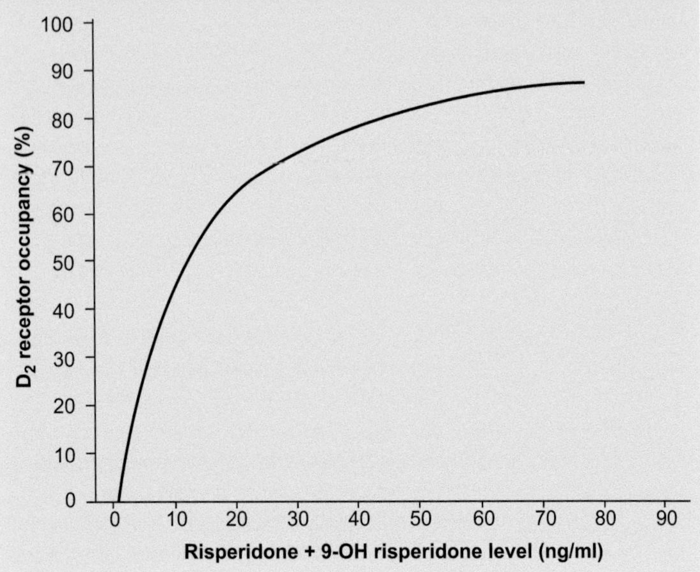

Adapted from: G. Remington, D. Mamo, A. Labelle, *et al.* [2006]. A PET study evaluating dopamine D2 receptor occupancy for long-acting injectable risperidone. *Am J Psychiatry*, 163, 396–401.)

[3]. When the maximal D_2 receptor occupancy for the active moiety was calculated at 88.0% ± 2.1% using an unconstrained, one site occupancy model, the estimated EC_{50} was a much lower value of 4.9 ng/ml; however, when the maximal occupancy was constrained to 100%, the estimated EC_{50} was 8.2 ng/ml [3]. Using the EC_{50} value of 4.9 ng/ml, the 65% D_2 occupancy threshold is 9.1 ng/ml, equivalent to an oral dose of only 1.3 mg/d; however, using the EC_{50} value of 8.2 ng/ml, the 65% D_2 occupancy threshold is 15.23 ng/ml, equivalent to an oral dose of 2.2 mg/d. While the authors assert that the data were better explained by the unconstrained model, the absence of any positive clinical data for oral risperidone doses < 2 mg/d calls the low EC_{50} estimate of 4.9 ng/ml into question. The constrained EC_{50} appears consistent with the clinical data as analyzed by Leucht in 2014, and places the response threshold at 15 ng/ml.

3 Clinical Evidence for a Therapeutic Threshold for Paliperidone

In the 2014 paper on minimum effective doses, Leucht found seven fixed-dose, placebo-controlled paliperidone trials at doses between 1.5 and 15 mg/d [4]. While no ROC analysis was performed, Leucht found that a daily paliperidone dose of 6 mg met criteria for a minimum effective dose using the sensitivity analysis that demands separation from placebo in two RCTs; the 3 mg/d dose did separate in one trial, and qualified as a minimum effective dose with the less stringent definition of separation from placebo in one RCT. Although the 3 mg dose did meet the lesser threshold, this corresponds to what appears to be an ineffective oral risperidone dose of ≤ 1.5 mg/d, so a minimum oral paliperidone dose in the range of 4.5–6 mg/d appears more consistent with the accumulated clinical data on risperidone and paliperidone. Using the plasma level conversion factor of 4.09 for oral paliperidone, the response threshold is likely in the range of 18–24 ng/ml [10]. It is also worth noting that the manufacturer-recommended monthly maintenance dose of paliperidone palmitate for schizophrenia is 117 mg (equivalent to 75 mg paliperidone), which corresponds to a plasma level of 19.25 ng/ml [39, 51]. As with risperidone, the aggregated information is consistent with the AGNP/ASCP consensus paper that sets a lower bound for the paliperidone therapeutic range at 20 ng/ml, although their rationale for choosing that value is not explicitly delineated [6].

4 Imaging Evidence for a Therapeutic Threshold for Paliperidone

Paliperidone has higher affinity for the PGP efflux transporter than does risperidone, so the relationship between peripheral plasma levels and striatal D_2 occupancy will not necessarily be identical for the active moiety plasma level achieved from risperidone treatment and for plasma paliperidone levels from directly administered paliperidone. Unfortunately, there is relatively limited data correlating paliperidone plasma levels and D_2 occupancy. In a small study of healthy volunteers administered single oral doses of immediate release (1 mg, n = 3) or extended release (6 mg, n = 4) paliperidone, the estimated plasma level to achieve 65% D_2 receptor occupancy was 9.1 ng/ml [60]. A more generalizable estimate can be gleaned from a study of 13 male schizophrenia patients imaged at steady state on stable oral paliperidone doses ranging from 3 to 15 mg/d [11]. The investigators calculated EC_{50} at 6.65 ng/ml, which translates to a plasma level of 12.4 ng/ml to achieve 65% D_2 receptor occupancy, a level identical to that achievable with 3 mg/d oral risperidone (Figure 14.10) [11, 10]. Given the sparse PET data in schizophrenia patients, greater weight should be given to the plasma level response thresholds derived from clinical studies rather than one inferred from a single study of 13 subjects.

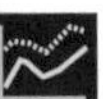

Figure 14.10 Fitted D_2 occupancy curve for plasma paliperidone levels from paliperidone oral dosing [11]

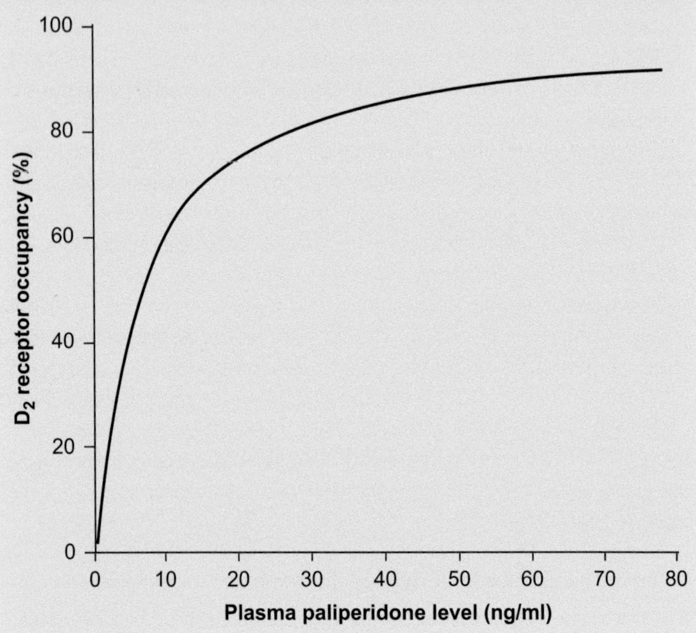

(Adapted from: R. Arakawa, H. Ito, A. Takano, *et al.* [2008]. Dose-finding study of paliperidone ER based on striatal and extrastriatal dopamine D2 receptor occupancy in patients with schizophrenia. *Psychopharmacology*, 197, 229–235.)

The Point of Futility for Risperidone and Paliperidone

1 Clinical Evidence for a Point of Futility for Risperidone

As with most potent D_2 antagonists, a trial of risperidone may be terminated due to neurological adverse effects associated with excessive D_2 blockade ***for that patient*** (see Chapter 5 for discussion of clinical endpoints). Defining the point of futility addresses an important question for treating extremely ill schizophrenia patients, and creates an easily understood concept: further titration beyond this point is of limited value with an estimated < 5% chance of response (Chapter 2). For first-generation antipsychotics, the point of futility typically appears when more than 90%

of patients find treatment intolerable, and this correlates with > 90% D_2 receptor occupancy. Risperidone is a potent serotonin $5HT_{2A}$ antagonist, and thus possesses an inherent mechanism to mitigate neurological adverse effects despite high levels of D_2 occupancy [33]. This improved adverse effect profile compared to FGAs alters the assumed relationship between D_2 occupancy and the point where 90% or more of subjects experience intolerability. One method of analyzing the clinical trials data was discussed in Chapter 2, and involves identifying antipsychotic doses that produce 95% of the maximum symptom reduction in chronic schizophrenia patients with acute exacerbation [61]. While this is not the same as identifying the dose at which probability of response in nonresponders is < 5%, it does provide some useful information. Professor Leucht's 2020 meta-analysis of 68 placebo-controlled, dose-finding antipsychotic studies noted that the daily risperidone dose which produces 95% of expected possible symptom reduction is 6.3 mg/d [61]. The risperidone result of 6.3 mg maps very closely to the plasma level associated with 80% D_2 occupancy, and indicates that for many patients higher dosages might not yield greater symptom reduction. However, many patients are not average, and not only tolerate higher levels of D_2 antagonism without neurological adverse effects, but require this level of D_2 blockade for optimal positive symptom control.

Another way to address the question of the point of futility is to examine the results from the early fixed-dose studies, three of which included arms with risperidone 16 mg/d, a dose that vastly exceeds the active moiety exposure provided by approved doses of LAI risperidone or studied with oral or LAI paliperidone. As noted in the InfoBox and graphed in Figure 14.3, the estimated active moiety plasma level for risperidone 16 mg/d is 16 x 7.0 = 112 ng/ml. A responder analysis for the three trials noted risperidone 16 mg/d consistently underperformed lower dosages in the range of 4–8 mg/d, bearing in mind that in clinical practice a candidate for 16 mg/d would be an individual who tolerates and fails to respond to lower dosages. In the international study (n = 1362), the highest response rate (defined as ≥ 20% decrease in the Positive and Negative Syndrome Scale [PANSS]) was seen in the risperidone 4 mg and 8 mg groups (63.4% and 65.8%); however, the response rate was only slightly lower, at 58.7%, for the 16 mg cohort [55]. The pivotal North American trials reported US and Canadian data separately. In the US study (n = 388) the highest response rate (defined as ≥ 20% decrease in the Brief Psychiatric Rating Scale [BPRS]) was seen in the risperidone 6 mg group (57%), but was comparable, at 54%, for the 16 mg arm [54]. For the Canadian study (n = 135), the highest response rate (defined as ≥ 20% decrease in BPRS) was seen in the risperidone 6 mg group (45%), but for the 16 mg cohort it was only 21% [53]. Using the need for antiparkinsonian medication as a proxy for intolerability, the rates for 16 mg/d were 26%, 39%, and 50% for the international, US, and Canadian studies, respectively [53–55]. Study dropout rates reflect a complex mixture of inefficacy and intolerability, but were consistent across risperidone dosages from 1 to 16 mg, comparable to haloperidol 10 mg in the international study, and significantly lower than for haloperidol 20 mg in the North American studies [53–55]. The 16 mg/d dose thus appears tolerable to 50% or more of patients even without extended titration to assess tolerability, but the clinical trials data unfortunately do not provide an exact answer to the question regarding the proportion of patients who might respond to dosages above 16 mg/d.

2 Imaging Evidence for a Point of Futility for Risperidone

Given the limitations from the clinical trials data, identification of the plasma level associated with 90% D_2 receptor occupancy becomes an acceptable substitute for a point of futility. Extrapolating from the graphical depiction in Figure 14.9, one can estimate that an active moiety level of 112 ng/ml generates at least 90% D_2 blockade; however, a more accurate assessment can be calculated using the EC_{50}. The 2011 paper arrived at an EC_{50} of 8.2 ng/ml when the maximal occupancy was constrained to 100%, and earlier papers found a mean EC_{50} of 10.48 ng/ml [59, 41, 2, 3, 8]. With an active moiety level of 112 ng/ml, the estimated D_2 occupancy for these two EC_{50} values ranges from 91% to 93%. As there is no evidence that dosages > 16 mg/d are more effective in nonresponders, the 112 ng/ml active moiety plasma level emerges as a reasonable point to consider other antipsychotic options (e.g. clozapine), based on the expectation that > 90% D_2 occupancy has been achieved. This corresponds very closely to the AGNP/ASCP laboratory alert level of 120 ng/ml (see Chapter 2 for discussion of the AGNP/ASCP definition for the laboratory alert level) [6].

3 Clinical Evidence for a Point of Futility for Paliperidone

There is no data on high-dose paliperidone exposure from which to draw conclusions about a point of futility, or to arrive at any estimate that might differ substantially from the estimates for risperidone. Pharmacokinetic modeling studies indicate that the 90% prediction interval for patients on the maximum monthly dose of paliperidone palmitate 234 mg (150 mg paliperidone equivalent) might extend to 100 ng/ml, but there is no systematic data on psychiatric response or tolerability outcomes at that level [62]. As with risperidone, imaging data is more instructive as it permits estimation of a plasma level associated with > 90% D_2 receptor occupancy.

4 Imaging Evidence for a Point of Futility for Paliperidone

With the absence of high plasma level clinical data, one is left to estimate a point of futility by calculating the paliperidone plasma level needed for 90% receptor occupancy from the EC_{50} value (6.65 ng/ml) obtained in schizophrenia patients [11]. From that EC_{50} estimate, the calculated paliperidone plasma level to achieve 90% D_2 receptor occupancy is 60 ng/ml. Given the lack of other EC_{50} estimates in schizophrenia patients, the similar pharmacodynamic properties for risperidone and paliperidone, and the significant discrepancy between this finding and that found with risperidone exposure, the value arrived at for the risperidone active moiety should be given greater weight and used in clinical practice. The AGNP/ASCP consensus paper also lists the same laboratory alert level of 120 ng/ml for paliperidone as for risperidone (see Chapter 2 for discussion of the AGNP/ASCP definition for the laboratory alert level) [6].

Summary Points

a Risperidone is the most widely used second-generation antipsychotic, with a wealth of information on dosing and expected plasma levels. The active metabolite 9-OH risperidone (paliperidone) is reported by most laboratories, and this permits calculation of the active moiety level (the sum of risperidone + paliperidone) and the ratio of risperidone to paliperidone. The latter can be used to assess risperidone drug metabolism. Both risperidone and paliperidone are the antipsychotics with the highest risk for hyperprolactinemia.

b Risperidone is available in two LAI formulations, with the older risperidone microspheres largely avoided due to its kinetic limitations. The subcutaneous formulation requires no loading or oral bridging coverage.

c There is no reason to use oral paliperidone, but the LAI paliperidone palmitate has a well-defined loading regimen and a 3-month formulation for those who have been on the monthly version for at least 4 months.

d The therapeutic threshold of 15 ng/ml for risperidone is consistent with clinical and imaging data, and is very close to the estimate for paliperidone (20 ng/ml), noting that there is much less data for the latter. The point of futility for risperidone is less well defined, but is estimated to be around 112 ng/ml for the active moiety (corresponding to 16 mg/d of oral risperidone), based on the PET data that associates this level with > 90% D_2 occupancy. There is no data for high plasma levels of paliperidone, and very limited imaging data. Given the similar pharmacodynamic properties for risperidone and paliperidone, the point of futility for the risperidone active moiety should be used for management of paliperidone-treated schizophrenia patients.

References

1. **de Leon, J., Wynn, G., and Sandson, N. B. (2010).** The pharmacokinetics of paliperidone versus risperidone. *Psychosomatics*, 51, 80–88.
2. **Remington, G., Mamo, D., Labelle, A., *et al.* (2006).** A PET study evaluating dopamine D2 receptor occupancy for long-acting injectable risperidone. *Am J Psychiatry*, 163, 396–401.
3. **Uchida, H., Takeuchi, H., Graff-Guerrero, A., *et al.* (2011).** Predicting dopamine D2 receptor occupancy from plasma levels of antipsychotic drugs: a systematic review and pooled analysis. *J Clin Psychopharmacol*, 31, 318–325.
4. **Leucht, S., Samara, M., Heres, S., *et al.* (2014).** Dose equivalents for second-generation antipsychotics: the minimum effective dose method. *Schizophr Bull*, 40, 314–326.
5. **Schoretsanitis, G., Spina, E., Hiemke, C., *et al.* (2017).** A systematic review and combined analysis of therapeutic drug monitoring studies for long-acting risperidone. *Expert Rev Clin Pharmacol*, 10, 965–981.
6. **Schoretsanitis, G., Kane, J. M., Correll, C. U., *et al.* (2020).** Blood levels to optimize antipsychotic treatment in clinical practice; a joint consensus statement of the American Society of Clinical Psychopharmacology (ASCP) and the Therapeutic Drug Monitoring (TDM) Task Force of the Arbeitsgemeinschaft für Neuropsychopharmakologie und Pharmakopsychiatrie (AGNP). *J Clin Psychiatry*, 81, https://doi.org/10.4088/JCP.4019cs13169.
7. **Ezewuzie, N. and Taylor, D. (2006).** Establishing a dose-response relationship for oral risperidone in relapsed schizophrenia. *J Psychopharmacol*, 20, 86–90.
8. **Ikai, S., Remington, G., Suzuki, T., *et al.* (2012).** A cross-sectional study of plasma risperidone levels with risperidone long-acting injectable: implications for dopamine D2 receptor occupancy during maintenance treatment in schizophrenia. *J Clin Psychiatry*, 73, 1147–1152.
9. **Meyer, J. M. (2014).** A rational approach to employing high plasma levels of antipsychotics for violence associated with schizophrenia: case vignettes. *CNS Spectr*, 19, 432–438.
10. **Schoretsanitis, G., Spina, E., Hiemke, C., *et al.* (2018).** A systematic review and combined analysis of therapeutic drug monitoring studies for oral paliperidone. *Expert Rev Clin Pharmacol*, 11, 625–639.
11. **Arakawa, R., Ito, H., Takano, A., *et al.* (2008).** Dose-finding study of paliperidone ER based on striatal and extrastriatal dopamine D2 receptor occupancy in patients with schizophrenia. *Psychopharmacology*, 197, 229–235.
12. **Kapur, S., Zipursky, R., Remington, G., *et al.* (1997).** PET evidence that loxapine is an equipotent blocker of 5-HT2 and D2 receptors: implications for the therapeutics of schizophrenia. *Am J Psychiatry*, 154, 1525–1529.
13. **Barnas, C., Quiner, S., Tauscher, J., *et al.* (2001).** In vivo (123)I IBZM SPECT imaging of striatal dopamine 2 receptor occupancy in schizophrenic patients. *Psychopharmacology (Berl)*, 157, 236–242.
14. **Tauscher, J., Kufferle, B., Asenbaum, S., *et al.* (2002).** Striatal dopamine-2 receptor occupancy as measured with [123I]iodobenzamide and SPECT predicted the occurrence of EPS in patients treated with atypical antipsychotics and haloperidol. *Psychopharmacology*, 162, 42–49.
15. **Nyberg, S., Farde, L., Eriksson, L., *et al.* (1993).** 5-HT2 and D2 dopamine receptor occupancy in the living human brain: a PET study with risperidone. *Psychopharmacology*, 110, 265–272.
16. **Ereshefsky, L. and Mascarenas, C. A. (2003).** Comparison of the effects of different routes of antipsychotic administration on pharmacokinetics and pharmacodynamics. *J Clin Psychiatry*, 64, 18–23.
17. **Samtani, M. N., Vermeulen, A., and Stuyckens, K. (2009).** Population pharmacokinetics of intramuscular paliperidone palmitate in patients with schizophrenia: a novel once-monthly, long-acting formulation of an atypical antipsychotic. *Clin Pharmacokinet*, 48, 585–600.

18. **Gomeni, R., Heidbreder, C., Fudala, P. J., *et al.* (2013).** A model-based approach to characterize the population pharmacokinetics and the relationship between the pharmacokinetic and safety profiles of RBP-7000, a new, long-acting, sustained-released formulation of risperidone. *J Clin Pharmacol*, 53, 1010–1019.
19. **Kapur, S., Zipursky, R. B., and Remington, G. (1999).** Clinical and theoretical implications of 5-HT2 and D2 receptor occupancy of clozapine, risperidone, and olanzapine in schizophrenia. *Am J Psychiatry*, 156, 286–293.
20. **Huhn, M., Nikolakopoulou, A., Schneider-Thoma, J., *et al.* (2019).** Comparative efficacy and tolerability of 32 oral antipsychotics for the acute treatment of adults with multi-episode schizophrenia: a systematic review and network meta-analysis. *Lancet*, 394, 939–951.
21. **Gaebel, W., Riesbeck, M., von Wilmsdorff, M., *et al.* (2010).** Drug attitude as predictor for effectiveness in first-episode schizophrenia: results of an open randomized trial (EUFEST). *Eur Neuropsychopharmacol*, 20, 310–316.
22. **Boulton, D. W., DeVane, C. L., Liston, H. L., *et al.* (2002).** In vitro P-glycoprotein affinity for atypical and conventional antipsychotics. *Life Sciences*, 71, 163–169.
23. **Nakagami, T., Yasui-Furukori, N., Saito, M., *et al.* (2005).** Effect of verapamil on pharmacokinetics and pharmacodynamics of risperidone: in vivo evidence of involvement of P-glycoprotein in risperidone disposition. *Clin Pharmacol Ther*, 78, 43–51.
24. **Wang, R., Sun, X., Deng, Y. S., *et al.* (2018).** ABCB1 1199G > A polymorphism impacts transport ability of P-gp-mediated antipsychotics. *DNA Cell Biol*, 37, 325–329.
25. **Linnet, K. and Ejsing, T. B. (2008).** A review on the impact of P-glycoprotein on the penetration of drugs into the brain: focus on psychotropic drugs. *Eur Neuropsychopharmacol*, 18, 157–169.
26. **Hartter, S., Huwel, S., Lohmann, T., *et al.* (2003).** How does the benzamide antipsychotic amisulpride get into the brain? – An in vitro approach comparing amisulpride with clozapine. *Neuropsychopharmacology*, 28, 1916–1922.
27. **Janssen Pharmaceuticals Inc. (2019).** Invega package insert. Titusville, NJ.
28. **Janssen Pharmaceuticals Inc. (2020).** Risperdal package insert. Titusville, NJ.
29. **O'Brien, F. E., Dinan, T. G., Griffin, B. T., *et al.* (2012).** Interactions between antidepressants and P-glycoprotein at the blood-brain barrier: clinical significance of in vitro and in vivo findings. *Br J Pharmacol*, 165, 289–312.
30. **Zanger, U. M. and Schwab, M. (2013).** Cytochrome P450 enzymes in drug metabolism: regulation of gene expression, enzyme activities, and impact of genetic variation. *Pharmacol Ther*, 138, 103–141.
31. **de Leon, J., Sandson, N. B., and Cozza, K. L. (2008).** A preliminary attempt to personalize risperidone dosing using drug–drug interactions and genetics, Part II. *Psychosomatics*, 48, 347–361.
32. **Verbeeck, R. K. (2008).** Pharmacokinetics and dosage adjustment in patients with hepatic dysfunction. *Eur J Clin Pharmacol*, 64, 1147–1161.
33. **Meyer, J. M. (2018).** Pharmacotherapy of psychosis and mania. In L. L. Brunton, R. Hilal-Dandan and B. C. Knollmann, eds., *Goodman & Gilman's The Pharmacological Basis of Therapeutics*, 13th edn. Chicago, IL: McGraw-Hill, pp. 279–302.
34. **Selmin, F., Blasi, P., and DeLuca, P. P. (2012).** Accelerated polymer biodegradation of risperidone poly(D, L-lactide-co-glycolide) microspheres. *AAPS PharmSciTech*, 13, 1465–1472.
35. **Fleischhacker, W. W., Eerdekens, M., Karcher, K., *et al.* (2003).** Treatment of schizophrenia with long-acting injectable risperidone: a 12-month open-label trial of the first long-acting second-generation antipsychotic. *J Clin Psychiatry*, 64, 1250–1257.
36. **Wilson, W. H. (2004).** A visual guide to expected blood levels of long-acting injectable risperidone in clinical practice. *J Psychiatr Pract*, 10, 393–401.

37. **Kane, J. M., Eerdekens, M., Lindenmayer, J. P., *et al.* (2003).** Long-acting injectable risperidone: efficacy and safety of the first long-acting atypical antipsychotic. *Am J Psychiatry*, 160, 1125–1132.
38. **Meltzer, H. Y., Lindenmayer, J. P., Kwentus, J., *et al.* (2014).** A six month randomized controlled trial of long acting injectable risperidone 50 and 100mg in treatment resistant schizophrenia. *Schizophr Res*, 154, 14–22, https://doi.org/10.1016/j.schres.2014.1002.1015.
39. **Schoretsanitis, G., Spina, E., Hiemke, C., *et al.* (2018).** A systematic review and combined analysis of therapeutic drug monitoring studies for long-acting paliperidone. *Expert Rev Clin Pharmacol*, 11, 1237–1253.
40. **Janssen Pharmaceuticals Inc. (2020).** Risperdal Consta package insert. Titusville, NJ.
41. **Gefvert, O., Eriksson, B., Persson, P., *et al.* (2005).** Pharmacokinetics and D2 receptor occupancy of long-acting injectable risperidone (Risperdal Consta) in patients with schizophrenia. *Int J Neuropsychopharmacol*, 8, 27–36.
42. **Janssen Pharmaceuticals Inc. (2019).** Invega Trinza package insert. Titusville, NJ.
43. **Haddad, P., Lambert, T., and Lauriello, J., eds. (2016).** *Antipsychotic Long-Acting Injections*, 2nd edn. New York: Oxford University Press.
44. **Nasser, A. F., Henderson, D. C., Fava, M., *et al.* (2016).** Efficacy, safety, and tolerability of RBP-7000 once-monthly risperidone for the treatment of acute schizophrenia: an 8-week, randomized, double-blind, placebo-controlled, multicenter phase 3 study. *J Clin Psychopharmacol*, 36, 130–140.
45. **Ivaturi, V., Gopalakrishnan, M., Gobburu, J. V. S., *et al.* (2017).** Exposure-response analysis after subcutaneous administration of RBP-7000, a once-a-month long-acting Atrigel formulation of risperidone. *Br J Clin Pharmacol*, 83, 1476–1498.
46. **Southard, G. L., Dunn, R. L., and Garrett, S. (1998).** The drug delivery and biomaterial attributes of the ATRIGEL technology in the treatment of periodontal disease. *Expert Opin Investig Drugs*, 7, 1483–1491.
47. **Meyer, J. M. (2018).** Risperidone extended-release injectable suspension. *Curr Psychiatr*, 17, 23–33.
48. **Laffont, C. M., Gomeni, R., Zheng, B., *et al.* (2014).** Population pharmacokinetics and prediction of dopamine D2 receptor occupancy after multiple doses of RBP-7000, a new sustained-release formulation of risperidone, in schizophrenia patients on stable oral risperidone treatment. *Clin Pharmacokinet*, 53, 533–543.
49. **Laffont, C. M., Gomeni, R., Zheng, B., *et al.* (2015).** Population pharmacokinetic modeling and simulation to guide dose selection for RBP-7000, a new sustained-release formulation of risperidone. *J Clin Pharmacol*, 55, 93–103.
50. **Indivior Inc. (2019).** Perseris package insert. North Chesterfield, VA 23235.
51. **Janssen Pharmaceuticals Inc. (2019).** Invega Sustenna package insert. Titusville, NJ.
42. **Janssen Pharmaceuticals Inc. (2019).** Invega Trinza package insert. Titusville, NJ.
52. **Pandina, G. J., Lindenmayer, J. P., Lull, J., *et al.* (2010).** A randomized, placebo-controlled study to assess the efficacy and safety of 3 doses of paliperidone palmitate in adults with acutely exacerbated schizophrenia. *J Clin Psychopharmacol*, 30, 235–244, https://doi.org/210.1097/JCP.1090b1013e3181dd3103.
53. **Chouinard, G., Jones, B., Remington, G., *et al.* (1993).** A Canadian multicenter placebo-controlled study of fixed doses of risperidone and haloperidol in the treatment of chronic schizophrenic patients. *J Clin Psychopharmacol*, 13, 25–40.
54. **Marder, S. R. and Meibach, R. C. (1994).** Risperidone in the treatment of schizophrenia. *Am J Psychiatry*, 151, 825–835.
55. **Peuskens, J. (1995).** Risperidone in the treatment of patients with chronic schizophrenia: a multi-national, multi-centre, double-blind, parallel-group study versus haloperidol. Risperidone Study Group. *Br J Psychiatry*, 166, 712–726; discussion 727–733.

56. **Merlo, M. C., Hofer, H., Gekle, W., *et al.* (2002).** Risperidone, 2 mg/day vs. 4 mg/day, in first-episode, acutely psychotic patients: treatment efficacy and effects on fine motor functioning. *J Clin Psychiatry*, 63, 885–891.

57. **Li, C., Xia, J., and Wang, J. (2009).** Risperidone dose for schizophrenia. *Cochrane Database Syst Rev*, CD007474.

58. **Kapur, S., Zipursky, R., Jones, C., *et al.* (2000).** Relationship between dopamine D(2) occupancy, clinical response, and side effects: a double-blind PET study of first-episode schizophrenia. *Am J Psychiatry*, 157, 514–520.

59. **Remington, G., Kapur, S., and Zipursky, R. (1998).** The relationship between risperidone plasma levels and dopamine D2 occupancy: a positron emission tomographic study. *J Clin Psychopharmacol*, 18, 82–83.

60. **Karlsson, P., Hargarter, L., Dencker, E., *et al.* (2007).** Pharmacokinetics and dopamine D2 and serotonin 5-HT2a receptor occupancy of paliperidone in healthy subjects: two open-label, single-dose studies (PAL-115). *Pharmacopsychiatry*, 40, A106.

61. **Leucht, S., Crippa, A., Siafis, S., *et al.* (2020).** Dose-response meta-analysis of antipsychotic drugs for acute schizophrenia. *Am J Psychiatry*, 177, 342–353.

62. **Samtani, M. N., Gopal, S., Gassmann-Mayer, C., *et al.* (2011).** Dosing and switching strategies for paliperidone palmitate: based on population pharmacokinetic modelling and clinical trial data. *CNS Drugs*, 25, 829–845.

15 Olanzapine and Olanzapine Pamoate

QUICK CHECK

PRINCIPLES

- Olanzapine provides an inexpensive method of delivering D_2 antagonism, with extensive plasma level data, and a long-acting injectable (LAI) preparation (olanzapine pamoate).
- When treatment resistance is strictly defined using all three Kane criteria, treatment-resistant schizophrenia patients have a 5%–7% response rate to higher plasma levels of olanzapine in double-blind conditions, compared to < 5% for most antipsychotics, and 40%–60% for clozapine.
- While minimally more effective than other antipsychotics, olanzapine should not be used as initial treatment in first-episode schizophrenia patients due to the significant problem with weight gain and metabolic dysfunction. Because of this marked propensity for metabolic dysfunction in all patients, olanzapine is considered a third-line agent for the treatment of schizophrenia.
- The LAI preparation, olanzapine pamoate, provides up to the equivalent of 20 mg/d of oral olanzapine. Use is extremely limited due to the need for patients to be observed after each injection for at least 3 hours in a registered facility to monitor for post-injection delirium/sedation syndrome.

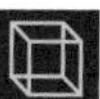

InfoBox Oral Olanzapine Plasma Level Essentials

Oral dose correlation (bedtime dosing, 12h trough)	Level of evidence	Therapeutic threshold	Level of evidence	Point of futility	Level of evidence
Nonsmoker: 10 mg = 20 ng/ml Smoker: 14 mg = 20 ng/ml [1, 2] **Smoker: multiply oral dose by 1.43** **Nonsmoker: multiply oral dose by 2.0** [a, b] (see Table 15.1 for effects of CYP inhibitors/inducers on this relationship)	High	23 ng/ml [3, 4]	High	150 ng/ml [5, 6]	Moderate

[a] The predicted trough plasma olanzapine level for a given dose is increased by 26%–38% in females compared with males, primarily ascribed to lower CYP 1A2 activity [7, 8].

[b] In general, the plasma trough plasma olanzapine level for a given dose is approximately 50% higher for nonsmokers than for smokers [7, 8].

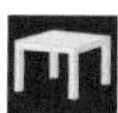

Table 15.1 Oral olanzapine kinetic facts [27, 28]

Basic facts	Inhibition effects	Induction effects
US FDA approval: Sept. 30, 1996 Absolute oral bioavailability: 60% $T_{1/2}$ 30 (21–54) hours T_{max} 6 hours Metabolism: Direct glucuronidation via UGT 1A4 or UGT 2B10, or CYP 1A2 mediated oxidation to *N*-desmethylolanzapine [29] **Formulations:** Tablets, oral dissolving tablets (also acute intramuscular)	The mean increase in olanzapine AUC following fluvoxamine exposure is 52% and 108%, respectively, in female nonsmokers and male smokers, but the effect is dependent on the fluvoxamine dose Fluvoxamine 100 mg/day for 8 weeks resulted in an increase in trough olanzapine levels from 31 ± 15 ng/ml to 56 ± 31 ng/ml (81%), with a range of 12%–112% [30]. A smaller fluvoxamine dose (25 mg/d) increased exposure only 26% [31]	Carbamazepine use increases clearance by 50%. The olanzapine concentration–dose ratio is at least 30% lower in smokers, and may be 50% lower in some patients

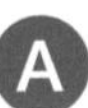

Basic Pharmacokinetic Information for Oral and Long-Acting Injectable Olanzapine

Olanzapine is among the more extensively studied second-generation antipsychotics (SGAs), partly due to its approval 25 years ago (1996), and also due to its penchant for significant metabolic adverse effects [9, 10]. Olanzapine distinguished itself by its efficacy profile (Figure 15.1), combined with lower rates of hyperprolactinemia and neurological adverse effects than first-generation antipsychotics (FGAs) and risperidone [11]. In the US Clinical Antipsychotic Trials of Intervention Effectiveness (CATIE) schizophrenia study, the primary outcome measure was time to all-cause discontinuation, and olanzapine outperformed other antipsychotics in phase 1 [12].

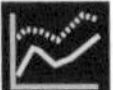

Figure 15.1 Standardized mean difference (SMD) from placebo in positive psychosis symptom improvement during oral antipsychotic treatment for adults with acutely relapsed schizophrenia [11]

	SMD (95% CrI)
AMI (n = 626)	−0.69 (−0.86 to −0.52)
RIS (n = 3351)	−0.61 (−0.68 to −0.54)
CLO (n = 31)	−0.64 (−1.09 to −0.19)
OLA (n = 4227)	−0.53 (−0.60 to −0.46)
PAL (n = 1373)	−0.53 (−0.65 to −0.42)
HAL (n = 3042)	−0.49 (−0.56 to −0.41)
ASE (n = 734)	−0.47 (−0.63 to −0.32)
PERPH (n = 734)	−0.45 (−0.66 to −0.24)
ZIP (n = 1102)	−0.43 (−0.53 to −0.32)
QUE (n = 2935)	−0.40 (−0.49 to −0.31)
ARI (n = 1451)	−0.38 (−0.48 to −0.28)
LUR (n = 1165)	−0.33 (−0.45 to −0.20)
CAR (n = 999)	−0.30 (−0.45 to 0.16)
ILO (n = 918)	−0.30 (−0.43 to −0.17)
BRE (n = 1180)	−0.17 (−0.31 to 0.04)
PBO (n = 6489)	0.00 (0.00 to 0.00)

AMI - Amisulpride; RIS - Risperidone; CLO - Clozapine; OLA - Olanzapine; PAL - Paliperidone; HAL - Haloperidol; ASE - Asenapine; PERPH - Perphenazine; ZIP - Ziprasidone; QUE - Quetiapine; ARI - Aripiprazole; LUR - Lurasidone; CAR - Cariprazine; ILO - Iloperidone; BRE - Brexpiprazole; PBO - Placebo.

(Adapted from: M. Huhn, A. Nikolakopoulou, J. Schneider-Thoma, *et al.* [2019]. Comparative efficacy and tolerability of 32 oral antipsychotics for the acute treatment of adults with multi-episode schizophrenia: a systematic review and network meta-analysis. *Lancet*, 394, 939–951.)

However, the CATIE trial also highlighted that olanzapine treatment is associated with markedly greater metabolic risk than every antipsychotic except clozapine, but lacked clozapine's efficacy among nonresponders enrolled in phase 2 [12, 13, 9]. Subsequent meta-analyses have confirmed olanzapine's adverse effect on metabolic parameters (Figure 15.2) [14]. From the finding that olanzapine outperformed other medications in phase 1 of CATIE, a misperception arose that olanzapine is markedly more effective than other antipsychotics and might rival clozapine's efficacy in treatment-resistant patients [15]. This misperception was fueled by studies that enrolled treatment-resistant schizophrenia patients based solely on the historical failure of two antipsychotics, but did not confirm the lack of adequate response through a prospective antipsychotic trial [16]. While more time-consuming, this last step is crucial in differentiating treatment

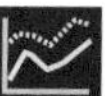

Figure 15.2 Mean difference from placebo in weight gain (in kg units) during oral antipsychotic treatment for adults with acutely relapsed schizophrenia [14]

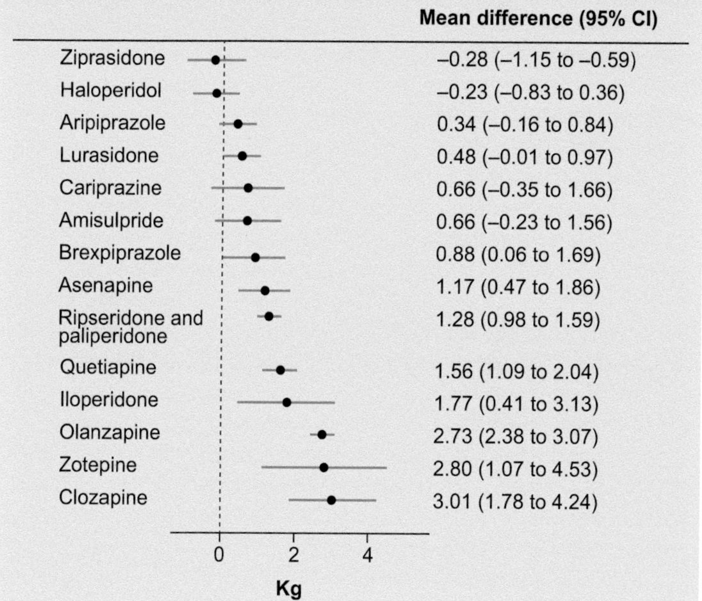

(Adapted from: T. Pillinger, R. A. McCutcheon, L. Vano, *et al.* [2020]. Comparative effects of 18 antipsychotics on metabolic function in patients with schizophrenia, predictors of metabolic dysregulation, and association with psychopathology: a systematic review and network meta-analysis. *Lancet Psychiatry*, 7, 64–77.)

resistance from nonadherence or kinetic failures, and was used by Professor John Kane as one of the necessary criteria for defining treatment-resistant patients who were eligible for the pivotal clozapine trial [17, 18]. Fewer than 2% of patients met response criteria in the prospective haloperidol arm of the Kane 1988 clozapine study (mean dose 61 mg/d), while 80% were nonresponders and 18% were intolerant of high dose haloperidol [17]. This element of the Kane 1988 criteria (Box 15.1) is central to a research definition of treatment resistance; studies using "modified Kane criteria" that omit this step report unrealistically high response rates for atypical antipsychotics other than clozapine [19]. The enormous impact of criterion 3 can be seen in the three double-blind studies of olanzapine for treatment-resistant schizophrenia. Response rates to olanzapine at doses up to 50 mg/d were 0%, 5%, and 7% in the studies that included criterion 3 [20–22], but response to olanzapine was 50% when this was omitted [16]. When the olanzapine nonresponders from the studies reporting 5% and 7% response rates were transitioned to clozapine, 41% met response criteria [21].

Although amisulpride is not available in the US and Canada, it is marketed in most European countries, the UK, and Australia (see Chapter 17). As seen in Figure 15.1, amisulpride ranks at the top in terms of efficacy versus placebo, although the overlapping confidence intervals imply that, like olanzapine, any differences with most agents are small [11]. Nonetheless, this logic was used to examine amisulpride as the first phase of a multinational adult schizophrenia trial to study the effectiveness of amisulpride, olanzapine, and clozapine for inducing remission [23]. Remission criteria are much more stringent than for response, and included mild severity (rating of 3 or less on a 7-point scale) for eight specific schizophrenia symptoms on the PANSS (items P1, P2, P3, N1, N4, N6, G5, and G9). In this three-phase design, adult patients (18–40 years) who met criteria for a schizophrenia spectrum disorder were started on open-label amisulpride up to 800 mg/d for 4 weeks. Those who failed to remit were randomized in a double-blind manner to remain on amisulpride or switch to olanzapine (up to 20 mg/d) for 6 weeks. Patients who were not in remission after 10 combined weeks of treatment were given open-label clozapine (up to 900 mg/d) for an additional 12 weeks. Of the 446 subjects who started the study, 83% completed open-label amisulpride treatment, of which 56% achieved remission; 93 patients who were not in remission on amisulpride continued to the 6-week double-blind switch arm, and 72 (77%) completed that portion of the trial (olanzapine n = 39, amisulpride n = 33). In the double-blind phase of the study, switching to olanzapine was not superior to continuing on amisulpride, with both arms reporting nearly identical remission rates: olanzapine 44%, amisulpride 45% [23]. Although there was some concern that the maximum olanzapine dose was 20 mg/d, the mean olanzapine dose for individuals who met remission criteria was 14.4 ± 5.6 mg/d. Moreover, the mean dose of remitters was not significantly different than for patients who did not achieve remission (17.5 ± 6.3 mg/d; p = 0.12) [23]. Within the context of this study design, olanzapine did not demonstrate any added benefit over amisulpride.

There is a subgroup of patients who do respond to olanzapine after having failed more metabolically benign antipsychotics, and, like 50% of all schizophrenia patients, are expected to have inadequate oral medication adherence. For this patient cohort, a long-acting injectable (LAI) formulation was created (olanzapine pamoate) and approved in the US on December 11, 2009. However, cases surfaced during the clinical trials in which patients experienced extremely high plasma olanzapine levels and severe sedation shortly after the injection. The median onset time was 25 minutes post injection, but some did not manifest symptoms until 3–5 hours after the injection [24]. As noted in the product label, symptoms included sedation (ranging from mild in severity to coma) and/or delirium (including confusion, disorientation, agitation, anxiety, and other cognitive impairment). Other adverse effects included extrapyramidal symptoms, dysarthria, ataxia, aggression, dizziness, weakness, hypertension, and convulsion [25]. The majority required hospitalization and supportive care, including intubation in several cases, but all largely recovered by 72 hours [25]. Based on approximately 45,000 olanzapine long-acting injectable (LAI) injections given to 2054 patients in clinical trials, **post-injection delirium/sedation syndrome occurred** in approximately 0.07% of injections, or 1.4% of patients [24]. The recognition that this syndrome can occur with any injection resulted in a mandatory risk mitigation program. Prior to dispensing olanzapine pamoate, the prescriber, healthcare facility, patient, and pharmacy must be enrolled in the distribution program, and **after each injection the patient must be observed for at least 3 hours in a registered facility with ready access to emergency response services** [25]. Although the LAI formulation sees very limited use due to the onerous monitoring

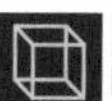

Box 15.1 Essential Components of the Kane Definition of Treatment-Resistant Schizophrenia for Patients Enrolled in the Pivotal Clozapine Trial [17]

1. At least three periods of treatment in the preceding 5 years with antipsychotics (from at least two different chemical classes) at dosages equivalent to or greater than 1000 mg/d of chlorpromazine for a period of 6 weeks, each without significant symptomatic relief.
2. No period of good functioning within the preceding 5 years.
3. Failure to respond to a **prospective high dose trial** of a typical antipsychotic (haloperidol at doses up to 60 mg/d or higher, administered with benztropine 6 mg/d). Response was defined as a 20% decrease in the BPRS total score, plus either a post-treatment CGI severity rating of mildly ill (≤ 3) or a post-treatment BPRS score ≤ 35.

requirements, oral olanzapine is widely prescribed, and olanzapine was assigned a Level 1 recommendation (strongly recommended) for use of plasma level monitoring in the 2020 consensus paper authored jointly by the Therapeutic Drug Monitoring (TDM) task force of the German Arbeitsgemeinschaft für Neuropsychopharmakologie und Pharmakopsychiatrie (AGNP) and the American Society for Clinical Psychopharmacology (ASCP) [26].

B Essential Information for Oral and Long-Acting Injectable Olanzapine

1 Essential Oral Olanzapine Information

The oral olanzapine concentration–dose relationship presented in the InfoBox is based on results from multiple studies, and assumes that the patient is an extensive metabolizer at relevant cytochrome P450 (CYP) enzymes, and is not exposed to CYP inhibitors or inducers. An active metabolite, *N*-desmethylolanzapine, is generated by CYP 1A2 but is not routinely measured. As CYP 1A2 is partly responsible for olanzapine's metabolism, smoking cigarettes (or cannabis) creates aryl hydrocarbons from the burnt plant matter that induce CYP 1A2 expression [1]. Vaping, which involves inhalation of a heated water-based solution, does not burn any organic matter, and does not induce CYP 1A2 [32]. It is worth noting that the impact of smoking on olanzapine levels is not as great as for clozapine since a substantial proportion of olanzapine's clearance is not dependent on phase I CYP metabolism but on direct glucuronidation [29]. This phase 2 process, mediated by the enzymes UGT 1A4 and UGT 2B10, produces 10-*N*-glucuronide and, to a lesser extent, 4'-*N*-glucuronide, with 10-*N*-glucuronide having steady state plasma levels 44% of those of olanzapine [33]. The active metabolite *N*-desmethylolanzapine is present at a concentration 10%–30% of the parent drug [33, 26]. Because two phase 2 enzymes mediate olanzapine glucuronidation, use of the UGT 1A4 inhibitor valproate alters dose-adjusted olanzapine exposure, but the reduction is < 20% on average, although the effect may be slightly greater in smokers [34]. There is no impact of valproate on LAI olanzapine clearance, suggesting that presystemic processes are impacted during first pass metabolism of the oral formulation [34]. In addition to the impact of smoking behavior on the concentration–dose relationship, there is also an influence of gender, with women having 26%–38% higher levels compared with men, primarily due to lower CYP 1A2 activity [7, 8]. The average 12h trough plasma level for nonsmokers is an easily remembered conversion factor of 2.0, so a patient at steady state on 15 mg QHS should have a trough level of approximately 30 ng/ml (Figure 15.3).

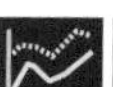

Figure 15.3 Relationship between mean steady state plasma olanzapine level and oral dose. Dotted lines represent 95% confidence intervals [2]

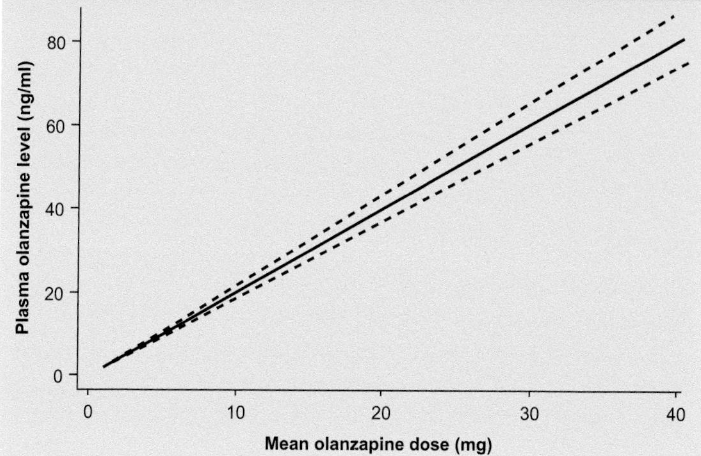

(Adapted from: D. Bishara, O. Olofinjana, A. Sparshatt, *et al.* [2013]. Olanzapine: a systematic review and meta-regression of the relationships between dose, plasma concentration, receptor occupancy, and response. *J Clin Psychopharmacol*, 33, 329–335.)

An interesting feature of oral olanzapine is the long time to maximum plasma levels (C_{max}), estimated at 6 hours, compared to 0.5–2 hours for most orally administered antipsychotics [27, 28]. For acutely symptomatic or agitated patients, this long C_{max} is undesirable, but there is an acute intramuscular (IM) formulation with a concentration of 5 mg/ml when reconstituted with 2.1 ml sterile water [35]. In schizophrenia patients, acute IM olanzapine has a T_{max} of 30 minutes, with a mean C_{max} of 21–33 ng/ml in several trials using the 10 mg IM dose, although the range is surprisingly large (4.9–75.1 ng/ml) [35].

2 Essential Long-Acting Injectable Olanzapine Information

As noted previously, use of olanzapine pamoate is associated with post-injection delirium/sedation syndrome in approximately 0.07% of injections or 1.4% of patients [24, 36]. Use of LAI olanzapine is thus restricted to facilities, providers, and patients that are enrolled in the risk mitigation program designed to insure compliance with continuous monitoring in a healthcare facility for 3 hours after each injection. Olanzapine pamoate has a T_{max} under 7 days (Figure 15.4), and can be loaded using a strategy devised by the manufacturer (Table 15.2) [37]. The maximum olanzapine exposure is provided by a maintenance dose of 300 mg/2 weeks, equivalent to 20 mg/d oral olanzapine, and this LAI dose is associated with a steady state plasma olanzapine level of at least 45 ng/ml (10th–90th percentile range: 20–67 ng/ml) [37]. A more general plasma level conversion formula based on the ***daily dose*** (i.e. the monthly dose divided by 30) is: 2.25 x dose (mg/d). As seen in Figures 15.5a and 15.5b, initiating olanzapine pamoate at 300 mg IM every 2 weeks for 8 weeks without oral coverage generates a plasma level close to 23 ng/ml by week 4, and near 40 ng/ml by week 8 [38]. For less stable patients transitioning from 20 mg/d oral, consideration can be given to supplementation with 10 mg oral olanzapine during the first 2 weeks of therapy.

By viewing the expected plasma levels with various olanzapine pamoate loading regimens (Figures 15.5a, 15.5b), and the single-dose kinetics of 405 mg (Figure 15.4), one can appreciate the magnitude of the problem underlying the development of

Figure 15.4 Single-dose kinetic profile for olanzapine pamoate 405 mg IM [37]

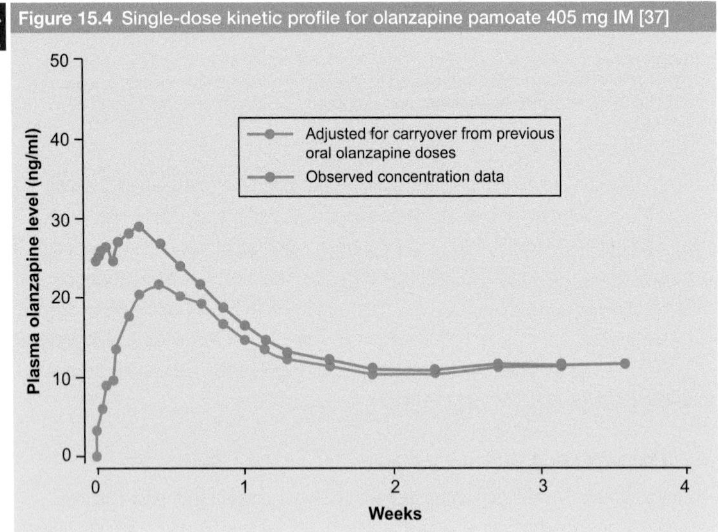

(Adapted from: S. Heres, S. Kraemer, R. F. Bergstrom, *et al.* [2014]. Pharmacokinetics of olanzapine long-acting injection: the clinical perspective. *Int Clin Psychopharmacol*, 29, 299–312.)

Table 15.2 Olanzapine pamoate essentials [37, 25]

Vehicle	Concentration	Dosage	T_{max} (days)	$T_{1/2}$ (days) multiple dosing	Able to be loaded	Maintenance dose: oral equivalence [38, 25]
Water	210 mg/1.3 ml 300 mg/1.8 ml 405 mg/2.3 ml	150–300 mg/2 weeks 300–405 mg/4 weeks **Max:** 300 mg/2 weeks	6–7	30	Yes	10 mg/d = 300 mg/4 weeks 15 mg/d = 405 mg/4 weeks 20 mg/d = 300 mg/2 weeks

Steady state trough plasma level conversion formula: using the olanzapine pamoate ***daily dose*** (i.e. the monthly dose divided by 30): **2.25 x daily dose (mg/d)** [37].

Example 1: Patient on 300 mg/2 weeks

Daily dose: 600 mg/month divided by 30 = 20 mg/d. 20 x 2.25 = 45 ng/ml.

Example 2: Patient on 405 mg/4 weeks

Daily dose: 405 mg/month divided by 30 = 13.5 mg/d. 13.5 x 2.25 = 30.375 ng/ml.

Note: The package labeling notes that patients are at risk for post-injection delirium/sedation syndrome **after each injection**, and must be observed for at least 3 hours in a registered facility with ready access to emergency response services (see Figure 15.6) [25].

Table 15.3 Based on relapse rates at 6 months, manufacturer-recommended strategies for switching patients from oral olanzapine 10–20 mg/d to olanzapine pamoate without oral bridging coverage [38]

Oral dose	Olanzapine pamoate IM dose in first 8 weeks	Maintenance dose: oral equivalence
10 mg/d	210 mg/2 weeks	300 mg/4 weeks
15 mg/d	300 mg/2 weeks	405 mg/4 weeks
20 mg/d	300 mg/2 weeks	300 mg/2 weeks

(For further reading about use of LAI antipsychotics, please see the comprehensive edited book ***Antipsychotic Long-Acting Injections***, now in its 2nd edition [49].)

post-injection delirium/sedation syndrome. Even with the carryover from prior oral therapy, maximal plasma olanzapine levels from a single injection of 405 mg are typically < 50 ng/ml including values one standard deviation above the mean [37]. Figure 15.6 presents a detailed analysis of post-injection delirium/sedation syndrome cases illustrating that olanzapine plasma levels exceeding 500 ng/ml were seen in multiple instances [24]. Olanzapine pamoate is not widely available worldwide, but has

Figure 15.5a, 15.5b Kinetic profile for initiating olanzapine pamoate to obtain monthly maintenance doses of 300 mg or 405 mg [38]

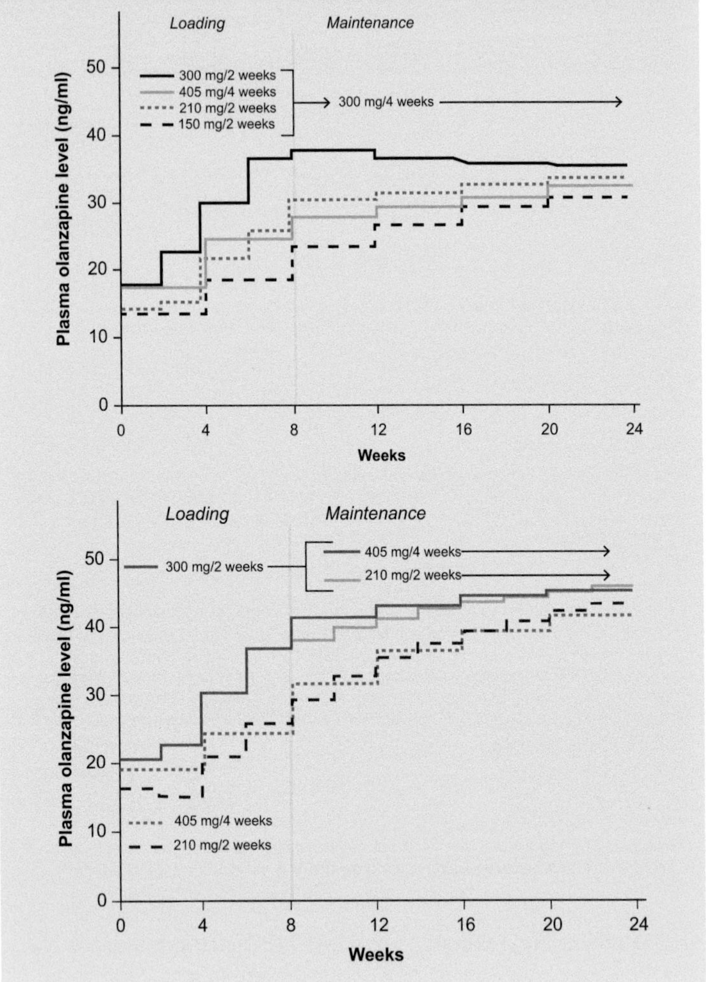

(Adapted from: H. C. Detke, F. Zhao, P. Garhyan, *et al.* [2011]. Dose correspondence between olanzapine long-acting injection and oral olanzapine: recommendations for switching. *Int Clin Psychopharmacol*, 26, 35–42.)

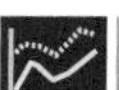

Figure 15.6 Plasma olanzapine levels in cases of post-injection delirium/sedation syndrome following olanzapine pamoate injection [36]

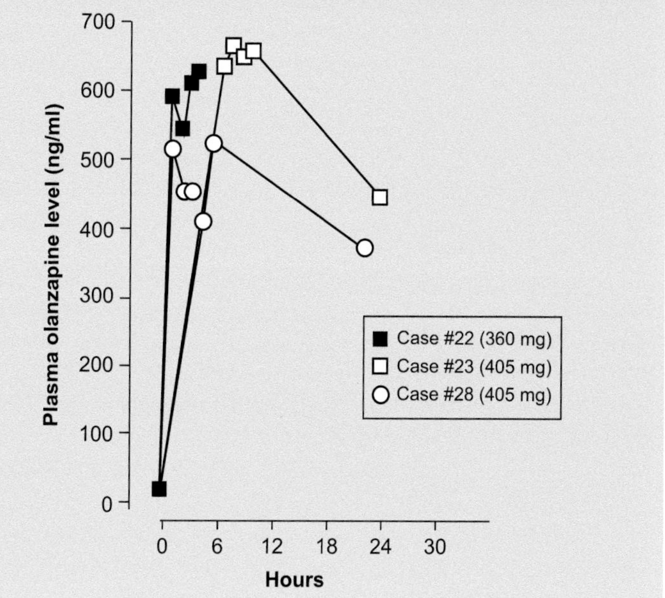

(Adapted from: D. P. McDonnell, H. C. Detke, R. F. Bergstrom, *et al.* [2010]. Post-injection delirium/sedation syndrome in patients with schizophrenia treated with olanzapine long-acting injection, II: investigations of mechanism. *BMC Psychiatry*, 10, 45–54.)

approval in the US, UK, and Australia, with risk mitigation programs as mandated by local authorities. Given the concerns about post-injection delirium/sedation syndrome, doses above 300 mg/2 weeks or 405 mg/4 weeks have not been studied and should not be used.

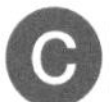

C The Therapeutic Threshold for Olanzapine

1 Clinical Evidence for a Therapeutic Threshold

Clinical evidence, especially from fixed-dose, prospective, randomized trials, is the most important tool we have for estimation of plasma level response thresholds (see Chapter 2). There are three receiver operating characteristic (ROC) analyses available for olanzapine – one fixed-dose study, one flexible dose study, and one cross-sectional study – all of which show a remarkable degree of agreement despite varying methodologies [3, 39, 4]. As noted in Chapter 2, ROC analysis is ideal for establishing a cutpoint below which the proportion of false positives is higher, and thus presents an initial treatment target for patients with inadequate response. The fixed dose ROC analysis utilized endpoint plasma levels from the 6-week North American Double-Blind Olanzapine Trial in which patients were randomly assigned to one of three daily dose ranges: 5 ± 2.5 mg/d, 10 ± 2.5 mg/d, or 15 ± 2.5 mg/d on a once daily dosing schedule [3]. Response was defined as ≥ 20% decrease in the total Brief Psychiatric Rating Scale (BPRS), and an endpoint clinical global impression (CGI) severity score ≤ 3 or an endpoint BPRS score ≤ 35. Olanzapine plasma concentrations used in the ROC analysis were from patients on the same dosage for at least 2 weeks, with time from last dose between 10 and 16 hours (mean 11.7 ± 1.7 hours) [3]. Of 198 patients randomized at study entry, 101 had plasma levels that were valid for the analysis. Using those response criteria, an olanzapine 12h trough plasma level of 23.2 ng/ml was identified as the response threshold. Patients with olanzapine levels ≥ 23.2 ng/ml had a response rate of 52%, while those with endpoint levels < 23.2 ng/ml only had a 25% response rate. This cutpoint had high specificity of 81%, with acceptable sensitivity of 44%.

A subsequent open-label, 6-week, two-site Australian trial examined the plasma level response threshold in adults with schizophrenia flexibly dosed in the range of 5–30 mg/d, with the oral dose administered between 8 and 10 PM [39]. All patients were rated with the Positive and Negative Syndrome Scale (PANSS) at baseline and at the week 6 endpoint, and dosing changes were avoided starting week 5 (unless clinically necessary). Patients were classified as responders based on a ≥ 20% decrease in admission PANSS total score, with analysis of subscore changes for positive, negative, and general psychopathology items. Of 108 patients who commenced the study, 53 had endpoint olanzapine plasma levels that were valid for this analysis, with a median time of 13.5 hours post-dose. Noncompleters were demographically similar but had higher mean baseline PANSS scores than completers (79 ± 19 versus 69 ± 21) [39]. Despite the open-label design and higher drop-out rate among more ill patients, the ROC analysis identified a cutpoint of 23 ng/ml for responders, using the PANSS criteria [39]. Sensitivity and specificity were not reported. In the secondary analysis, a cutpoint of 24 ng/ml was identified, based on reduction of positive psychotic symptoms.

Lastly, investigators in Taiwan examined 12h trough plasma level data from 151 adult patients with schizophrenia (aged 18–60 years) on a stable olanzapine dose

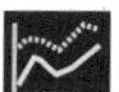

Figure 15.7 Receiver operating characteristic (ROC) curve of the plasma olanzapine level required to be rated as mildly ill (PANSS score ≤ 58) from a cohort of Taiwanese schizophrenia patients (n = 151) [4]

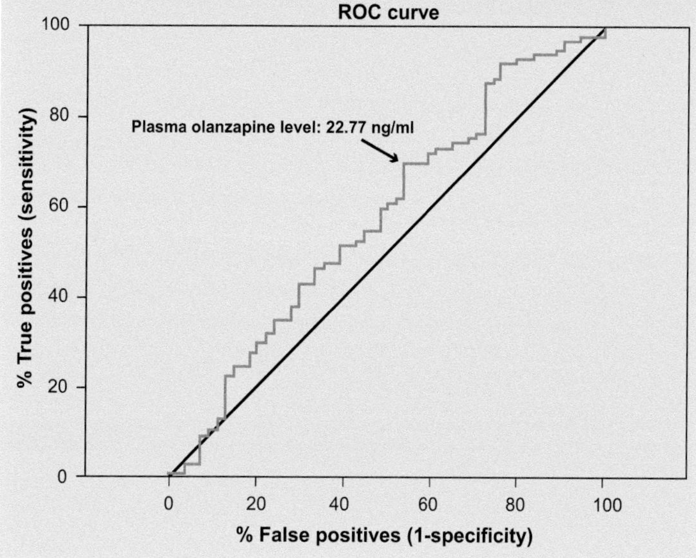

(Adapted from: M. L. Lu, Y. X. Wu, C. H. Chen, *et al.* [2016]. Application of plasma levels of olanzapine and N-desmethyl-olanzapine to monitor clinical efficacy in patients with schizophrenia. *PLoS One*, 11, e0148539.)

for at least 3 months, all of whom were rated using the PANSS [4]. None of the patients had previously been on clozapine, and samples were excluded from patients on medications that had kinetic interactions with olanzapine, except for cigarette smoking. Based on the known correlation between CGI-severity ratings and the PANSS score (see Chapter 5) [40], a PANSS total score of 58 was used in the ROC analysis to determine the plasma olanzapine level required to be rated as mildly ill [4]. In this cross-sectional analysis of stable patients, a trough plasma olanzapine level cutpoint of 22.77 ng/ml best discriminated those schizophrenia patients rated as mildly ill, with a sensitivity of 70.1% and specificity of 46.3% (Figure 15.7) [4].

The ROC analysis from a fixed-dose trial is always weighted more heavily than other study designs, but the consistency of therapeutic thresholds obtained from these three studies is remarkable and points to 23 ng/ml as the response threshold for olanzapine. For a nonsmoker, this corresponds to an oral dose of 11.5 mg/d, and for a smoker, 16.1 mg/d. This conclusion is very consistent with that from the 2020 AGNP/ASCP consensus paper which proposes a 20 ng/ml threshold [26].

2 Imaging Evidence for a Therapeutic Threshold

Given the larger sample sizes and consistency of the ROC findings, the clinical evidence for a therapeutic threshold is compelling, but there are several Positron Emission Tomography (PET) imaging studies that can be used to explore correlations between striatal D_2 occupancy and olanzapine plasma levels. As discussed in Chapter 2, antipsychotic response with D_2 antagonists starts at 65% D_2 occupancy, and one can calculate the level needed for that threshold from papers that provide an estimated plasma concentration for 50% occupancy (the EC_{50}). EC_{50} values ranging from 7.1–11.0 ng/ml are reported [41–44, 2], with graphical representations of fitted D_2 occupancy curves shown here based on dose (Figure 15.8), or plasma olanzapine

Figure 15.8 Fitted D_2 occupancy curve for oral olanzapine doses [2]

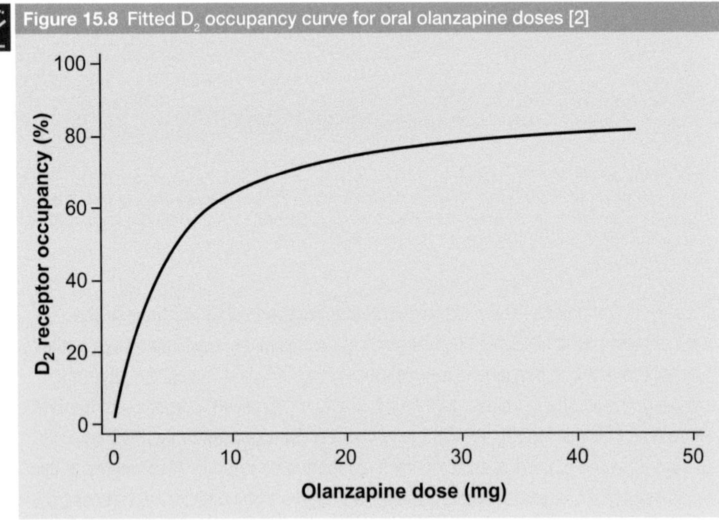

(Adapted from: D. Bishara, O. Olofinjana, A. Sparshatt, *et al.* [2013]. Olanzapine: a systematic review and meta-regression of the relationships between dose, plasma concentration, receptor occupancy, and response. *J Clin Psychopharmacol*, 33, 329–335.)

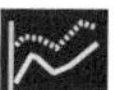

Figure 15.9 Fitted D_2 occupancy curve for plasma olanzapine levels [41]

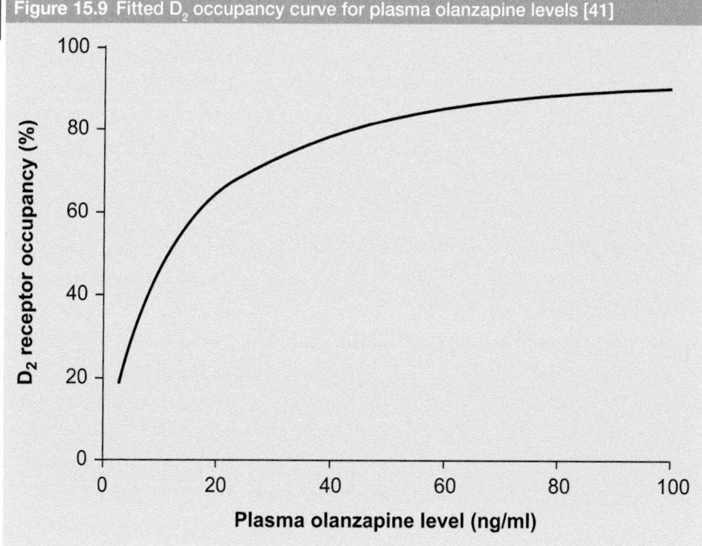

(Adapted from: D. Mamo, S. Kapur, M. Keshavan, *et al*. [2008]. D2 receptor occupancy of olanzapine pamoate depot using positron emission tomography: an open-label study in patients with schizophrenia. *Neuropsychopharmacology*, 33, 298–304.)

level (Figure 15.9). From these values, the plasma levels associated with 65% striatal D_2 occupancy range from 13.2–20.4 ng/ml. The lower estimate of 13.2 ng/ml equals an oral dose in a nonsmoker < 7 mg/d, while the upper end of the range is approximately equal to that found in the ROC analyses and is a dose of 10 mg/d for a nonsmoker. In this instance, the imaging data are not inconsistent with the ROC analyses from clinical studies, but the latter should be viewed as having more solid support.

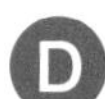

D The Point of Futility for Olanzapine

1 Clinical Evidence for a Point of Futility

The level where the average patient might respond or achieve maximum symptom reduction is important, but the question of futility revolves around when further titration should stop for nonresponders in the absence of dose-limiting side effects

[45]. Given the high $5HT_{2A}$ binding affinity that decreases rates of neurological adverse effects, olanzapine titration will not necessarily end at one of the hard clinical endpoints (intolerability) from parkinsonism or akathisia, or the unpleasant, dysphoric subjective experience associated with excessive D_2 blockade ***for that patient*** (see Chapter 5 for discussion of clinical endpoints) [46, 47]. There is no question that outstanding tolerability is a significant factor in defining olanzapine's point of futility, as patients may be more likely to tolerate plasma levels that exceed the point where the chance of response is extremely limited.

Evidence for an endpoint beyond which response is small can be derived from three studies of high-dose olanzapine in rigorously defined treatment-resistant schizophrenia patients, all of whom had failed a prospective high-dose antipsychotic trial based on Kane's criteria (Box 15.1). Two trials included double-blind and open-label periods of olanzapine at 25 mg/d, and this dose was associated with response rates of 5%–7% based on a response definition of ≥ 20% improvement in BPRS total score ***and*** a final BPRS score of < 35 or a 1-point improvement on the CGI-Severity scale [20, 21]. Unfortunately, no plasma level data was reported. When olanzapine nonresponders (n = 27) were transitioned to clozapine, 41% met response criteria [21]. A double-blind cross-over design of olanzapine 50 mg/d versus clozapine 450 mg/d provides the best source from which to estimate a point of futility [22]. For the assigned arm, patients were titrated over 2 weeks with the option of reduction to 30 mg/d olanzapine if needed for tolerability, with response defined based on the same criteria as in the 25 mg/d trials [22]. A total of 13 olanzapine treatment episodes were recorded, and 0% were associated with response, while 6 of 13 (46%) olanzapine-treated patients discontinued the study [22]. Of note, none of the clozapine-treated patients discontinued the study medication and the eventual response rate was 30%, despite dosing not being tied to plasma clozapine levels. At 8 weeks, women had mean steady state olanzapine levels of 278 ± 62 ng/ml, while men had mean levels of 127 ± 47 ng/ml [22]. Despite the extremely high plasma olanzapine levels, with multiple subjects exceeding 200 ng/ml and one > 300 ng/ml, significant akathisia was not reported. Olanzapine-treated patients did experience high rates of anticholinergic effects such as dry mouth (80%), constipation (60%), and blurred vision (40%) [48].

From these studies, we have evidence that plasma levels associated with 50 mg/d are not more effective than treatment with 25 mg/d, but D_2-related adverse effects such as akathisia may not be the limiting factor as levels > 200 ng/ml are clearly tolerated by a large subgroup of the patients who remained in the high-dose 50 mg/d olanzapine trial [22, 5]. No unusual safety concerns emerged during the 2-week titration to 50 mg/d, and the dropout rate was only 46%, implying that the remaining 54% could tolerate the anticholinergic burden, though without clinical benefit. While perhaps not more effective, evidence that high plasma levels are not inherently unsafe comes from a therapeutic drug monitoring analysis of data from the UK and Ireland for 1999–2009 [8]. Among the sample of 5856 patients, 1556 provided the time since last dose, of which 80% (1221) were obtained in the window of 6–18 hours post-dose [8]. There were 99 samples with trough olanzapine levels ≥ 150 ng/ml, with a median value of 190 ng/ml (10th–90th percentile range: 155–327 ng/ml) in those with dosing information. One woman on a prescribed dose of 30 mg/d with a history of nonadherence had a plasma level of 480 ng/ml. In attempting to estimate a point of futility, we know that 25 mg/d produced a response rate of 7% in treatment-resistant patients, and that mean levels ≥ 127 ng/ml in males on 50 mg/d produced no responders. The next issue to decide is the expected upper range of plasma levels for 25 mg/d, especially in nonsmoking females. In addressing this, we have to account for the exaggerated difference between men and women in the concentration–dose relationship at 50 mg/d, with women experiencing mean trough levels almost six times the oral dose, while for men mean levels are close to the expected value of two times the dose [5]. As women generally have lower levels of CYP 1A2 function, this marked difference is likely due to saturation of the low-capacity enzyme CYP 1A2. Although there is limited data on plasma levels for nonsmoking females on 25 mg/d, if we assume that the concentration might indeed be as high as six times the oral dose, a plasma level of 150 ng/ml is a reasonable estimate of the point of futility, and accurately embodies the concept that higher levels might be tolerable but are unlikely to be effective in > 90% of patients. The 2020 AGNP/ASCP consensus paper proposes a 100 ng/ml laboratory alert level, although the rationale is not made explicit [26]. As noted previously, levels exceeding 200 ng/ml do not appear unsafe, although they are not necessarily effective.

2 Imaging Evidence for a Point of Futility

For first-generation antipsychotics (FGAs), tolerability decreases markedly when D_2 receptor occupancy exceeds 80%, and the rates of neurological adverse effects significantly increase. This is projected to be true for second-generation agents, but the high-dose olanzapine studies and the UK/Ireland data set suggest that plasma levels associated with extremely high D_2 occupancy are more tolerable than with FGAs, likely due to the presence of significant $5HT_{2A}$ antagonism that helps to reduce the incidence of neurological adverse effects. While a range of EC_{50} results have been published in olanzapine PET studies, the EC_{50} value of 11.0 ng/ml discussed previously resulted in a calculated plasma level of 20 ng/ml to reach 65% D_2 occupancy, very close to the clinically derived response threshold of 23 ng/ml [41]. Using this EC_{50}

15

value of 11.0 ng/ml for the sake of consistency, a plasma level of 44.0 ng/ml is needed to achieve 80% D_2 receptor occupancy. That akathisia was not seen among the female cohort in the 50 mg/d study despite a mean plasma level of 278 ± 62 ng/ml is confirmation that near saturation of the $5HT_{2A}$ receptor markedly reduces D_2-related adverse effects, although one could hypothesize that certain patients may have dropped out due to akathisia-related symptoms such as dysphoria or symptomatic worsening [5]. Nonetheless, a plasma level of 278 ng/ml is associated with 96% D_2 occupancy, a level of striatal postsynaptic antagonism that would be intolerable to > 95% of patients exposed to FGAs. This high degree of tolerability limits the ability to define a point of futility for olanzapine from imaging studies alone, leaving the clinically based conclusions as the better source of information to define this important treatment endpoint.

Summary Points

a The correlation between olanzapine plasma levels and schizophrenia response has been widely studied. The suggested therapeutic response threshold is 23 ng/ml, and the point of futility is 150 ng/ml. The 2020 AGNP/ASCP consensus paper strongly recommends plasma level monitoring.

b The oral olanzapine concentration–dose relationship is well established, with approximately 50% higher levels in nonsmokers for a given dose: nonsmokers 10 mg at bedtime = 20.0 ng/ml; smokers 14 mg at bedtime = 20.0 ng/ml (12h trough).

c When treatment resistance is rigorously defined, response rates to high-dose olanzapine are 7% or less. It should not be considered a substitute for clozapine, although it shares with clozapine the penchant for significant weight gain and other metabolic adverse effects.

d The maximum monthly maintenance dose of the long-acting injectable olanzapine pamoate is 300 mg/2 weeks, and this provides the equivalent of 20 mg/d oral olanzapine. Due to the risk for post-injection delirium/sedation syndrome **after each injection**, prescribers, patients, and facilities must register in most countries with a risk mitigation program, and patients must be observed for at least 3 hours in a registered facility with ready access to emergency response services **after each injection**.

References

1. **Haslemo, T., Eikeseth, P. H., Tanum, L., *et al.* (2006).** The effect of variable cigarette consumption on the interaction with clozapine and olanzapine. *Eur J Clin Pharmacol*, 62, 1049–1053.
2. **Bishara, D., Olofinjana, O., Sparshatt, A., *et al.* (2013).** Olanzapine: a systematic review and meta-regression of the relationships between dose, plasma concentration, receptor occupancy, and response. *J Clin Psychopharmacol*, 33, 329–335.
3. **Perry, P. J., Lund, B. C., Sanger, T., *et al.* (2001).** Olanzapine plasma concentrations and clinical response: acute phase results of the North American Olanzapine Trial. *J Clin Psychopharmacol*, 21, 14–20.
4. **Lu, M. L., Wu, Y. X., Chen, C. H., *et al.* (2016).** Application of plasma levels of olanzapine and N-desmethyl-olanzapine to monitor clinical efficacy in patients with schizophrenia. *PLoS One*, 11, e0148539.
5. **Kelly, D. L., Richardson, C. M., Yang, Y., *et al.* (2006).** Plasma concentrations of high-dose olanzapine in a double-blind crossover study. *Hum Psychopharmacol*, 21, 393–398.
6. **Meyer, J. M. (2014).** A rational approach to employing high plasma levels of antipsychotics for violence associated with schizophrenia: case vignettes. *CNS Spectr*, 19, 432–438.
7. **Bigos, K. L., Pollock, B. G., Coley, K. C., *et al.* (2008).** Sex, race, and smoking impact olanzapine exposure. *J Clin Pharmacol*, 48, 157–165.
8. **Patel, M. X., Bowskill, S., Couchman, L., *et al.* (2011).** Plasma olanzapine in relation to prescribed dose and other factors: data from a therapeutic drug monitoring service, 1999–2009. *J Clin Psychopharmacol*, 31, 411–417.
9. **Meyer, J. M., Davis, V. G., Goff, D. C., *et al.* (2008).** Change in metabolic syndrome parameters with antipsychotic treatment in the CATIE Schizophrenia Trial: prospective data from phase 1. *Schizophr Res*, 101, 273–286.
10. **Meyer, J. M. (2010).** Antipsychotics and metabolics in the post-CATIE era. *Curr Top Behav Neurosci*, 4, 23–42.
11. **Huhn, M., Nikolakopoulou, A., Schneider-Thoma, J., *et al.* (2019).** Comparative efficacy and tolerability of 32 oral antipsychotics for the acute treatment of adults with multi-episode schizophrenia: a systematic review and network meta-analysis. *Lancet*, 394, 939–951.
12. **Lieberman, J. A., Stroup, T. S., McEvoy, J. P., *et al.* (2005).** Effectiveness of antipsychotic drugs in patients with chronic schizophrenia. *N Engl J Med*, 353, 1209–1223.
13. **McEvoy, J. P., Lieberman, J. A., Stroup, T. S., *et al.* (2006).** Effectiveness of clozapine versus olanzapine, quetiapine, and risperidone in patients with chronic schizophrenia who did not respond to prior atypical antipsychotic treatment. *Am J Psychiatry*, 163, 600–610.
14. **Pillinger, T., McCutcheon, R. A., Vano, L., *et al.* (2020).** Comparative effects of 18 antipsychotics on metabolic function in patients with schizophrenia, predictors of metabolic dysregulation, and association with psychopathology: a systematic review and network meta-analysis. *Lancet Psychiatry*, 7, 64–77.
15. **Meyer, J. M. and Stahl, S. M. (2019).** *The Clozapine Handbook*. Cambridge: Cambridge University Press.
16. **Meltzer, H. Y., Bobo, W. V., Roy, A., *et al.* (2008).** A randomized, double-blind comparison of clozapine and high-dose olanzapine in treatment-resistant patients with schizophrenia. *J Clin Psychiatry*, 69, 274–285.
17. **Kane, J., Honigfeld, G., Singer, J., *et al.* (1988).** Clozapine for the treatment-resistant schizophrenic: a double-blind comparison with chlorpromazine. *Arch Gen Psychiatry*, 45, 789–796.
18. **Samara, M. T., Dold, M., Gianatsi, M., *et al.* (2016).** Efficacy, acceptability, and tolerability of antipsychotics in treatment-resistant schizophrenia: a network meta-analysis. *JAMA Psychiatry*, 73, 199–210.

19. **Howes, O. D., McCutcheon, R., Agid, O., *et al.* (2017).** Treatment-resistant schizophrenia: Treatment Response and Resistance in Psychosis (TRRIP) working group consensus guidelines on diagnosis and terminology. *Am J Psychiatry*, 174, 216–229.
20. **Conley, R. R., Tamminga, C. A., Bartko, J. J., *et al.* (1998).** Olanzapine compared with chlorpromazine in treatment-resistant schizophrenia. *Am J Psychiatry*, 155, 914–920.
21. **Conley, R. R., Tamminga, C. A., Kelly, D. L., *et al.* (1999).** Treatment-resistant schizophrenic patients respond to clozapine after olanzapine non-response. *Biol Psychiatry*, 46, 73–77.
22. **Conley, R. R., Kelly, D. L., Richardson, C. M., *et al.* (2003).** The efficacy of high-dose olanzapine versus clozapine in treatment-resistant schizophrenia: a double-blind crossover study. *J Clin Psychopharmacol*, 23, 668–671.
23. **Kahn, R. S., Winter van Rossum, I., Leucht, S., *et al.* (2018).** Amisulpride and olanzapine followed by open-label treatment with clozapine in first-episode schizophrenia and schizophreniform disorder (OPTiMiSE): a three-phase switching study. *Lancet Psychiatry*, 5, 797–807.
24. **Detke, H. C., McDonnell, D. P., Brunner, E., *et al.* (2010).** Post-injection delirium/sedation syndrome in patients with schizophrenia treated with olanzapine long-acting injection, I: analysis of cases. *BMC Psychiatry*, 10,
25. **Eli Lilly and Company (2020).** Relprevv package insert. Indianapolis, IN.
26. **Schoretsanitis, G., Kane, J. M., Correll, C. U., *et al.* (2020).** Blood levels to optimize antipsychotic treatment in clinical practice: a joint consensus statement of the American Society of Clinical Psychopharmacology (ASCP) and the Therapeutic Drug Monitoring (TDM) Task Force of the Arbeitsgemeinschaft für Neuropsychopharmakologie und Pharmakopsychiatrie (AGNP). *J Clin Psychiatry*, 81, https://doi.org/10.4088/JCP.4019cs13169.
27. **Meyer, J. M. (2018).** Pharmacotherapy of psychosis and mania. In L. L. Brunton, R. Hilal-Dandan and B. C. Knollmann, eds., *Goodman & Gilman's The Pharmacological Basis of Therapeutics*, 13th edn. Chicago, IL: McGraw-Hill, pp. 279–302.
28. **Eli Lilly and Company (2020).** Zyprexa Tablet, Intramuscular Injection package insert. Indianapolis, IN.
29. **Soderberg, M. M. and Dahl, M. L. (2013).** Pharmacogenetics of olanzapine metabolism. *Pharmacogenomics*, 14, 1319–1336.
30. **Hiemke, C., Peled, A., Jabarin, M., *et al.* (2002).** Fluvoxamine augmentation of olanzapine in chronic schizophrenia: pharmacokinetic interactions and clinical effects. *J Clin Psychopharmacol*, 22, 502–506.
31. **Albers, L. J., Ozdemir, V., Marder, S. R., *et al.* (2005).** Low-dose fluvoxamine as an adjunct to reduce olanzapine therapeutic dose requirements: a prospective dose-adjusted drug interaction strategy. *J Clin Psychopharmacol*, 25, 170–174.
32. **Khorassani, F., Kaufman, M., and Lopez, L. V. (2018).** Supratherapeutic serum clozapine concentration after transition from traditional to electronic cigarettes. *J Clin Psychopharmacol*, 38, 391–392.
33. **Patteet, L., Morrens, M., Maudens, K. E., *et al.* (2012).** Therapeutic drug monitoring of common antipsychotics. *Ther Drug Monit*, 34, 629–651.
34. **Tveito, M., Smith, R. L., Høiseth, G., *et al.* (2019).** The effect of valproic acid on olanzapine serum concentration: a study including 2791 patients treated with olanzapine tablets or long-acting injections. *J Clin Psychopharmacol*, 39, 561–566.
35. **Food and Drug Administration Center for Drug Evaluation and Research (2003).** Olanzapine for injection pharmacology/clinical pharmacology and biopharmaceutics review.
36. **McDonnell, D. P., Detke, H. C., Bergstrom, R. F., *et al.* (2010).** Post-injection delirium/sedation syndrome in patients with schizophrenia treated with olanzapine long-acting injection, II: investigations of mechanism. *BMC Psychiatry*, 10, 45–54.

37. **Heres, S., Kraemer, S., Bergstrom, R. F., *et al.* (2014).** Pharmacokinetics of olanzapine long-acting injection: the clinical perspective. *Int Clin Psychopharmacol*, 29, 299–312.

38. **Detke, H. C., Zhao, F., Garhyan, P., *et al.* (2011).** Dose correspondence between olanzapine long-acting injection and oral olanzapine: recommendations for switching. *Int Clin Psychopharmacol*, 26, 35–42.

39. **Fellows, L., Ahmad, F., Castle, D. J., *et al.* (2003).** Investigation of target plasma concentration–effect relationships for olanzapine in schizophrenia. *Ther Drug Monit*, 25, 682–689.

40. **Leucht, S., Kane, J. M., Kissling, W., *et al.* (2005).** What does the PANSS mean? *Schizophr Res*, 79, 231–238.

41. **Mamo, D., Kapur, S., Keshavan, M., *et al.* (2008).** D2 receptor occupancy of olanzapine pamoate depot using positron emission tomography: an open-label study in patients with schizophrenia. *Neuropsychopharmacology*, 33, 298–304.

42. **Lataster, J., van Os, J., de Haan, L., *et al.* (2011).** Emotional experience and estimates of D2 receptor occupancy in psychotic patients treated with haloperidol, risperidone, or olanzapine: an experience sampling study. *J Clin Psychiatry*, 72, 1397–1404.

43. **Uchida, H., Takeuchi, H., Graff-Guerrero, A., *et al.* (2011).** Predicting dopamine D2 receptor occupancy from plasma levels of antipsychotic drugs: a systematic review and pooled analysis. *J Clin Psychopharmacol*, 31, 318–325.

44. **Mizuno, Y., Bies, R. R., Remington, G., *et al.* (2012).** Dopamine D2 receptor occupancy with risperidone or olanzapine during maintenance treatment of schizophrenia: a cross-sectional study. *Prog Neuropsychopharmacol Biol Psychiatry*, 37, 182–187.

45. **Giegling, I., Drago, A., Schafer, M., *et al.* (2010).** Interaction of haloperidol plasma level and antipsychotic effect in early phases of acute psychosis treatment. *J Psychiatr Res*, 44, 487–492.

46. **de Haan, L., van Bruggen, M., Lavalaye, J., *et al.* (2003).** Subjective experience and D2 receptor occupancy in patients with recent-onset schizophrenia treated with low-dose olanzapine or haloperidol: a randomized, double-blind study. *Am J Psychiatry*, 160, 303–309.

47. **Veselinović, T., Scharpenberg, M., Heinze, M., *et al.* (2019).** Dopamine D2 receptor occupancy estimated from plasma concentrations of four different antipsychotics and the subjective experience of physical and mental well-being in schizophrenia: results from the randomized NeSSy Trial. *J Clin Psychopharmacol*, 39, 550–560.

48. **Kelly, D. L., Conley, R. R., Richardson, C. M., *et al.* (2003).** Adverse effects and laboratory parameters of high-dose olanzapine vs. clozapine in treatment-resistant schizophrenia. *Ann Clin Psychiatry*, 15, 181–186.

49. **Haddad, P., Lambert, T., and Lauriello, J., eds. (2016).** *Antipsychotic Long-Acting Injections*, 2nd edn. New York: Oxford University Press.

16 Aripiprazole, Aripiprazole Monohydrate, and Aripiprazole Lauroxil

QUICK CHECK

PRINCIPLES

- Aripiprazole was the first approved dopamine partial agonist, with numerous indications beyond schizophrenia. It exists in oral and in two long-acting injectable (LAI) versions.
- There is an extensive database of plasma level information and imaging studies. As a dopamine partial agonist, aripiprazole works in a range of 83%–100% dopamine D_2 receptor occupancy for schizophrenia, with a therapeutic threshold of 110 ng/ml. The point of futility is defined when one reaches a plasma level associated with 100% D_2 occupancy, approximately 500 ng/ml.
- The two LAI versions differ in kinetics, the method of initiation, and guidelines around cytochrome P450 interactions and missed doses. Aripiprazole monohydrate (Abilify Maintena®) requires 2 weeks of oral bridging therapy when starting treatment. When starting aripiprazole lauroxil (Aristada®), one can use 3 weeks of oral bridging therapy, or an initiation regimen involving a single 30 mg oral aripiprazole dose and a single injection of aripiprazole lauroxil nanocrystal suspension (Aristada Initio®).

InfoBox Oral Aripiprazole Plasma Level Essentials

Oral dose correlation (bedtime dosing, 12h trough)	Level of evidence	Therapeutic threshold	Level of evidence	Point of futility	Level of evidence
10 mg = 110 ng/ml [1] **Multiply oral dose by 11.0** (see Table 16.1 for effects of CYP inhibitors/inducers on this relationship)	High	110 ng/ml	High	500 ng/ml	High

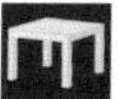

Table 16.1 Oral aripiprazole kinetic facts [8, 26]

Basic facts	Inhibition effects	Induction effects
US FDA approval: Nov. 15, 2002 $T_{1/2}$ 75 hours $T_{1/2}$ 94 hours (dehydroaripiprazole) Bioavailability: 87% T_{max} 3–5 hours Metabolism: CYP 2D6 and to a lesser extent CYP 3A4. The active metabolite dehydroaripiprazole is present at plasma levels approximately 36% that of aripiprazole [16, 1, 17]* **Formulations:** Tablets, oral dissolving tablets, oral solution	CYP 2D6 poor metabolizers (PM) experience 80% increase in aripiprazole AUC, and 30% decrease in metabolite AUC (net effect is 60% increase in AUC for active moiety). Aripiprazole half-life is 146 hours in CYP 2D6 PM Strong 2D6 inhibitors increase aripiprazole AUC by 112% and decrease the metabolite AUC by 35% Ketoconazole increases AUC of a single 15 mg aripiprazole dose and its active metabolite by 63% and 77%, respectively	3A4/PGP induction decreases the AUC of aripiprazole and its metabolite by 70%

* Dehydroaripiprazole contributes to the activity, but most laboratories do not report this level, and efficacy correlates well with the plasma aripiprazole level. Moreover, only aripiprazole levels are increased significantly during exposure to a strong CYP 2D6 inhibitor, or when administered to CYP 2D6 poor metabolizers, while these circumstances have a modest effect on dehydroaripiprazole levels [27, 28].

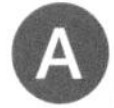

A Basic Pharmacokinetic Information for Oral Aripiprazole and Long-Acting Injectable Aripiprazole Monohydrate and Aripiprazole Lauroxil

Aripiprazole has been available since 2002, with long-acting injectable versions approved in 2013 and 2015. Aside from clozapine, all antipsychotics approved prior to aripiprazole acted principally via postsynaptic dopamine D_2 receptor antagonism in the associative striatum [2, 3]. While D_2 antagonist antipsychotics are very useful, excessively high levels of striatal D_2 occupancy (i.e. ≫ 80% reduction in the postsynaptic dopamine signal) resulted in higher rates of adverse neurological effects (e.g. parkinsonism, akathisia), subjective complaints of dysphoria or decreased well-being, and occasionally symptomatic worsening [4, 5]. The idea behind a dopamine D_2 partial agonist is to modulate D_2-related neurotransmission with limited risk for excessive reduction in the postsynaptic D_2 signal (Figure 16.1) [7]. Although aripiprazole has been available for nearly 20 years, and there are now three approved partial agonist antipsychotics, how this mechanism translates into antipsychotic activity requires some explanation. Based on *in vitro* assays, aripiprazole is postulated to have approximately 25% of the intrinsic activity of dopamine itself at D_2 receptors [7]. Figure 16.2 illustrates two important points: (a) A partial agonist like

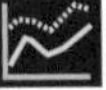

Figure 16.1 The differential relationship between subjective well-being score and ventral striatal D_2 receptor occupancy in patients treated with dopamine antagonist or partial agonist antipsychotics [22]

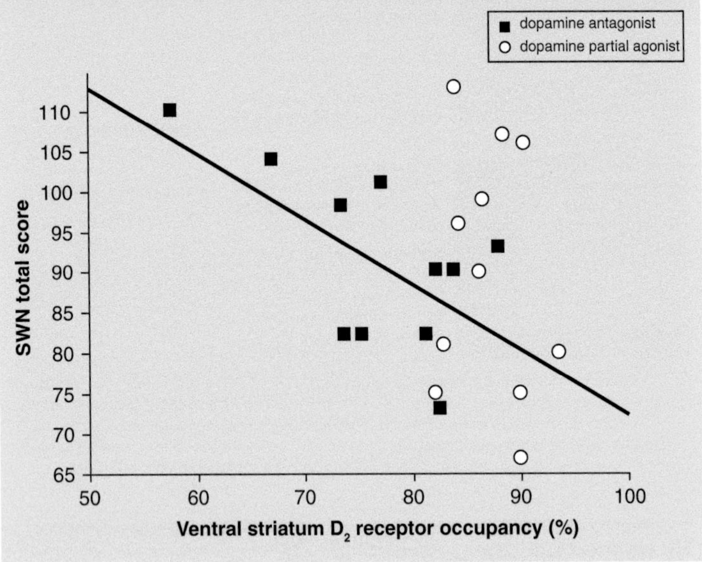

(Adapted from: R. Mizrahi, D. Mamo, P. Rusjan, *et al*. [2009]. The relationship between subjective well-being and dopamine D2 receptors in patients treated with a dopamine partial agonist and full antagonist antipsychotics. *Int J Neuropsychopharmacol*, 12, 715–721.)

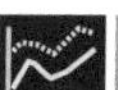

Figure 16.2 How the partial agonist aripiprazole acts as an antipsychotic at D_2 receptors

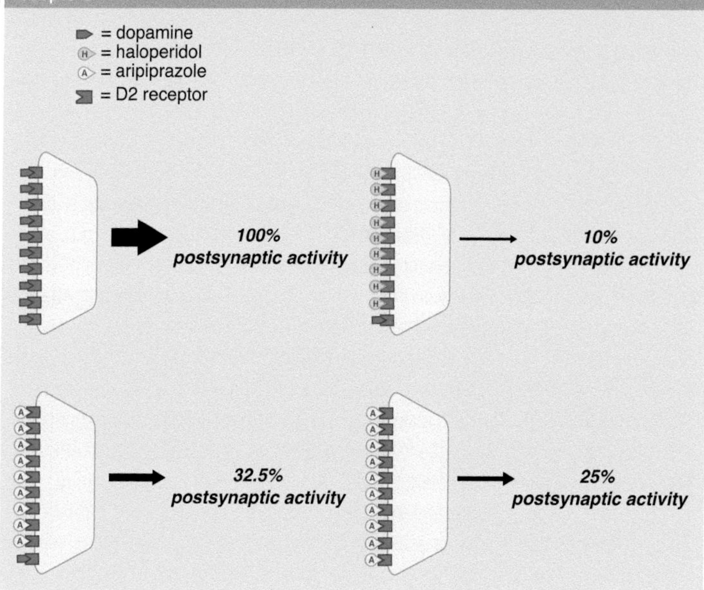

The full postsynaptic signal is seen when dopamine binds to all D_2 receptors. What happens if haloperidol or aripiprazole occupy some of these receptors?

[a] (Upper left): A neuron with ten D_2 receptors, each of which has dopamine binding to the receptor. Each receptor contributes a 100% signal x 10/10. Net is 100% postsynaptic activity.

[b] (Upper right): A neuron with ten D_2 receptors, nine of which have haloperidol and one with dopamine binding to the receptor. The haloperidol-bound receptors contribute no signal, and the dopamine-bound receptor contributes 100% signal x 1/10 = 10%. Net is 10% postsynaptic activity (i.e. a decrease of 90%).

[c] (Lower left): A neuron with ten D_2 receptors, nine of which have aripiprazole and one with dopamine binding to the receptor. The aripiprazole-bound receptors each have a 25% signal: 25% x 9/10 = 22.5%. The one dopamine-bound receptor contributes a 100% signal: 100% x 1/10 = 10%. Net is 22.5% + 10% = 32.5% postsynaptic activity (i.e. a decrease of 67.5%).

[d] (Lower right): A neuron with ten D_2 receptors, all of which have aripiprazole binding to the receptor. The aripiprazole-bound receptors each have a 25% signal: 25% x 10/10 = 25% total. Net is 25% postsynaptic activity (i.e. a decrease of 75%).

aripiprazole with 25% intrinsic activity will be an effective agent only at very high levels of striatal D_2 occupancy (e.g. 83%–100%), higher than that for a D_2 antagonist; and (b) even when pushed to 100% receptor occupancy, the postsynaptic dopamine signal will be sufficient to limit neurological adverse effects in most patients. Parkinsonism and dystonia are therefore uncommon, but akathisia does occur during aripiprazole therapy and is postulated to be a result of D_2 partial agonism as opposed to excessive D_2 antagonism [8]. Aripiprazole's high affinity for the D_2 receptor and the fact that it operates at extremely high levels of D_2 receptor occupancy can result in situations where addition of aripiprazole to a potent D_2 antagonist (e.g. first-generation antipsychotics, risperidone > 6 mg/d, olanzapine > 25 mg/d, etc.) can result in symptomatic worsening as D_2 receptor antagonism is replaced with partial agonism [9]. Conversely, symptom exacerbation is unlikely to occur when aripiprazole (or another partial agonist antipsychotic) is added to modest levels of D_2 antagonism. In a clinical trial, adjunctive aripiprazole (mean dose 10.3 mg/d) was added to patients on a mean risperidone dose of 4.7 mg/d, or a mean quetiapine dose of 515 mg/d, but did not cause symptom exacerbation [10]. Aripiprazole has also been successfully added to clozapine, a weaker D_2 antagonist whose efficacy likely relates to other mechanisms [11, 12]. Aripiprazole also has high affinity for the dopamine D_3 receptor, and this is hypothesized to be one of the primary antidepressant mechanisms for aripiprazole, brexpiprazole, and cariprazine, with the latter having the greatest affinity among the three partial agonist antipsychotics (Ki 0.085 nM) [13, 14].

Unlike D_2 antagonists, aripiprazole tends to lower serum prolactin values [10]; moreover, aripiprazole has relatively low risk for metabolic adverse effects, both of which are features that offer tolerability advantages over other second-generation antipsychotics [15]. Aripiprazole's metabolic pathways and oral concentration–dose relationships are also well characterized. There is an active metabolite dehydroaripiprazole present at levels approximately 36% that of the parent compound, although few laboratories report the metabolite levels [16, 1, 17]. In addition to extensive clinical data for schizophrenia treatment, multiple Positron Emission Tomography (PET) imaging studies have been performed correlating response and D_2 receptor occupancy [18–23, 5, 24]. Aripiprazole was assigned a Level 2 recommendation (recommended) for use of plasma level monitoring in the 2020 consensus paper authored jointly by the Therapeutic Drug Monitoring (TDM) task force of the German Arbeitsgemeinschaft für Neuropsychopharmakologie und Pharmakopsychiatrie (AGNP) and the American Society for Clinical Psychopharmacology (ASCP) [25].

Essential Information for Oral Aripiprazole and Long-Acting Injectable Aripiprazole Monohydrate and Aripiprazole Lauroxil

1 Essential Oral Aripiprazole Information

Aripiprazole has a long half-life of 75 hours, and the active metabolite dehydroaripiprazole has an even longer half-life of 95 hours [8]. Not surprisingly, the half-life is sufficiently long to support once daily dosing, and it should always be administered at bedtime for reasons of tolerability (see Chapter 5) and to insure that the morning trough is approximately 12h from the last dose. Aripiprazole is metabolized via cytochrome P450 (CYP) 2D6 and CYP 3A4, but more so through CYP 2D6. Patients receiving strong CYP 2D6 inhibitors or those who are CYP 2D6 poor metabolizers will have higher aripiprazole levels, but with limited change in metabolite levels (although few laboratories report dehydroaripiprazole at the present time) [16, 1, 17]. Strong CYP 3A4 inhibitors have less of an impact on drug exposure than strong CYP 2D6 inhibitors, but strong CYP 3A4 inducers (e.g. carbamazepine, phenytoin, rifampin) lower plasma levels by 70% [8]. The absolute oral bioavailability of aripiprazole is 87%, and large therapeutic drug monitoring studies indicate that trough plasma aripiprazole levels are approximately 11.0 times the oral dose [16, 1, 26].

2 Essential Long-Acting Injectable Aripiprazole Monohydrate Information

Aripiprazole monohydrate was the first approved LAI aripiprazole formulation, and has been available in the US since 2013. Although aripiprazole monohydrate has a short T_{max} of approximately 7 days, loading studies were not performed by the manufacturer, so initiation requires 2 weeks of oral bridging therapy, and steady state is achieved after 4 monthly injections (Table 16.2, Figure 16.3) [29, 30]. The missed dose guidelines reflect this and mandate 2 weeks of oral therapy when a patient is more than 7 days late for the injection if they have not yet received the fourth monthly injection (Table 16.3). The maximum dose of 400 mg/month provides the equivalent of 20 mg/d oral aripiprazole at steady state, with adjustments needed based on patient tolerance and CYP interactions (Table 16.3) [29]. No specific dose equivalence is provided for lower monthly dosages, but one can estimate that 300 mg/month is equivalent to 15 mg/d from steady state plasma levels. The inability to load aripiprazole monohydrate or initiate without extended oral bridging therapy, the lack of dosing interval options beyond 4 weeks, and the fact that aripiprazole monohydrate cannot be used in the presence of CYP 3A4 inducers are limiting factors.

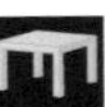

Table 16.2 Aripiprazole monohydrate, aripiprazole lauroxil, and aripiprazole lauroxil nanocrystal suspension essential information [31, 32, 30]

	Vehicle	Concentration	Dosage[a]	T_{max} (days)	$T_{1/2}$ (days) multiple dosing	Able to be loaded	Maintenance dose: oral equivalence
Aripiprazole monohydrate (Abilify Maintena®)	Water	300 mg/1.5 ml 400 mg/1.9 ml	300–400 mg/4 weeks **Max:** 400 mg/4 weeks	6.5–7.1 days	29.9–46.5 days	**No[b]**	400 mg/4 weeks = 20 mg/d oral
Aripiprazole lauroxil (Aristada®)[c]	Water	441 mg/1.6 ml 662 mg/2.4 ml 882 mg/3.2 ml 1064 mg/3.9 ml	441 mg, 662 mg, or 882 mg/4 weeks 882 mg/6 weeks 1064/8 weeks **Max:** 882 mg/4 weeks	41 days (single dose) [33] 24.4–35.2 days (repeated dosing) [34]	53.9–57.2 days	**See below[c]**	441 mg/4 weeks = 10 mg/d 662 mg/4 weeks = 15 mg/d 882 mg/6 weeks = 15 mg/d 1064 mg/8 weeks ≤ 15 mg/d 822 mg/4 weeks = 20 mg/d
Aripiprazole lauroxil nanocrystal (Aristada Initio®)[d]	Water	675 mg/2.4 ml	675 mg once	27 days (range: 16 to 35 days)	15–18 days (single dose)	–	N/A

[a] See Tables 16.3 and 16.4 for dosing adjustments in the presence of strong CYP 2D6 or 3A4 inhibitors, in CYP 2D6 poor metabolizers, or with use of strong CYP 3A4 inducers.

[b] Requires 14 days oral overlap.

[c] Requires 21 days oral overlap unless starting with aripiprazole lauroxil nanocrystal 675 mg IM + a single 30 mg oral dose.

[d] Aripiprazole lauroxil nanocrystal (AL_{NC}) is only used for initiation of treatment with aripiprazole lauroxil, or for resumption of treatment. It is always administered together with the clinician-determined dose of aripiprazole lauroxil, although the latter can be given ≤ 10 days after the aripiprazole lauroxil nanocrystal injection.

(For further reading about use of LAI antipsychotics, please see the comprehensive edited book ***Antipsychotic Long-Acting Injections***, now in its 2nd edition [35]).

Figure 16.3 Plasma aripiprazole levels following administration of aripiprazole monohydrate with 2 weeks of oral aripiprazole 10 mg/day overlap [29]

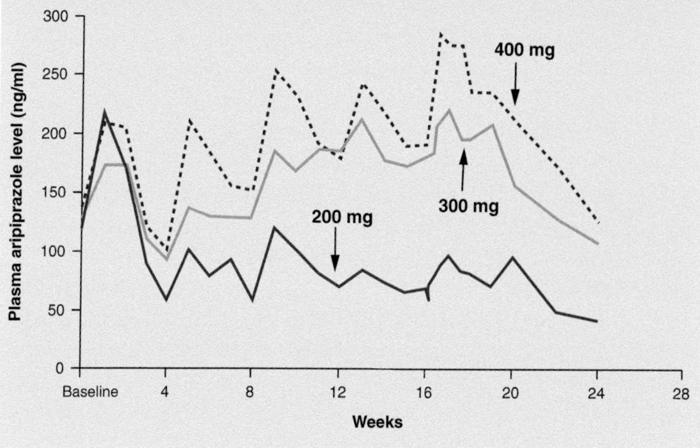

(Adapted from: J. M. Meyer [2017]. Converting oral to long acting injectable antipsychotics: a guide for the perplexed. *CNS Spectr*, 22, 14–28.)

Table 16.3 Aripiprazole monohydrate cytochrome P450 (CYP) dosing adjustments and missed dose guidelines [30]

CYP 450 dosing adjustments		Missed dose guidelines
Patients taking 400 mg		*If the 2nd or 3rd doses are missed:*
CYP2D6 poor metabolizers	300 mg	If more than 4 wks and less than 5 wks have elapsed since the last injection, administer the injection as soon as possible.
CYP2D6 poor metabolizers taking concomitant CYP3A4 inhibitors	200 mg	**If more than 5 wks have elapsed since the last injection, restart concomitant oral aripiprazole for 14 days with the next administered injection.**
Patients taking 400 mg		
Strong CYP2D6 **or** CYP3A4 inhibitors	300 mg	*If the 4th or subsequent doses are missed:*
CYP2D6 **and** CYP3A4 inhibitors	200 mg	If more than 4 wks and less than 6 wks have elapsed since the last injection, administer the injection as soon as possible.
CYP3A4 inducers	Avoid use	
Patients taking 300 mg		
Strong CYP2D6 **or** CYP3A4 inhibitors	200 mg	**If more than 6 wks have elapsed since the last injection, restart concomitant oral aripiprazole for 14 days with the next administered injection.**
CYP2D6 **and** CYP3A4 inhibitors	160 mg	
CYP3A4 inducers	**Avoid use**	

16

3 Essential Long-Acting Injectable Aripiprazole Lauroxil and Aripiprazole Lauroxil Nanocrystal Suspension

Aripiprazole lauroxil was approved in 2015, and has a different kinetic profile than aripiprazole monohydrate, with a long T_{max} and a longer half-life (Table 16.2, Figure 16.4). The slow systemic delivery of aripiprazole results in missed dose guidelines that in some circumstances allow a patient to be up to 4 weeks late for an injection without the need for any supplemental aripiprazole (Table 16.4a, 16.4b); moreover, the sustained plasma levels permit use with CYP 3A4 inducers, and with no dose adjustment except for those patients on the lowest dose of 441 mg/month. There are also multiple dosage strengths tied directly to oral equivalents from 10 mg/d to 20 mg/d, and both 6-week and 8-week dosage intervals (Tables 16.4a, 16.4b). When initially approved, the long T_{max} necessitated 3 weeks of oral bridging therapy, but a formulation with nanomolecular size crystals was approved in 2018 to obviate the need for extended oral coverage when starting or reinitiating aripiprazole lauroxil [32]. The combination of a single 675 mg IM injection of this nanocrystal suspension and a single 30 mg oral dose replicates what would be achieved with 3 weeks of oral aripiprazole, and this combination is administered at the same time as the clinician-chosen maintenance dose of aripiprazole lauroxil (Figure 16.4). Patients, carers, and other clinical staff may require education that this initiation regimen is comparable to 21 days of oral coverage when co-administered with the maintenance dose of aripiprazole lauroxil, as the milligram dosages involved may seem large (e.g. 882 mg + 675 mg). The kinetic study in Figure 16.4 demonstrates this equivalence and may

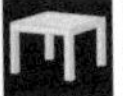

Tables 16.4a and 4b Aripiprazole lauroxil cytochrome P450 (CYP) dosing adjustments and missed dose guidelines [31, 32]

CYP 450 dosing adjustments	
Concomitant medicine	**Dose change**
Strong 3A4 inhibitor	Reduce the dose to next lower strength.* No adjustment in pts taking 441 mg, if tolerated. For CYP2D6 PM: reduce dose to 441 mg from 662 mg, 882 mg, or 1064 mg. No adjustment in pts taking 441, mg if tolerated.
Strong 2D6 inhibitor	Reduce the dose to next lower strength.* No adjustment in pts taking 441 mg, if tolerated. For CYP2D6 PM: no adjustment required.
Strong 2D6 and 3A4 inhibitor	Avoid 662 mg, 882 mg, or 1064 mg doses. No adjustment in pts taking 441 mg, if tolerated.
3A4 inducers	No dose adjustment for 662 mg, 882 mg, or 1064 mg dose. For those on 441 mg, increase to 662 mg.

* For 882 mg/6 weeks and 1064 mg/8 weeks, the next lower strength is 441 mg/4 weeks.

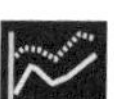

Figure 16.4 Plasma aripiprazole levels following an initiation regimen of 675 mg IM aripiprazole lauroxil nanocrystal (AL_{NC}), a single 30 mg oral dose, and simultaneous administration of 882 mg IM aripiprazole lauroxil, compared to levels from 21 days of 15 mg oral aripiprazole with 882 mg IM aripiprazole lauroxil [36]

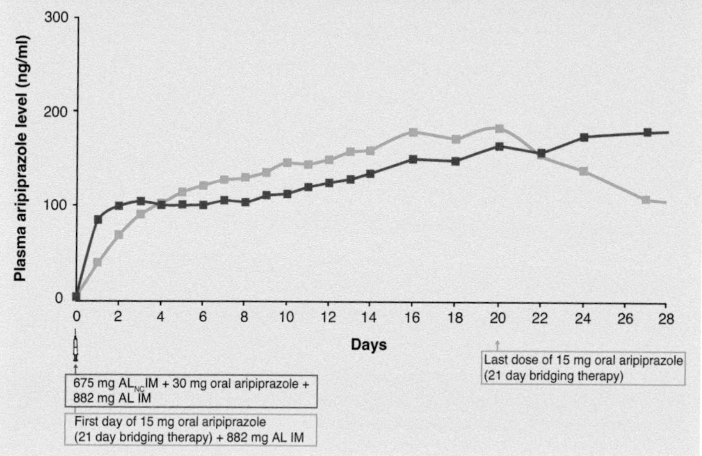

(Adapted from: R. Jain, J. M. Meyer, A. Y. Wehr, *et al.* [2020]. Size matters: the importance of particle size in a newly developed injectable formulation for the treatment of schizophrenia. *CNS Spectr*, 25, 323–330.)

be very helpful in reassuring those who express concern about the total dosage being administered.

The 30 mg oral dose which is part of the initiation regimen helps provide clinically relevant aripiprazole exposure (equivalent to 10 mg/d) by day 4 of treatment until levels increase from the nanocrystal suspension injection (Figure 16.5) [36]. Failure to administer the 30 mg oral dose means that relevant plasma levels are not achieved until day 11 [36]. The aripiprazole lauroxil formulation used for maintenance dosing has a long T_{max} related to the slow dissolution of its micron-sized crystals, and thus provides limited drug levels during the first few weeks [36]. The maintenance formulation contributes so little early on that it can be administered up to 10 days after the nanocrystal suspension injection + 30 mg oral dose combination; however, the nanocrystal suspension has a shorter T_{max} and much shorter half-life, so failure to administer the maintenance dose will result in subtherapeutic levels once the plasma levels rapidly decline from the nanocrystal suspension injection [32, 31]. The nanocrystal suspension can also be used to reinitiate treatment according to the missed dose guidelines. In circumstances where the patient refuses an injection of the nanocrystal suspension when starting or resuming treatment with aripiprazole lauroxil, oral bridging therapy is used.

C The Therapeutic Threshold for Aripiprazole

1 Clinical Evidence for a Therapeutic Threshold for Aripiprazole

Extensive fixed-dose aripiprazole studies have been performed with oral and LAI formulations, but no publication has performed a receiver operating curve (ROC) analysis to calculate a threshold response plasma level. Despite this, the abundant body of data points to an oral dose of 10 mg/d as representing a response threshold, the evidence for which is summed in a 2010 review [1]. From the larger therapeutic drug monitoring studies, 10 mg at bedtime (QHS) of oral aripiprazole equals a 12h trough plasma level of 110 ng/ml, but threshold levels of 100 ng/ml are also cited in the literature, including the AGNP/ASCP consensus paper [1, 25]. The D_2 occupancy curve becomes very flat after this point, and there is less efficacy separation in the range of

Figure 16.5 Plasma aripiprazole levels from the combination of one injection of aripiprazole lauroxil nanocrystal suspension (AL_{NC}) (675 mg), a single 30 mg oral aripiprazole dose, and aripiprazole lauroxil (1064 mg). Highlighted are the contributions of the individual components [36]

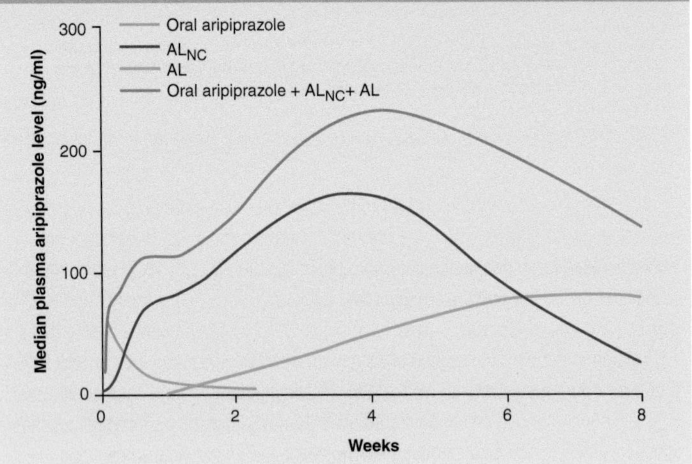

(Adapted from: R. Jain, J. M. Meyer, A. Y. Wehr, *et al.* [2020]. Size matters: the importance of particle size in a newly developed injectable formulation for the treatment of schizophrenia. *CNS Spectr*, 25, 323–330.)

Dose of last aripiprazole lauroxil maintenance injection	Missed dose guidelines Length of time since last injection*	
441 mg	> 6 and ≤ 7 weeks	> 7 weeks
662 mg or 882 mg	> 8 and ≤ 12 weeks	> 12 weeks
1064 mg	> 10 and ≤ 12 weeks	> 12 weeks
Dosage and administration for reinitiation of aripiprazole lauroxil	Supplement with a single dose of AL_{NC}**	Supplement with a single dose of AL_{NC} and a single dose of oral aripiprazole 30 mg***

* Patients should receive their maintenance injection of aripiprazole lauroxil in addition to any supplementation.

** If the patient refuses the injection of aripiprazole lauroxil nanocrystal, supplement with 7 days of oral aripiprazole.

*** If the patient refuses the injection of aripiprazole lauroxil nanocrystal + 30 mg oral dose, supplement with 21 days of oral aripiprazole.

10–30 mg/d than one might expect for a three-fold difference in drug exposure (Table 16.5, Figure 16.6); even the pivotal aripiprazole lauroxil trial in acutely exacerbated schizophrenia patients found nearly identical symptom reduction from the 441 mg/month dose (equivalent to 10 mg/d oral) and the 882 mg/month dose (equivalent to 20 mg/d oral) after 12 weeks of treatment [37]. While cross-sectional data make it hard to distinguish the efficacy differences between dosages above the equivalent of 10 mg/d, for any individual patient this may not be true, and ongoing titration should be pursued using the precepts in Chapter 5. The longer time to steady state compared to most oral antipsychotics (15.6 d) does not have an impact on response trajectory (Figure 16.7), so the 2-week rule on early nonresponse applies [38].

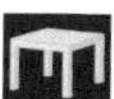

Table 16.5 Estimated dopamine D_2 receptor occupancy by aripiprazole oral dose [1]

Oral dose (mg)	D_2 receptor occupancy	Estimated plasma level
0.5	33.7%	5.5 ng/ml
1	57.2%	11 ng/ml
2	71.6%	22 ng/ml
10	85.3%	110 ng/ml
18.8	83–85%	207 ng/ml
30	86.4%	330 mg/ml
40	96.8%	440 ng/ml

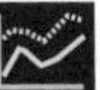

Figure 16.6 Fitted D_2 occupancy curve for aripiprazole in the dosage range of 10–30 mg/d, and the corresponding plasma levels [19]

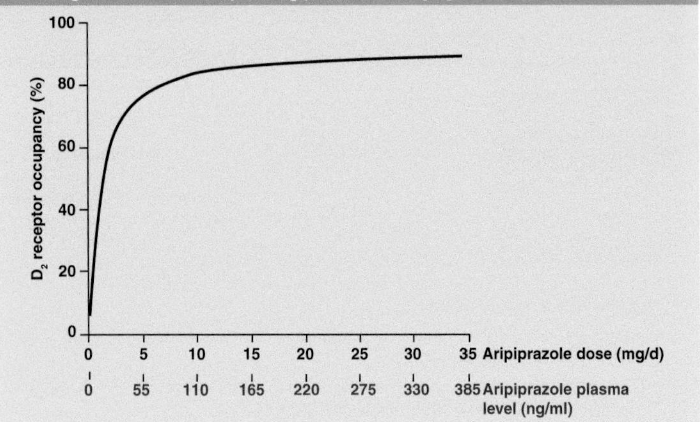

(Adapted from: D. Mamo, A. Graff, R. Mizrahi, *et al.* [2007]. Differential effects of aripiprazole on D(2), 5-HT(2), and 5-HT(1A) receptor occupancy in patients with schizophrenia: a triple tracer PET study. *Am J Psychiatry*, 164, 1411–1417.)

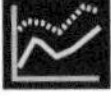

Figure 16.7 Mean change in Positive and Negative Syndrome Scale (PANSS) total score from baseline (week 0) to week 4 of treatment with aripiprazole (20 mg/d or 30 mg/d), risperidone (6 mg/d), or placebo [38]

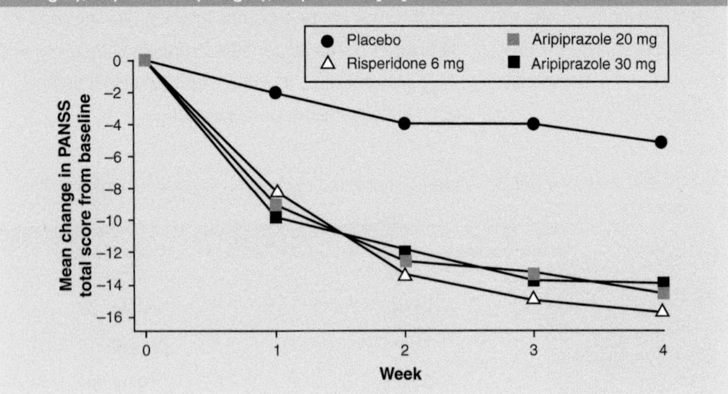

(Adapted from: S. G. Potkin, A. R. Saha, M. J. Kujawa, *et al.* [2003]. Aripiprazole, an antipsychotic with a novel mechanism of action, and risperidone vs placebo in patients with schizophrenia and schizoaffective disorder. *Arch Gen Psychiatry*, 60, 681–690.)

2 Imaging Evidence for a Therapeutic Threshold for Aripiprazole

As illustrated in Figure 16.2, a partial dopamine agonist with 25% intrinsic activity should require > 80% D_2 receptor occupancy to act as an antipsychotic. Based on the calculations shown with Figure 16.2, with 84% D_2 occupancy from aripiprazole the estimated postsynaptic D_2 activity is 37%, implying a 63% reduction. This 63% reduction in the postsynaptic D_2 signal is very close to the 65% occupancy threshold seen with D_2 antagonist antipsychotics for which occupancy is mathematically identical to the reduction in D_2 activity [8]. The curve in Figure 16.6 was based on dose, and 10 mg/d generates the D_2 occupancy required for aripiprazole antipsychotic efficacy [19]. From this, we can calculate the estimated plasma level for a response threshold of 110 ng/ml [1, 23].

D The Point of Futility for Aripiprazole

1 Clinical Evidence for a Point of Futility for Aripiprazole

Unlike D_2 antagonist antipsychotics, the point of futility for partial agonists is better defined by PET data than by the clinical data since there is a disconnect between the plasma level at which the biologically useful mechanism (D_2 blockade) is exhausted at 100% receptor occupancy, and the fact that many patients can have plasma levels pushed beyond this point. As has been shown, one could potentially titrate aripiprazole to the point of 100% D_2 receptor occupancy and even higher where other aspects of the molecule (e.g. alpha$_1$-adrenergic antagonism, histamine H_1 antagonism) might not be prominent enough to limit tolerability [16]. Based on the calculations shown with Figure 16.2, 100% D_2 occupancy from aripiprazole equals 25% postsynaptic D_2 activity, implying a 75% reduction. For most patients, the threshold for inducing neurological adverse effects starts at 80% reduction of postsynaptic D_2 activity, so parkinsonism and dystonia are much less likely to occur with aripiprazole compared to a situation when high D_2 occupancy is achieved with antagonist antipsychotics, although akathisia may occur due to aripiprazole's partial agonist properties [39]. Confusing the issue is the fact that aripiprazole is tolerated even in overdose situations. Among 239 aripiprazole overdose cases reported to the Danish Poison Information Centre from June 2007 to May 2015, 86 involved single-drug exposure to aripiprazole, with a median ingested dose of 105 mg (interquartile range: 50–1680 mg) [40]. The most commonly reported symptom in this group was light sedation, occurring in 63%. Given the fact that D_2-related adverse neurological effects may not be limiting, there have been clinical reports of high-dose aripiprazole use [41]. The most systematic data was collected in a 2-week, double-blind, five-arm study of 40 stable adult schizophrenia spectrum patients (mean baseline PANSS total score range: 43–64): 30 mg/d (n = 12),

45 mg/d (n = 7), 60 mg/d (n = 7), 75 mg/d (n = 7), and 90 mg/d (n = 7) [39]. Only four discontinued treatment due to adverse effects: two in the 30 mg/d group, and two in the 60 mg/d group. The 90 mg/d group did experience more adverse effects than the other treatment groups in the form of akathisia (57%) and tachycardia (71%), but these were not severe enough to cause study discontinuation [39]. Plasma aripiprazole levels increased linearly with dose and there were no clinically significant ECG changes [39]; however, higher dosages were not necessarily more effective. The paucity of other systematic data for doses > 30 mg/d limits conclusions from clinical trials regarding a point of futility for high-dose aripiprazole, but our understanding of the point of futility is better defined by the imaging findings.

2 Imaging Evidence for a Point of Futility for Aripiprazole

Aripiprazole's known mechanism of action is related to modulation of postsynaptic striatal D_2 activity, and thus will be maximized at the plasma level which achieves 100% receptor occupancy. While patients may tolerate higher drug exposure [39], the laws of mass action preclude occupying more than 100% of available receptors; therefore, plasma antipsychotic levels associated with saturation of the D_2 receptor become the defined points of futility as further modulation of D_2-mediated neurotransmission is literally impossible [19, 1, 13]. Extrapolating from the available PET studies [21, 1, 23], one can estimate that close to 100% striatal D_2 receptor occupancy will occur at a plasma level of 500 ng/ml, a level associated with an oral dose of 45 mg/d. While some patients may indeed tolerate a dose of 90 mg/d and the corresponding plasma level of 1000 ng/ml or more [39], the purpose of defining a point of futility around 500 ng/ml is to avoid a search for efficacy that prolongs patient suffering with little evidence for success.

Summary Points

a Aripiprazole is the prototypical dopamine partial agonist antipsychotic, whose usefulness is defined by lower rates of neurological adverse effects than D_2 antagonists, even at high plasma levels, low rates of endocrine and metabolic adverse effects, and the availability of two long-acting injectable formulations.

b Where available, aripiprazole lauroxil is the preferred LAI formulation for kinetic reasons, the availability of multiple doses including dosages that can be given every 6 or 8 weeks, the fact that it can be used with CYP 3A4 inducers, and the existence of an initiation regimen using a nanocrystal suspension of aripiprazole lauroxil that obviates the need for extended oral bridging coverage. Clinicians should be familiar with aripiprazole monohydrate as this formulation was approved earlier and is in more widespread use.

c The response threshold for aripiprazole is 110 ng/ml, equivalent to 10 mg/d of oral aripiprazole. Unlike D_2 antagonists, aripiprazole is so well tolerated that plasma levels can be pushed to doses beyond those expected to achieve 100% D_2 receptor occupancy. The point of futility is therefore not defined by tolerability, but by the plasma level estimated to be associated with 100% D_2 occupancy, which is approximately 500 ng/ml.

References

1. **Sparshatt, A., Taylor, D., Patel, M. X., *et al.* (2010).** A systematic review of aripiprazole – dose, plasma concentration, receptor occupancy, and response: implications for therapeutic drug monitoring. *J Clin Psychiatry*, 71, 1447–1556.
2. **Kegeles, L. S., Abi-Dargham, A., Frankle, W. G., *et al.* (2010).** Increased synaptic dopamine function in associative regions of the striatum in schizophrenia. *Arch Gen Psychiatry*, 67, 231–239.
3. **Kim, J. H., Son, Y. D., Kim, H. K., *et al.* (2011).** Antipsychotic-associated mental side effects and their relationship to dopamine D2 receptor occupancy in striatal subdivisions: a high-resolution PET study with [11C]raclopride. *J Clin Psychopharmacol*, 31, 507–511.
4. **Van Putten, T., Marder, S. R., Mintz, J., *et al.* (1992).** Haloperidol plasma levels and clinical response: a therapeutic window relationship. *Am J Psychiatry*, 149, 500–505.
5. **Veselinović, T., Scharpenberg, M., Heinze, M., *et al.* (2019).** Dopamine D2 receptor occupancy estimated from plasma concentrations of four different antipsychotics and the subjective experience of physical and mental well-being in schizophrenia: results from the randomized NeSSy Trial. *J Clin Psychopharmacol*, 39, 550–560.
6. **Burris, K. D., Molski, T. F., Xu, C., *et al.* (2002).** Aripiprazole, a novel antipsychotic, is a high-affinity partial agonist at human dopamine D2 receptors. *J Pharmacol Exp Ther*, 302, 381–389.
7. **Tadori, Y., Forbes, R. A., McQuade, R. D., *et al.* (2011).** In vitro pharmacology of aripiprazole, its metabolite and experimental dopamine partial agonists at human dopamine D2 and D3 receptors. *Eur J Pharmacol*, 668, 355–365.
8. **Meyer, J. M. (2018).** Pharmacotherapy of psychosis and mania. In L. L. Brunton, R. Hilal-Dandan and B. C. Knollmann, eds., *Goodman & Gilman's The Pharmacological Basis of Therapeutics*, 13th edn. Chicago, IL: McGraw-Hill, pp. 279–302.
9. **Takeuchi, H. and Remington, G. (2013).** A systematic review of reported cases involving psychotic symptoms worsened by aripiprazole in schizophrenia or schizoaffective disorder. *Psychopharmacology (Berl)*, 228, 175–185.
10. **Kane, J. M., Correll, C. U., Goff, D. C., *et al.* (2009).** A multicenter, randomized, double-blind, placebo-controlled, 16-week study of adjunctive aripiprazole for schizophrenia or schizoaffective disorder inadequately treated with quetiapine or risperidone monotherapy. *J Clin Psychiatry*, 70, 1348–1357.
11. **Cipriani, A., Accordini, S., Nose, M., *et al.* (2013).** Aripiprazole versus haloperidol in combination with clozapine for treatment-resistant schizophrenia: a 12-month, randomized, naturalistic trial. *J Clin Psychopharmacol*, 33, 533–537.
12. **Meyer, J. M. and Stahl, S. M. (2019).** *The Clozapine Handbook*. Cambridge: Cambridge University Press.
13. **Girgis, R. R., Slifstein, M., D'Souza, D., *et al.* (2016).** Preferential binding to dopamine D3 over D2 receptors by cariprazine in patients with schizophrenia using PET with the D3/D2 receptor ligand [(11)C]-(+)-PHNO. *Psychopharmacology (Berl)*, 233, 3503–3512.
14. **Stahl, S. M. (2017).** Drugs for psychosis and mood: unique actions at D3, D2, and D1 dopamine receptor subtypes. *CNS Spectr*, 22, 375–384.
15. **Stroup, T. S., McEvoy, J. P., Ring, K. D., *et al.* (2011).** A randomized trial examining the effectiveness of switching from olanzapine, quetiapine, or risperidone to aripiprazole to reduce metabolic risk: comparison of antipsychotics for metabolic problems (CAMP). *Am J Psychiatry*, 168, 947–956.
16. **Kirschbaum, K. M., Müller, M. J., Malevani, J., *et al.* (2008).** Serum levels of aripiprazole and dehydroaripiprazole, clinical response and side effects. *World J Biol Psychiatry*, 9, 212–218.
17. **Lin, S. K., Chen, C. K., and Liu, Y. L. (2011).** Aripiprazole and dehydroaripiprazole plasma concentrations and clinical responses in patients with schizophrenia. *J Clin Psychopharmacol*, 31, 758–762.

18. **Yokoi, F., Grunder, G., Biziere, K., *et al.* (2002).** Dopamine D2 and D3 receptor occupancy in normal humans treated with the antipsychotic drug aripiprazole (OPC 14597): a study using positron emission tomography and [11C]raclopride. *Neuropsychopharmacology*, 27, 248–259.
19. **Mamo, D., Graff, A., Mizrahi, R., *et al.* (2007).** Differential effects of aripiprazole on D(2), 5-HT(2), and 5-HT(1A) receptor occupancy in patients with schizophrenia: a triple tracer PET study. *Am J Psychiatry*, 164, 1411–1417.
20. **Grunder, G., Fellows, C., Janouschek, H., *et al.* (2008).** Brain and plasma pharmacokinetics of aripiprazole in patients with schizophrenia: an [18F]fallypride PET study. *Am J Psychiatry*, 165, 988–995.
21. **Kegeles, L. S., Slifstein, M., Frankle, W. G., *et al.* (2008).** Dose-occupancy study of striatal and extrastriatal dopamine D2 receptors by aripiprazole in schizophrenia with PET and [18F]fallypride. *Neuropsychopharmacology*, 33, 3111–3125.
22. **Mizrahi, R., Mamo, D., Rusjan, P., *et al.* (2009).** The relationship between subjective well-being and dopamine D2 receptors in patients treated with a dopamine partial agonist and full antagonist antipsychotics. *Int J Neuropsychopharmacol*, 12, 715–721.
23. **Takahata, K., Ito, H., Takano, H., *et al.* (2012).** Striatal and extrastriatal dopamine D2 receptor occupancy by the partial agonist antipsychotic drug aripiprazole in the human brain: a positron emission tomography study with [C]raclopride and [C]FLB457. *Psychopharmacology*, 222, 165–172.
24. **Kurose, S., Mimura, Y., Uchida, H., *et al.* (2020).** Dissociation in pharmacokinetic attenuation between central dopamine D2 receptor occupancy and peripheral blood concentration of antipsychotics: a systematic review. *J Clin Psychiatry*, 81, 19r13113.
25. **Schoretsanitis, G., Kane, J. M., Correll, C. U., *et al.* (2020).** Blood levels to optimize antipsychotic treatment in clinical practice: a joint consensus statement of the American Society of Clinical Psychopharmacology (ASCP) and the Therapeutic Drug Monitoring (TDM) Task Force of the Arbeitsgemeinschaft für Neuropsychopharmakologie und Pharmakopsychiatrie (AGNP). *J Clin Psychiatry*, 81, https://doi.org/10.4088/JCP.4019cs13169.
26. **Otsuka America Pharmaceutical Inc. (2020).** Abilify package insert. Rockville, MD.
27. **Nemoto, K., Mihara, K., Nakamura, A., *et al.* (2012).** Effects of paroxetine on plasma concentrations of aripiprazole and its active metabolite, dehydroaripiprazole, in Japanese patients with schizophrenia. *Ther Drug Monit*, 34, 188–192.
28. **Suzuki, T., Mihara, K., Nakamura, A., *et al.* (2014).** Effects of genetic polymorphisms of CYP2D6, CYP3A5, and ABCB1 on the steady-state plasma concentrations of aripiprazole and its active metabolite, dehydroaripiprazole, in Japanese patients with schizophrenia. *Ther Drug Monit*, 36, 651–655.
29. **Meyer, J. M. (2017).** Converting oral to long acting injectable antipsychotics: a guide for the perplexed. *CNS Spectr*, 22, 14–28.
30. **Otsuka America Pharmaceutical Inc. (2020).** Abilify Maintena package insert. Rockville, MD.
31. **Alkermes Inc. (2020).** Aristada package insert. Walltham, MA.
32. **Alkermes Inc. (2020).** Aristada Initio package insert. Walltham, MA.
33. **Hard, M. L., Mills, R. J., Sadler, B. M., *et al.* (2017).** Aripiprazole lauroxil: pharmacokinetic profile of this long-acting injectable antipsychotic in persons with schizophrenia. *J Clin Psychopharmacol*, 37, 289–295.
34. **Hard, M. L., Mills, R. J., Sadler, B. M., *et al.* (2017).** Pharmacokinetic profile of a 2-month dose regimen of aripiprazole lauroxil: a phase I study and a population pharmacokinetic model. *CNS Drugs*, 31, 617–624.
35. **Haddad, P., Lambert, T., and Lauriello, J., eds. (2016).** *Antipsychotic Long-Acting Injections*, 2nd edn. New York: Oxford University Press.
36. **Jain, R., Meyer, J. M., Wehr, A. Y., *et al.* (2020).** Size matters: the importance of particle size in a newly developed injectable formulation for the treatment of schizophrenia. *CNS Spectr*, 25, 323–330.

37. **Meltzer, H. Y., Risinger, R., Nasrallah, H. A., *et al.* (2015).** A randomized, double-blind, placebo-controlled trial of aripiprazole lauroxil in acute exacerbation of schizophrenia. *J Clin Psychiatry*, 76, 1085–1090.
38. **Potkin, S. G., Saha, A. R., Kujawa, M. J., *et al.* (2003).** Aripiprazole, an antipsychotic with a novel mechanism of action, and risperidone vs placebo in patients with schizophrenia and schizoaffective disorder. *Arch Gen Psychiatry*, 60, 681–690.
39. **Saha, A., Ali, M. W., Ingenito, G. G., *et al.* (2002).** P.4.E.026 – Safety and tolerability of aripiprazole at doses higher than 30 mg (abstract from the XXIII CINP Congress, Montréal, June 23–27, 2002). *Int J Neuropsychopharmacol*, 5, S185.
40. **Christensen, A. P., Boegevig, S., Christensen, M. B., *et al.* (2018).** Overdoses with aripiprazole: signs, symptoms and outcome in 239 exposures reported to the Danish Poison Information Centre. *Basic Clin Pharmacol Toxicol*, 122, 293–298.
41. **Chavez, B. and Poveda, R. A. (2006).** Efficacy with high-dose aripiprazole after olanzapine-related metabolic disturbances. *Ann Pharmacother*, 40, 2265–2268.

17 Amisulpride, Asenapine, Lurasidone, Brexpiprazole, Cariprazine

QUICK CHECK

PRINCIPLES

- Amisulpride is available in most countries except the US and Canada, but exists only in an oral formulation. Like olanzapine, amisulpride may be slightly more effective for schizophrenia than other antipsychotics, although it is not effective in treatment-resistant patients. Amisulpride also has antidepressant properties and low risk for drug–drug interactions, but is among the highest-risk agents for hyperprolactinemia.
- Asenapine is the only antipsychotic available in a sublingual form that relies completely on buccal absorption due to > 99% first pass metabolism if swallowed. To avoid the unique kinetic issues posed by the sublingual tablet, asenapine was developed as a transdermal patch, with much lower peak–trough plasma level variation, and a higher mean trough value. Due to the unique delivery methods, both forms of asenapine have a low risk for drug–drug interactions. While asenapine has binding properties that suggest antidepressant activity, this has not been extensively studied. Asenapine plasma levels are slowly becoming more available from laboratories.

- Lurasidone is extensively used due to its low risk for metabolic adverse effects and indications for schizophrenia and for bipolar I depression (as monotherapy, or adjunctive to lithium or valproate). Like ziprasidone, lurasidone drug exposure is doubled with food intake, but lurasidone only needs to be taken once daily. Lurasidone tolerability is greatly increased by dosing with an evening meal, so prescription orders should be very clear: take within 30 minutes of dinner. Lurasidone plasma levels are slowly becoming more available from laboratories.
- Brexpiprazole and cariprazine are the latest dopamine partial agonist antipsychotics to be approved, but with different indications and kinetic properties. Brexpiprazole is indicated for schizophrenia and adjunctively for unipolar major depression, while cariprazine is indicated for schizophrenia, acute manic or mixed episodes (as monotherapy), and bipolar I depression (as monotherapy). Cariprazine has a half-life of 31.6–68.4 hours and reaches steady state in 1–2 weeks, but it has an active metabolite with a half-life of 13–18 days, so steady state for the active moiety may not be achieved for 60–90 days. Very few laboratories run brexpiprazole or cariprazine assays, but over time this is likely to change.

The psychopharmacology field is moving toward a mechanism-based nomenclature to replace outmoded descriptors of molecules with multiple pharmacological properties. In addition to publications covering these efforts [15–17], a Neuroscience-Based Nomenclature website was created (https://nbn2r.com) where one can download a free smartphone app, and which posts twice-yearly glossary updates in May and September. For the sake of simplicity, the term second-generation antipsychotic (SGA) will be used in this chapter, but the antipsychotics described herein have a range of pharmacologic properties, and a wide variety of kinetic profiles. Moreover, with the exception of transdermal asenapine and cariprazine, the SGAs presented in this chapter represent a group that are generally available worldwide. As of this writing, plasma levels for each antipsychotic may not be available in certain countries, and none have a long-acting injectable (LAI) formulation. These important issues may limit use of specific agents as maintenance treatments for schizophrenia. (Though many antipsychotics are indicated for acute mania, it should be noted that lurasidone and cariprazine have indications for bipolar depression, and brexpiprazole for adjunctive use with antidepressants for unipolar major depression.) While cariprazine does not exist as an LAI, it has an active metabolite didesmethylcariprazine (DDCAR) that comprises over 60% of the active moiety at steady state and which has a half-life of 13–18 days; this

InfoBox Oral Antipsychotic Plasma Level Essentials for Amisulpride, Asenapine, Brexpiprazole, Cariprazine, Lurasidone

	Oral dose correlation (bedtime dosing, 12h trough)*	Level of evidence	Therapeutic threshold	Level of evidence	Point of futility	Level of evidence
Amisulpride	Females: 200 mg = 120 ± 90 ng/ml [1] Males: 200 mg = 92 ± 70 ng/ml [1] **Females: multiply dose by 0.60** **Males: multiply dose by 0.46**	High	100 ng/ml	Moderate	550–700 ng/ml	Low
Asenapine (oral)	Dose dependent due to decreasing buccal absorption at higher dosages: **5 mg BID trough level: 1.5 ng/ml** **10 mg BID trough level: 2.0 ng/ml**	High	1.0 ng/ml	Moderate	(Based on maximal licensed dose of 10 mg sublingual BID)	Low
Asenapine[a] (transdermal)	3.8 mg/24 hours x 0.53 = 2.0 ng/ml **Multiply transdermal dose by 0.53**	High	1.0 ng/ml[b]	Moderate	(Based on maximal licensed dose of 7.8 mg/24 hours)	Low
Brexpiprazole	CYP 2D6 EM 1 mg/d = 18 ng/ml [2] CYP 2D6 IM 1 mg/d = 46 ng/ml [2] **CYP 2D6 EM: multiply dose by 18** **CYP 2D6 IM: multiply dose by 46**	High	36 ng/ml	Low	(Based on maximal licensed dose of 4 mg QHS)	Low

	Oral dose correlation (bedtime dosing, 12h trough)*	Level of evidence	Therapeutic threshold	Level of evidence	Point of futility	Level of evidence
Cariprazine[c]	3 mg = 13.2 nmol/l = 5.62 ng/ml [3] 4.5 mg = 20.4 nmol/l = 8.74 ng/ml [3] **Multiply dose by 1.9**	High	5.6 ng/ml	High	(Based on maximal licensed dose of 6 mg QHS)	Low
Lurasidone[d]	80 mg with food = 14.0 ng/ml [4] 160 mg with food = 29.1 ng/ml [4] **Multiply dose by 0.18**	High	7.2 ng/ml	Moderate	(Based on maximal licensed dose of 160 mg with an evening meal)	Low

* See Table 17.1 for effects of CYP inhibitors/inducers on this relationship.

AUC_{0-24} = the area under the curve over 24 hours

[a] Although the lowest transdermal formulation dose of 3.8 mg/24 hours provides equivalent asenapine exposure over 24 hours to the sublingual dose of 5 mg BID (by AUC_{0-24}), trough levels for the sublingual dose are lower due to higher peak–trough variation (see Figure 17.8). The conversion factor of 0.53 is for the transdermal dose **per 24 hours**.

[b] The expected mean asenapine trough level for the lowest dose of the transdermal patch (3.8 mg/24 hours) is 2.0 ng/ml (see Figure 17.8).

[c] The values for cariprazine represent the parent compound only. At steady state on 6 mg/d the active moiety is: cariprazine 28%, DCAR 9%, and DDCAR 63% [5]. Very few laboratories have cariprazine assays, and none reports the metabolites at present. Should this change, the values represented will be nearly four-fold higher. For example, the steady state cariprazine level on 6 mg/d is 11.2 ng/ml, but the active moiety level will be approximately 40 ng/ml [3].

[d] The concentration–dose relationships for lurasidone are based on 12h trough values obtained at steady state (day 9 or later) and with lurasidone administered within 30 minutes of an evening meal of at least 350 kcal. This does not include the active metabolite ID-14283 (exohydroxylurasidone), which comprises 25% of the active moiety, but whose levels are not reported by commercial laboratories presently [6].

Table 17.1 Oral Kinetic Facts for Amisulpride, Asenapine, Brexpiprazole, Cariprazine, Lurasidone

	Basic facts	Inhibition effects	Induction effects
Amisulpride	Not approved in the US for schizophrenia treatment. $T_{1/2}$ 12 hours Absolute oral bioavailability: 48% [1] T_{max} There are two absorption peaks: 1 hour and 3–4 hours Metabolism: Primarily renally excreted unchanged via the P-glycoprotein (PGP) efflux transporter. **Formulations:** Tablets	No impact of cytochrome (CYP) inhibitors. Reports of increased dose corrected plasma levels in patients on lithium or clozapine [1]. As a PGP substrate, increased brain amisulpride levels may possibly be seen during concurrent use with strong PGP inhibitors (e.g. amiodarone, cyclosporine, nifedipine, verapamil) [7, 8]. This is best monitored by clinical observation and not plasma levels	No impact of smoking or CYP inducers
Asenapine (sublingual)	US FDA approval: Aug. 13, 2009 $T_{1/2}$ 24 hours Absolute oral bioavailability (with sublingual administration): 32%–40% after 10 minutes of buccal residence time. If water is given before 10 minutes, lower absorption is seen (see Figures 17.6 and 17.7) [9] T_{max} 1 hour Metabolism: Primarily CYP 1A2 and direct glucuronidation by the phase 2 enzyme UGT 1A4. CYP 3A4 and CYP 2D6 are minor pathways **Formulations:** Oral dissolving tablets	The strong CYP 1A2 inhibitor fluvoxamine at a dose of 25 mg BID had limited impact on drug levels, but a greater effect from higher fluvoxamine doses is possible. The asenapine dose may need to be adjusted in those circumstances [10] There is no impact from the strong CYP 2D6 inhibitor paroxetine, or the UGT 1A4 inhibitor valproate. Of note, asenapine increases paroxetine exposure two-fold, so paroxetine doses should be decreased by 50% [10]	There is no impact from the strong CYP 3A4 inducer carbamazepine [1]

	Basic facts	Inhibition effects	Induction effects
Asenapine (transdermal)	US FDA approval: Oct. 11, 2019 $T_{1/2}$ 30 hours [11] Relative bioavailability: the 3.8 mg/24 hours, 5.7 mg/24 hours, and 7.6 mg/24 hours doses are bioequivalent to the sublingual doses of 5 mg BID, 15 mg/d and 10 mg BID, respectively [11] T_{max} 12–24 hours [11] Metabolism: Primarily CYP 1A2 and direct glucuronidation by the phase 2 enzyme UGT 1A4. CYP 3A4 and CYP 2D6 are minor pathways **Formulations:** Transdermal patch	The strong CYP 1A2 inhibitor fluvoxamine at a dose of 25 mg BID had limited impact on drug levels, but a greater effect from higher fluvoxamine doses is possible. The asenapine dose may need to be adjusted in those circumstances [11] There is no impact from the strong CYP 2D6 inhibitor paroxetine, or the UGT 1A4 inhibitor valproate. Of note, asenapine increases paroxetine exposure two-fold, so paroxetine doses should be decreased by 50% [11]	There is no impact from the strong CYP 3A4 inducer carbamazepine [11]
Brexpiprazole	US FDA approval: July 10, 2015 $T_{1/2}$ 91 hours Absolute oral bioavailability: 95% T_{max} 4 hours Metabolism: CYP 2D6 and CYP 3A4 convert brexpiprazole to an inactive metabolite DM-3411. At steady state, exposure to DM-3411 is 23%–48% of brexpiprazole [2] **Formulations:** Tablets	Strong CYP 2D6 or CYP 3A4 inhibitors increase AUC_{0-24H} by two-fold. Combined use of a strong CYP 3A4 and 2D6 inhibitor (or with CYP 2D6 PM) increased AUC_{0-24H} 4.8–5.1-fold. Reduce the dose by 50% with strong 2D6 or 3A4 inhibitors, and by 75% with combined strong CYP 2D6/CYP 3A4 inhibitors [12] Reduce the dose by 50% in CYP 2D6 PM [12]	Strong 3A4 inducers reduce exposure AUC_{0-24H} by ~70%. Double the dose with strong CYP 3A4 inducers [12]

	Basic facts	Inhibition effects	Induction effects
Cariprazine	US FDA approval: Sept. 17, 2015 $T_{1/2}$ 31.6–68.4 hours (cariprazine) $T_{1/2}$ 29.7–39.5 hours (desmethylcariprazine – DCAR) $T_{1/2}$ 314–446 hours (didesmethylcariprazine – DDCAR) [13] **~50% of DDCAR is present 1 wk after discontinuation** Absolute oral bioavailability: 65% [14] T_{max} 3–6 hours Metabolism: CYP 3A4 converts cariprazine to its metabolites. CYP 2D6 is a minor pathway. At steady state on 6 mg/d the active moiety is: cariprazine 28%, DCAR 9%, and DDCAR 63% [5] **Formulations:** Capsules	The strong CYP 3A4 inhibitor ketoconazole at the dose of 400 mg/d increased cariprazine C_{max} and AUC_{0-24H} by 3.5- and 4.0-fold, respectively. Ketoconazole also increased DDCAR C_{max} and AUC_{0-24H} by 1.5-fold, and decreased DCAR C_{max} and AUC_{0-24H} by about one-third. **Reduce the dose by 50% with strong 3A4 inhibitors.** There is no impact from 2D6 inhibitors [13]	Not studied with inducers, and impact unknown. Not recommended with 3A4 inducers [13]
Lurasidone	US FDA approval: Oct. 28, 2010 $T_{1/2}$ 28.8–37.4 hours (at steady state) [6] $T_{1/2}$ 6–10 hours (ID-14283) Bioavailability: 9–19% 350 kcal of food increases AUC by 2.2-fold. **Lurasidone should be ordered to be given within 30 minutes of an evening meal. (Dosing with a morning meal decreases tolerability.) Administering lurasidone on an empty stomach decreases drug exposure by 50%** T_{max} 1–3 hours Metabolism: CYP 3A4 converts lurasidone to active metabolites exohydroxylurasidone (ID-14283) and ID-14326. ID-14283 is present at 25% of the lurasidone concentration, but ID-14326 only 3% [6] **Formulations:** Tablets	The strong CYP 3A4 inhibitor ketoconazole at a dose of 400 mg/day for 7 days in ten healthy volunteers increased AUC 9.3-fold from baseline. **Lurasidone cannot be used with strong CYP 3A4 inhibitors.** Exposure to the moderate CYP3A4 inhibitor diltiazem 240 mg/day for 7 days increased the single-dose AUC 2.2-fold for lurasidone and similarly for its metabolite ID-14283. **The lurasidone dose should be decreased by 50% with moderate CYP 3A4 inhibitors**	Rifampin, a strong CYP 3A4 inducer, decreased AUC by 80%. **Lurasidone cannot be used with strong CYP 3A4 inducers (e.g. rifampin, carbamazepine, phenytoin)**

extraordinarily long half-life has been shown to reduce relapse risk compared to other oral antipsychotics, all of which have much shorter half-lives [13, 18].

A number of other SGAs exist that are not covered here, as each has issues that result in low utilization for schizophrenia: iloperidone – prolonged titration to minimize orthostasis [19]; zotepine – regionally limited; sertindole – QT prolongation [20]; ziprasidone – multiple daily dosing and significant food kinetic effects [21, 22]; quetiapine – sedation, metabolic adverse effects, and efficacy concerns that preclude routine use as monotherapy for schizophrenia [23, 24]. Lumateperone is an SGA approved in the US in December 2019 with an interesting constellation of mechanisms; very low risk for metabolic, neurological, and endocrine adverse effects; and only one approved dosage form for schizophrenia (42 mg capsules) [25]. The approval of this one dose is due to the lack of separation of lower dosages (14 mg, 28 mg) and a higher dose (84 mg) from placebo, but this also limits the possibility of dose increases for those with lower than expected levels, since the licensed maximum dose is 42 mg/d [26, 27]. A lumateperone plasma level assay is not obtainable through commercial laboratories, but may be useful to track adherence once available.

Amisulpride

1 Oral Pharmacokinetic Information

Amisulpride is a benzamide antipsychotic approved for schizophrenia in most developed countries except for the United States and Canada. As with olanzapine, amisulpride may have slightly greater efficacy than other antipsychotics (Figure 17.1), but the difference from other agents is small, with no data supporting amisulpride's efficacy for treatment-resistant schizophrenia [28]. That amisulpride and olanzapine have similar effectiveness was demonstrated in a large first-episode schizophrenia trial (n = 446) in which patients who failed to remit after 4 weeks of open-label amisulpride up to 800 mg/d were randomized in a double-blind manner to 6 weeks of amisulpride continuation or a switch to olanzapine up to 20 mg/d [29]. In the open-label phase, 250 (56%) achieved remission, and 93 patients who were not in remission continued to the 6-week double-blind switching trial. In the double-blind phase of the study, nearly identical proportions attained remission on amisulpride (45%) and olanzapine (44%) [29].

Amisulpride was noted early in development to address depressive symptoms better than haloperidol [30], with subsequent studies relating this to high affinity for serotonin $5HT_7$ receptors, a property it shares with asenapine and lurasidone (Figure 17.2) [31–33]. Amisulpride also has high affinity for the dopamine D_3 receptor, and

Figure 17.1 Standardized mean difference (SMD) from placebo in positive psychosis symptom improvement during oral antipsychotic treatment for adults with acutely relapsed schizophrenia [28]

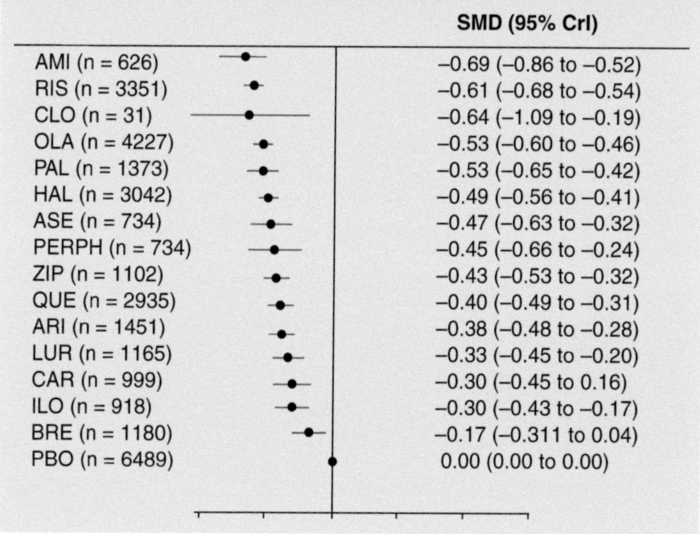

	SMD (95% CrI)
AMI (n = 626)	−0.69 (−0.86 to −0.52)
RIS (n = 3351)	−0.61 (−0.68 to −0.54)
CLO (n = 31)	−0.64 (−1.09 to −0.19)
OLA (n = 4227)	−0.53 (−0.60 to −0.46)
PAL (n = 1373)	−0.53 (−0.65 to −0.42)
HAL (n = 3042)	−0.49 (−0.56 to −0.41)
ASE (n = 734)	−0.47 (−0.63 to −0.32)
PERPH (n = 734)	−0.45 (−0.66 to −0.24)
ZIP (n = 1102)	−0.43 (−0.53 to −0.32)
QUE (n = 2935)	−0.40 (−0.49 to −0.31)
ARI (n = 1451)	−0.38 (−0.48 to −0.28)
LUR (n = 1165)	−0.33 (−0.45 to −0.20)
CAR (n = 999)	−0.30 (−0.45 to 0.16)
ILO (n = 918)	−0.30 (−0.43 to −0.17)
BRE (n = 1180)	−0.17 (−0.311 to 0.04)
PBO (n = 6489)	0.00 (0.00 to 0.00)

(Adapted from: M. Huhn, A. Nikolakopoulou, J. Schneider-Thoma, *et al*. [2019]. Comparative efficacy and tolerability of 32 oral antipsychotics for the acute treatment of adults with multi-episode schizophrenia: a systematic review and network meta-analysis. *Lancet*, 394, 939–951.)

this may contribute both to antidepressant effects and to efficacy at low doses for the negative symptoms of schizophrenia, via actions at striatal or cortical autoreceptors [34, 35]. Amisulpride can induce neurological adverse effects, but at rates much lower than for first-generation antipsychotics [30, 1]. The lower rates for neurological and metabolic side effects, combined with its antidepressant properties, are reasons why amisulpride is often chosen for first-episode schizophrenia trials, despite the lack of an LAI preparation [36]. Compared to its modest D_2 affinity, amisulpride disproportionately elevates serum prolactin in a manner seen with risperidone and its active metabolite 9-OH risperidone (paliperidone) (see Figure 17.3) [28]. The underlying mechanism for this effect is similar to that for risperidone and its metabolite: high affinity for the p-glycoprotein (PGP) efflux transporter at the blood–brain barrier [37, 38].

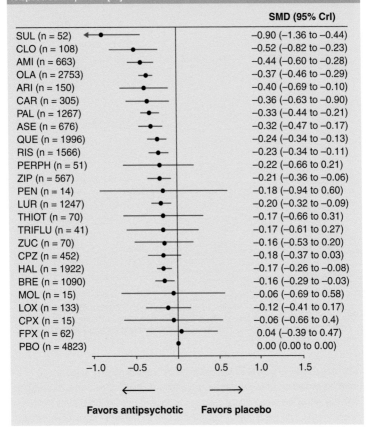

Figure 17.2 Standardized mean difference (SMD) from placebo in depressive symptom improvement during oral antipsychotic treatment for adults with acutely relapsed schizophrenia [28]

	SMD (95% CrI)
SUL (n = 52)	−0.90 (−1.36 to −0.44)
CLO (n = 108)	−0.52 (−0.82 to −0.23)
AMI (n = 663)	−0.44 (−0.60 to −0.28)
OLA (n = 2753)	−0.37 (−0.46 to −0.29)
ARI (n = 150)	−0.40 (−0.69 to −0.10)
CAR (n = 305)	−0.36 (−0.63 to −0.90)
PAL (n = 1267)	−0.33 (−0.44 to −0.21)
ASE (n = 676)	−0.32 (−0.47 to −0.17)
QUE (n = 1996)	−0.24 (−0.34 to −0.13)
RIS (n = 1566)	−0.23 (−0.34 to −0.11)
PERPH (n = 51)	−0.22 (−0.66 to 0.21)
ZIP (n = 567)	−0.21 (−0.36 to −0.06)
PEN (n = 14)	−0.18 (−0.94 to 0.60)
LUR (n = 1247)	−0.20 (−0.32 to −0.09)
THIOT (n = 70)	−0.17 (−0.66 to 0.31)
TRIFLU (n = 41)	−0.17 (−0.61 to 0.27)
ZUC (n = 70)	−0.16 (−0.53 to 0.20)
CPZ (n = 452)	−0.18 (−0.37 to 0.03)
HAL (n = 1922)	−0.17 (−0.26 to −0.08)
BRE (n = 1090)	−0.16 (−0.29 to −0.03)
MOL (n = 15)	−0.06 (−0.69 to 0.58)
LOX (n = 133)	−0.12 (−0.41 to 0.17)
CPX (n = 15)	−0.06 (−0.66 to 0.4)
FPX (n = 62)	0.04 (−0.39 to 0.47)
PBO (n = 4823)	0.00 (0.00 to 0.00)

(Adapted from: M. Huhn, A. Nikolakopoulou, J. Schneider-Thoma, *et al.* [2019]. Comparative efficacy and tolerability of 32 oral antipsychotics for the acute treatment of adults with multi-episode schizophrenia: a systematic review and network meta-analysis. *Lancet*, 394, 939–951.)

Amisulpride has been available for over 25 years, and its kinetic properties and concentration–dose relationships are well characterized (Figure 17.4) [1]. Amisulpride is minimally metabolized and is primarily excreted unchanged via renal mechanisms,

Figure 17.3 Standardized mean difference (SMD) from placebo in serum prolactin levels during oral antipsychotic treatment for schizophrenia [28]

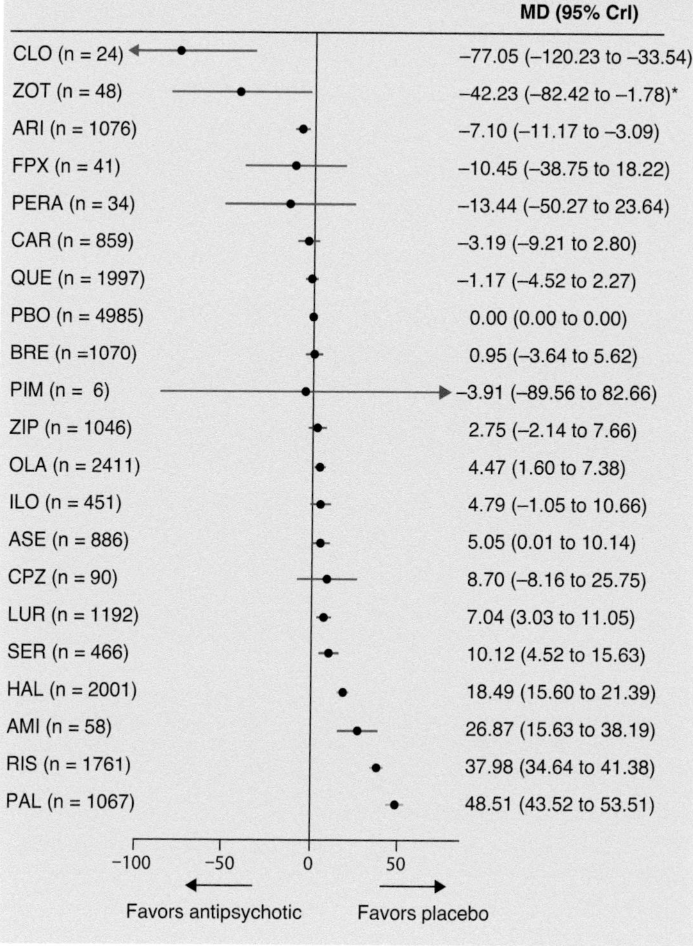

(Adapted from: M. Huhn, A. Nikolakopoulou, J. Schneider-Thoma, *et al*. [2019]. Comparative efficacy and tolerability of 32 oral antipsychotics for the acute treatment of adults with multi-episode schizophrenia: a systematic review and network meta-analysis. *Lancet*, 394, 939–951.)

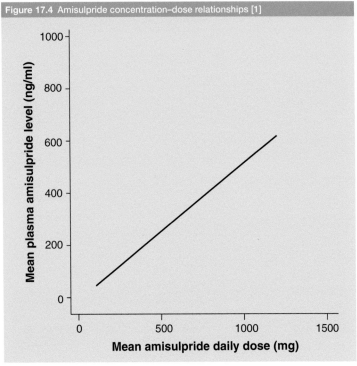

Figure 17.4 Amisulpride concentration–dose relationships [1]

(Adapted from: A. Sparshatt, D. Taylor, M. X. Patel, *et al*. [2009]. Amisulpride – dose, plasma concentration, occupancy and response: implications for therapeutic drug monitoring. *Acta Psychiatr Scand*, 120, 416–428.)

with modest differences for men and women in dose-corrected plasma levels [1]. Product labeling states that the amisulpride dose should be reduced by 50% in patients with creatinine clearance (CrCl) from 30–60 ml/min, and by two-thirds with CrCl 10–30 ml/min [39]. Manufacturer instructions also recommend twice daily dosing for total daily doses above 300 mg/d [39]. There are no significant drug–drug interactions, but two studies reported higher than expected amisulpride levels in lithium-treated patients, suggesting the impact of renal dysfunction [40, 41]. As a PGP substrate, there is also a theoretical risk for increased brain levels when exposed to known PGP inhibitors such as verapamil, but this effect (if it exists in humans) is best monitored by clinical inquiry for new adverse effects and not by plasma level monitoring [7, 8]. Despite its interesting clinical properties, amisulpride is not mentioned in the 2020 consensus paper authored jointly by the Therapeutic Drug Monitoring (TDM) task force of the German Arbeitsgemeinschaft für Neuropsychopharmakologie und Pharmakopsychiatrie (AGNP) and the American Society for Clinical Psychopharmacology (ASCP) [42].

2 Therapeutic Threshold and Point of Futility

Amisulpride has an extensive database of plasma level and imaging results from which to infer a therapeutic threshold with a high degree of confidence, but somewhat less so for a point of futility. The one fixed-dose, 4-week, double-blind study published in 1998 randomized subjects to amisulpride 100 mg/d, 400 mg/d, 800 mg/d, or 1200 mg/d, or haloperidol 16 mg/d [43]. The 100 mg dose was expected to be subtherapeutic and served as a negative control. Maximal response was seen for amisulpride doses of 400–800 mg/d, but no correlation between extent of symptom improvement and day 28 plasma levels was reported, and no responder analysis was conducted [43]. From these study results, a 2009 comprehensive review indicated that 200 ng/ml is the expected amisulpride plasma level for 400 mg/d, and that this could be considered as a lower limit for the optimal therapeutic window [1]. While naturalistic, a large study of 378 adult schizophrenia patients at steady state on amisulpride monotherapy performed a receiver operating characteristic (ROC) analysis to estimate the response threshold, and came to a result that is much lower [44]. This study used trough samples collected between 7 AM and 9 AM, with response defined by a clinician rating of 1–3 on the Clinical Global Impression (CGI) Improvement scale (1 – very good response; 2 – moderate response; 3 – slight improvement), and nonresponse by a CGI-I score of 4 (unchanged or worsened) or above. The ROC analysis did not find a significant correlation between dose and nonresponse, but plasma levels were clearly superior to dose and also predictive of response. Compared to trough amisulpride levels < 100 ng/ml, levels ≥ 100 ng/ml had a sensitivity of 84%, specificity of 54%, and a 95% positive predictive value for predicting response ($p < 0.05$) [44]. In weighing the conclusions from these two trials, the fixed-dose, double-blind design is more robust, but the absence of any responder analysis using plasma level data, and the lack of doses between 100 and 400 mg/d, limit the confidence in 200 ng/ml as an estimated response threshold. Moreover, the 2009 review provided a summary of amisulpride imaging studies (Figure 17.5) that appears to correlate a plasma level of 200 ng/ml with approximately 75% striatal D_2 receptor occupancy, significantly greater than the 65% occupancy values associated with the

Figure 17.5 Fitted dopamine D_2 occupancy curve for amisulpride [1]

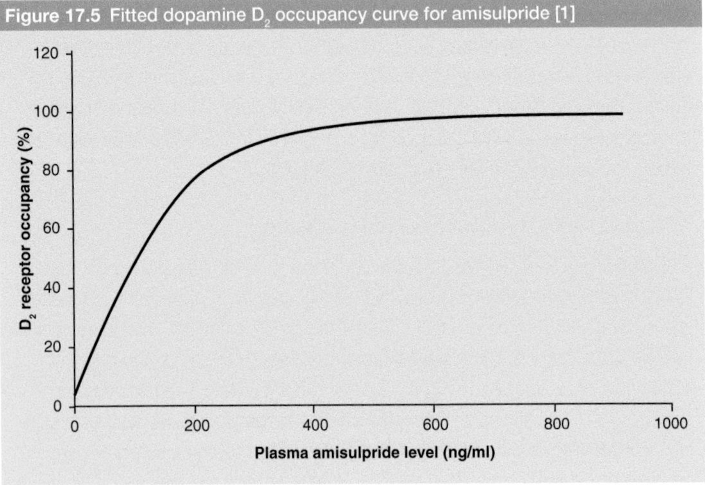

(Adapted from: A. Sparshatt, D. Taylor, M. X. Patel, *et al.* [2009]. Amisulpride – dose, plasma concentration, occupancy and response: implications for therapeutic drug monitoring. *Acta Psychiatr Scand*, 120, 416–428.)

response threshold for D_2 antagonists [1]. As the 200 ng/ml value is inferred from the 400 mg dose in the fixed-dose trial, while the threshold of 100 ng/ml is from an ROC analysis, the latter seems more plausible, and should be considered as an initial goal in nonresponders, with obvious consideration for higher levels in inadequate responders without adverse effects after 2 weeks at that level. The point of futility is unknown as doses above 1200 mg/d have not been studied extensively [45], although papers document daily dosages up to 1600 mg in clinical practice [46]. Since most countries limit dosing to the licensed maxima, the expected plasma level associated with 1200 mg/d is approximately 550 ng/ml for males, and 720 ng/ml for females [1]. As discussed previously, the 2020 AGNP/ASCP consensus paper does not discuss amisulpride [42].

B Asenapine

1 Oral and Transdermal Pharmacokinetic Information

Asenapine was initially developed by Organon, the same company which brought the antidepressants mianserin and mirtazapine to market. Those antidepressants had very high $5HT_{2C}$ affinity as one of the antidepressant mechanisms, and asenapine not only had higher affinity for that receptor (Ki 0.03 nM), but also possessed a second antidepressant mechanism in the form of nanomolar $5HT_7$ affinity (Ki 0.11 nM) [47, 48, 33]. Asenapine was approved in the US on August 13, 2009, for schizophrenia, and for manic or mixed episodes in bipolar I disorder (as monotherapy or adjunctive to lithium or valproate), but the potential to treat bipolar depression was not subsequently pursued despite efficacy signals from post hoc analyses and small prospective studies [49, 50]. Asenapine is as effective as other SGAs for adults with an acute exacerbation of schizophrenia [28], but has not been widely prescribed due to kinetic issues. While certain phenothiazines have oral bioavailability as low as 3% [51], asenapine experienced > 98% first pass metabolism when orally administered, an unfortunate kinetic problem that was solved through development of a sublingual formulation [52, 9, 53]. Orally dissolving tablet (ODT) antipsychotics have existed since the 1990s [54], and these formulations were designed to make it difficult for patients to spit out or cheek the medication. To achieve systemic exposure, ODT antipsychotics did not rely on buccal absorption but on the active ingredient eventually being swallowed. ODT antipsychotics approved prior to asenapine had the same kinetic parameters as regular tablets, and had no prohibition on drinking water after being placed in the mouth since the gastrointestinal tract was the site of drug absorption.

Unlike previously approved ODT antipsychotics, all of the systemic activity from sublingual asenapine is from buccal mucosal absorption since any swallowed medication is completely metabolized. The oral absorptive surface area is much smaller than that of the gastrointestinal tract and therefore can become saturated, leading to decreasing absorption with higher dosages (Figure 17.6) [9]. That the systemic exposure of asenapine 10 mg sublingual (SL) BID is not twice that of 5 mg SL BID was a novel concept for clinicians, and a source of some confusion [9]. The thornier clinical issue for SL asenapine derives from the fact that buccal absorption is highly time dependent (Figure 17.7). Maximal possible asenapine absorption requires 10 minutes of 'residence time' in the mouth [9]. Although other medications and ODT antipsychotics could be administered with water, patients had to be restricted from drinking after SL asenapine. Administering staff (or the patient, if self-administered) had to be instructed that SL asenapine should be placed in the mouth last after other medications were swallowed, and to abstain from drinking for 10 minutes. Asenapine absorption could thus be undone by an administration error or lack of patient cooperation, as any drug washed down into the gastrointestinal tract was completely metabolized. As shown in Figure 17.7, one could achieve 80% of the maximum possible absorption if the patient was restricted from drinking for just 2 minutes, diminishing the burden somewhat. When properly administered, the concentration–

Figure 17.6 Asenapine sublingual bioavailability by dose [9]

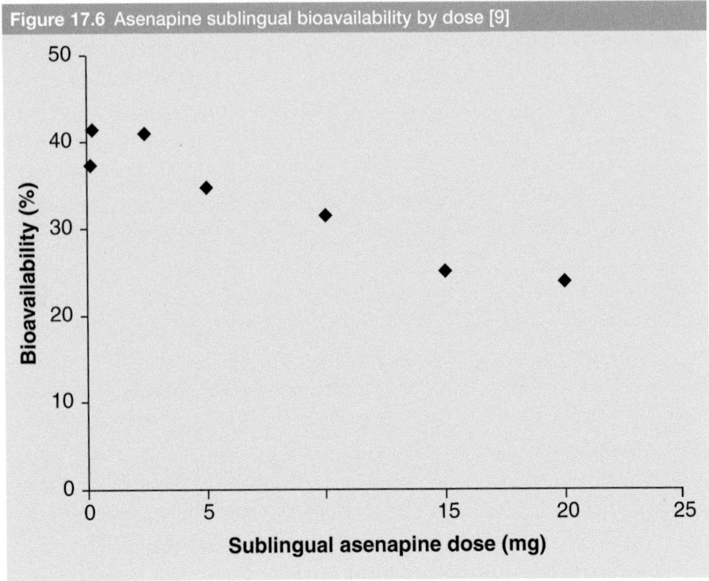

(Adapted from: J. A. Bartlett and K. van der Voort Maarschalk [2012]. Understanding the oral mucosal absorption and resulting clinical pharmacokinetics of asenapine. *AAPS PharmSciTech*, 13, 1110–1115.)

dose relationship is well established, allowing for monitoring of 12h trough plasma levels to track adherence (see InfoBox and Table 17.1). Asenapine is metabolized via CYP 1A2 and through direct phase 2 processes (UGT 1A4) in a manner akin to olanzapine [10]. Due to the multiple metabolic pathways and systemic delivery, there is lower risk for significant drug–drug interactions, with the caveat that exposure to high doses of the strong CYP 1A2 inhibitor fluvoxamine has not been studied, and that asenapine itself raises paroxetine levels two-fold [10]. Asenapine's risk for metabolic adverse effects is comparable to that for risperidone [55], with somnolence rates of 13%–15% in adult schizophrenia trials for asenapine SL 5 mg BID or 10 mg BID (compared to 7% for placebo) [10].

The complex procedure of sublingual administration, unlike that for any other orally administered psychotropic, limited use of asenapine SL, as did the occasional patient complaints of metallic taste, and diminished or odd taste sensations [10]. Nonetheless, asenapine was considered a sufficiently useful antipsychotic that several

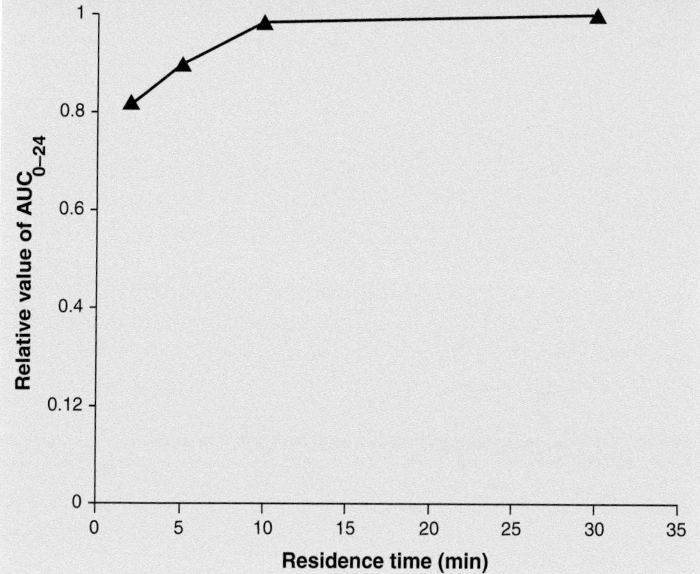

Figure 17.7 Asenapine sublingual drug exposure as a function of buccal residence time showing a plateau at 10 minutes. Even at 2 minutes 80% of the maximum absorption has occurred (triangle = AUC) [9]

(Adapted from: J. A. Bartlett and K. van der Voort Maarschalk [2012]. Understanding the oral mucosal absorption and resulting clinical pharmacokinetics of asenapine. *AAPS PharmSciTech*, 13, 1110–1115.)

entities pursued transdermal formulations to obviate issues related to sublingual administration, with Noven Therapeutics gaining US approval on October 11, 2019 [11]. Transdermal medications have some inherent disadvantages, including a long time to the maximal plasma level (T_{max}) of 12–24 hours [11], and the reality that an uncooperative patient can easily defeat the mechanism by removing the patch. However, for individuals who are motivated to try this formulation, there are significant kinetic advantages, including once daily application of the patch instead of twice daily sublingual dosing, and no concerns about water ingestion. As illustrated in Figure 17.8, plasma level variation throughout the day is markedly different between the two formulations, with a peak to trough ratio for transdermal asenapine of 1.5:1, compared to > 3:1 for sublingual administration [53]. The transdermal kinetic profile is an important factor in lessening peak plasma level adverse effects, particularly those experienced while awake following the morning sublingual dose [53]. The transdermal doses of 3.8 mg/24 hours, 5.7 mg/24 hours, and 7.6 mg/24 hours provide equivalent drug exposure to asenapine SL doses of 10 mg/d, 15 mg/d, and 20 mg/d respectively (defined by the area under the curve over 24 hours, or AUC_{0-24}), but it is important to note that trough levels differ between the two forms (Figure 17.8).

2 Therapeutic Threshold and Point of Futility

The sublingual clinical trials program for adults with schizophrenia utilized doses of 5 mg BID or 10 mg BID, establishing those dosages as effective and tolerable [56]. Despite numerous schizophrenia trials, there was a paucity of steady state plasma level data available for the sublingual preparation until comparative studies were performed as part of the transdermal approval process. As seen in Figure 17.8, the mean trough level for asenapine SL 5 mg BID in adults is 1.5 ng/ml. This is only slightly higher than the 12h trough values of approximately 1.0–1.25 ng/ml obtained for 5 mg BID in pediatric patients aged 10–17 years old [57]. Based on the phase 2

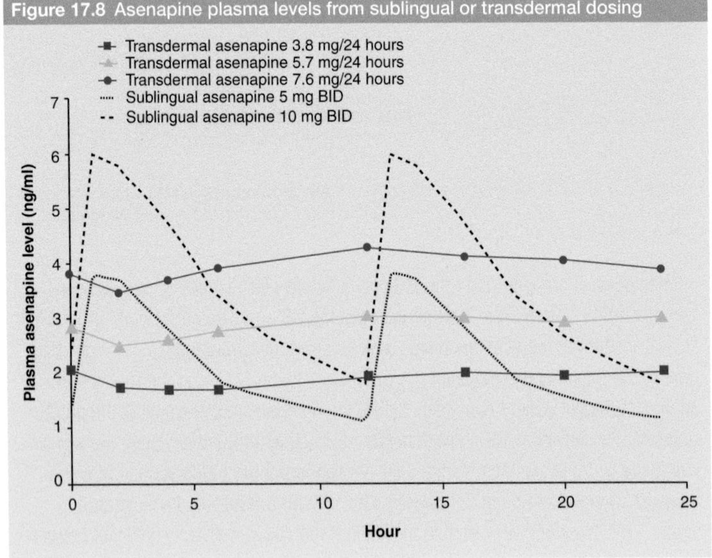

Figure 17.8 Asenapine plasma levels from sublingual or transdermal dosing

(Adapted from: Noven Therapeutics LLC, data on file.)

data showing that SL doses of 1.6 mg BID and 2.4 mg BID were less effective in adult schizophrenia than 5 mg BID, the clinical data supports 1.5 ng/ml as an estimated mean response threshold, but this estimate lacks the responder ROC analyses that provide a more evidence-based result [58]. As a dopamine antagonist, the threshold for response should be associated with plasma levels achieving 65% D_2 occupancy, and this can be used as a proxy for the lower response limit. The first published PET study used normal volunteers with asenapine SL doses of 0.1–0.6 mg/d and did not provide an asenapine concentration associated with 50% D_2 occupancy (the EC_{50}) [52], but a 2011 paper reviewed unpublished data in schizophrenia patients at doses up to 9.6 mg/d and estimated the EC_{50} at 0.528 ng/ml [58]. The FDA medical review of asenapine's preclinical program notes that a plasma level of 3.2 ng/ml achieved 80% D_2 occupancy, which equates to an EC_{50} of 0.80 ng/ml, but there is no discussion of the source of this data or presentation of other plasma levels and their associated receptor occupancy [59]. The lower EC_{50} value of 0.528 ng/ml in the 2011 review is the result of sophisticated modeling analyses performed on PET studies for multiple antipsychotics, with the rationale clearly delineated by the authors, so this will be given stronger weight [58]. From that value, an asenapine plasma level of 0.98 ng/ml is needed to achieve 65% D_2 blockade. For the sake of convenience, this will be rounded up to 1.0 ng/ml, a value very consistent with the lower therapeutic limit of 1 ng/ml proposed in the AGNP/ASCP 2020 consensus paper [42]. Asenapine plasma level monitoring was deemed potentially useful (level 4 recommendation) in the 2020 AGNP/ASCP consensus paper [42].

Use of asenapine SL or transdermal is limited by the licensed dose maximum of 10 mg BID or 7.6 mg/24 hours respectively, so discussions about a point of futility are to some extent an academic exercise since access to higher dosages is generally not possible, although one could potentially increase asenapine levels through use of a strong CYP 1A2 inhibitor such as fluvoxamine [48]. For most D_2 antagonist antipsychotics, tolerability diminishes as D_2 occupancy exceeds 80%, with the point of futility for SGAs occurring somewhere in the region of 90%–95% D_2 blockade. Using the EC_{50} of 0.528 ng/ml, the plasma levels corresponding to 90%–95% occupancy are 4.75–10.03 ng/ml. Where within this range the point of futility might lie will require studies with higher doses and corresponding plasma levels to ascertain the point at which the expectation of response (in those who tolerate such levels) is $< 5\%$. It is worth noting that the AGNP/ASCP 2020 consensus paper provides an upper limit of the therapeutic reference range of 5 ng/ml, and their laboratory alert level is arbitrarily defined as a drug concentration two-fold higher than the upper limit (i.e. 10 ng/ml) [60, 42]. Given the nonlinear kinetics from sublingual dosing, it might not be humanly possible to achieve a 12h trough close to 10 ng/ml, as QT studies with 20 mg BID demonstrate that steady state 12h trough asenapine levels one standard deviation above the mean were still under 5 ng/ml [61].

C Lurasidone

1 Oral Pharmacokinetic Information

Lurasidone is one of two antipsychotics whose absorption is significantly influenced by food intake, the other being ziprasidone [33]. Unlike ziprasidone, lurasidone can be dosed once daily, and when lurasidone is administered within 30 minutes of a meal consisting of a minimum 350 kcal, total drug exposure is doubled [32]. Lurasidone is one of few psychotropics with published data indicating decreased effectiveness after bariatric surgery, emphasizing the need to document a patient's 12h trough level prior to such procedures due to the unpredictable impact on drug absorption (see Chapter 3 for more information on plasma levels and bariatric surgery) [62]. Although lurasidone is recommended to be taken with food, there will be instances in which a patient prefers taking all medications at bedtime. In those circumstances, the dose can be doubled to avoid the need for a nighttime meal; however, clinicians will be limited by the maximum approved dose of 160 mg. If better symptom control necessitates doses higher than 160 mg on an empty stomach (equivalent to 80 mg with a 350 kcal meal), then there is no option but to educate the patient on taking lurasidone with food. As discussed extensively in Chapter 1, lurasidone tolerability is improved significantly by dosing with an evening meal instead of with a morning meal, based on differential adverse effect rates in the clinical trials. (See Chapter 1, Box 1.2, and Table 1.1 for discussion of tolerability with morning- versus evening-meal lurasidone dosing.) When prescribing lurasidone, the directions should be very explicit: take within 30 minutes of dinner. This avoids timing errors with respect to the dose, and misinterpretation of the vague parameter 'with food'. Lurasidone is one of three antipsychotics with an indication for bipolar I depression [63]. That indication, combined with lurasidone's lower risk for metabolic and endocrine adverse effects, and low risk for sedation and orthostasis, has led to approval in many countries in North and South America, the European Union and Asia, and also Australia.

When lurasidone is administered with an evening meal, the concentration–dose relationship is well established, with a 12h trough level 0.18 times the dose in adults [6, 4]. Lurasidone is metabolized via CYP 3A4, and concurrent use of strong 3A4 inhibitors is prohibited as they increase exposure nine-fold [64]; however, moderate CYP 3A4 inhibitors (e.g. diltiazem, verapamil, fluconazole) only double lurasidone exposure, so one can decrease the lurasidone dose by 50%, or administer the dose without food. Use of strong CYP 3A4 inducers is also prohibited as they decrease lurasidone exposure by 80% [64]. There is an active metabolite exohydroxylurasidone (ID-14283) which is present at levels 25% of the parent compound. Lurasidone plasma level assays are slowly becoming available, but no commercial laboratory provides metabolite levels.

2 Therapeutic Threshold and Point of Futility

Lurasidone has an extensive clinical trials program for adults with an acute exacerbation of schizophrenia, which established 40 mg as the minimum effective dose [64]. Although these were predominantly fixed-dose studies, there are no responder ROC analyses based on plasma level data, so one can only infer that the response threshold is the mean 12h trough plasma level expected for 40 mg with an evening meal, estimated at 7.2 ng/ml. As with other D_2 antagonist antipsychotics, the therapeutic threshold can also be inferred from imaging data that provide a plasma level correlate for 65% D_2 receptor occupancy. Unfortunately, the two PET studies used different ligands (raclopride, fallypride), different populations (healthy controls, schizophrenia spectrum patients), and different drug exposure (single dose, steady state), with three-fold variation in plasma level results [65, 66]. In the single-dose study using healthy male volunteers (mean age 27.7 years), four subjects each were scanned at doses of 10 mg, 20 mg, 40 mg, 60 mg, and 80 mg, all of which were ingested with a meal. The threshold of 65% D_2 occupancy was achieved for scans obtained 90 minutes after the 40 mg dose, with a mean lurasidone level of 18.00 ng/ml, and an ID-14283 level of 5.49 ng/ml (Figure 17.9) [65]. Unfortunately, the lurasidone active moiety level needed for 65% D_2 occupancy from that study (18.00 + 5.49 = 23.49 ng/ml) is one-third of the value obtained from a study of 17 schizophrenia spectrum patients (mean age 39.4 years) randomly assigned to doses of 80 mg, 120 mg, or 160 mg with food after washout of prior antipsychotic [66]. From PET scans obtained approximately 26 hours post-dose after 1 week, the estimated active moiety level associated with 65% D_2 receptor occupancy was 70 ng/ml. With this marked discrepancy between the two imaging studies, the consistent clinical evidence that 40 mg with food is an effective lurasidone dose for adult schizophrenia patients makes 7.2 ng/ml a more solid estimate for the therapeutic threshold. The AGNP/ASCP 2020 consensus paper lists 15 ng/ml as the therapeutic threshold, although the reasons for that choice are not made explicit. Nonetheless, lurasidone plasma level monitoring is considered useful (level 3 recommendation) in the 2020 AGNP/ASCP consensus paper [42].

As with many recently marketed antipsychotics, lurasidone prescribing is limited by the licensed maximum dose of 160 mg with food, so discussions about the

Figure 17.9 Fitted dopamine D_2 occupancy curve for lurasidone and its active metabolite exohydroxylurasidone (ID-14283) [65]

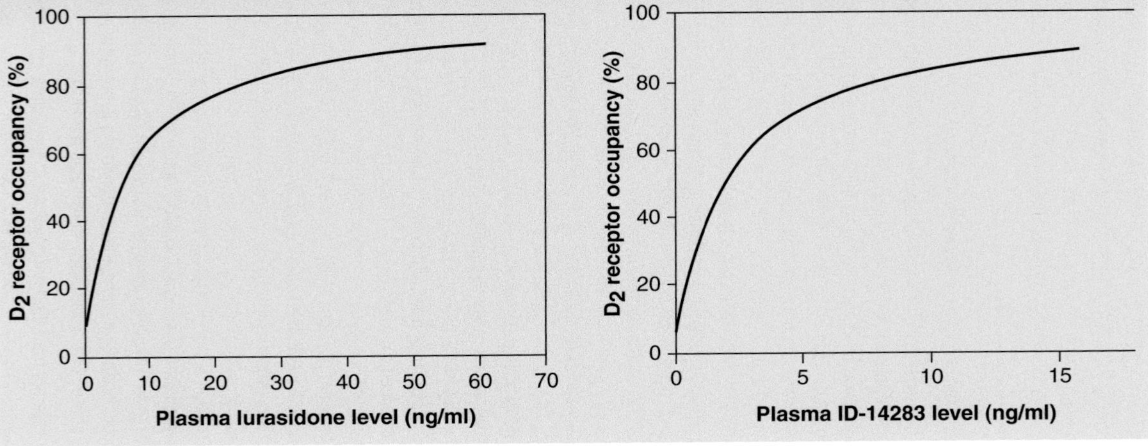

(Adapted from: D. F. Wong, H. Kuwabara, J. R. Brašić, *et al*. [2013]. Determination of dopamine D2 receptor occupancy by lurasidone using positron emission tomography in healthy male subjects. *Psychopharmacology*, 229, 245–252.)

point of futility are mostly an academic exercise since access to higher dosages is generally not possible. There is also insufficient high dose information from clinical trials: the maximum dose with efficacy data is 160 mg. When 160 mg was dosed with an evening meal, it produced akathisia in only 7% of patients, and other extrapyramidal adverse effects in only 13%, so higher dosages might still be tolerated by a significant proportion of the patient population [64]. Generally, one can estimate the plasma level associated with 90%–95% D_2 antagonism from EC_{50} estimates, but the three-fold difference in EC_{50} values from the two PET studies makes these calculations problematic. The AGNP/ASCP consensus paper provides an upper limit for the therapeutic threshold of 40 ng/ml, and a laboratory alert level of 120 ng/ml, but the logic underlying these choices is not known [42]. A plasma level of 40 ng/ml obtained as a 12h trough would be expected for a dose of 240 mg, beyond what is usually permissible until lurasidone becomes a generic product. In the PET study using schizophrenia spectrum patients, active moiety levels of 110 ng/ml were seen in two subjects. Although patients were supposed to be scanned at 26h troughs, levels > 100 ng/ml are only seen with peak plasma levels obtained 2–3 hours after ingesting 120–160 mg with food [6].

D Brexpiprazole

1 Oral Pharmacokinetic Information

Brexpiprazole was the second dopamine partial agonist antipsychotic developed by Otsuka Pharmaceutical, and was approved in the US on July 10, 2015, for adults with schizophrenia, and for adjunctive use with antidepressants in adults with unipolar major depression [12]. Scientists at Otsuka modified the core structure of aripiprazole to arrive at a new molecule with several pharmacodynamic differences, including higher affinity for $5HT_{1A}$, $5HT_{2A}$, and $5HT_7$ receptors than aripiprazole, and less intrinsic dopamine agonism [67, 68]. As noted in Chapter 16, aripiprazole is estimated to have 25% of the intrinsic activity of dopamine at human D_2 receptors [69], while brexpiprazole's activity is 18% [68]. Consistent with less intrinsic dopamine agonism than aripiprazole, brexpiprazole had low rates of akathisia [70, 71]. Brexpiprazole does have sufficient dopamine partial agonism to generate two important outcomes: (a) there is low risk for neurological adverse effects, with rates of extrapyramidal symptoms (excluding akathisia) in schizophrenia trials of 5% for brexpiprazole versus 4% for placebo, and, for akathisia, 6% for brexpiprazole versus 5% for placebo [12]; (b) the relationship between D_2 receptor occupancy and therapeutic response in schizophrenia is different than that for dopamine antagonists [72]. Like aripiprazole, brexpiprazole has a long half-life (91 hours) and is metabolized through

CYP 2D6 and CYP 3A4, but its metabolite does not appear to contribute significantly to central nervous system activity [12]. The concentration–dose relationship is well established for brexpiprazole, bearing in mind that a substantial portion of metabolism is via CYP 2D6, an enzyme with functional genetic variations. As seen in Figure 17.10, intermediate metabolizers at CYP 2D6 experience more than double the expected exposure, and similar effects are seen in poor metabolizers, leading to the manufacturer recommendation to decrease the dose by 50% in the latter group [2]. Brexpiprazole plasma level monitoring is considered useful (level 3 recommendation) in the 2020 AGNP/ASCP consensus paper [42].

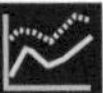

Figure 17.10 Dose normalized brexpiprazole plasma levels (per mg) at steady state by CYP 2D6 metabolizer status (EM = extensive metabolizer; IM = intermediate metabolizer) [2]

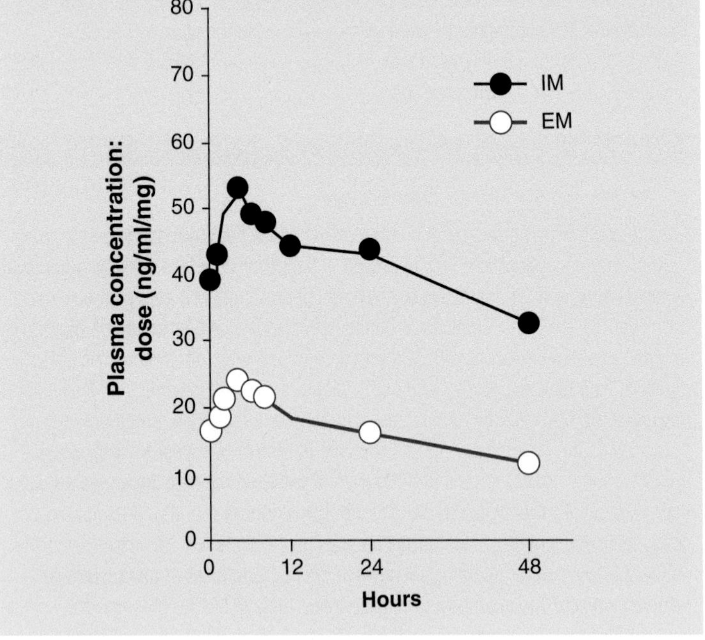

(Adapted from: J. Ishigooka, S. Iwashita, K. Higashi, *et al.* [2018]. Pharmacokinetics and safety of brexpiprazole following multiple-dose administration to Japanese patients with schizophrenia. *J Clin Pharmacol*, 58, 74–80.)

2 Therapeutic Threshold and Point of Futility

Brexpiprazole's recommended dosing was derived from an extensive clinical trials program for adults with an acute exacerbation of schizophrenia that established 2 mg as the minimum effective dose [64]. Despite the availability of fixed-dose studies, there are no responder ROC analyses from plasma level data, so one can only infer that the response threshold is the mean 12h trough plasma level for 2 mg, estimated at 36 ng/ml [2]. This value is very close to the threshold of 40 ng/ml suggested in the 2020 AGNP/ASCP consensus paper [42]. If brexpiprazole was a D_2 antagonist antipsychotic, the therapeutic threshold could also be inferred from imaging data that provides a plasma level correlate for 65% D_2 receptor occupancy. For a partial agonist like brexpiprazole, effectiveness will only be seen at higher levels of striatal D_2 occupancy (e.g. > 80%). As illustrated in Chapter 16, Figure 16.2, even with 100% D_2 receptor occupancy, the postsynaptic dopamine signal will not be 0%, but will reflect the agonist properties of brexpiprazole. With its 18% intrinsic activity, the dopamine signal at 100% receptor occupancy is estimated at 18%, a net 82% reduction and very close to the point (80% reduction) where neurological adverse effects are seen with D_2 antagonists. Using the same calculations as Figure 16.2, but substituting 18% in lieu of aripiprazole's 25% activity, the net reduction in postsynaptic D_2 activity is estimated at 65.6% when brexpiprazole occupies 80% of D_2 receptors, and 73.8% reduction with 90% D_2 occupancy. Brexpiprazole's high affinity for the D_2 receptor and the fact that it operates at extremely high levels of D_2 receptor occupancy may possibly result in the types of situations described with aripiprazole in which addition of the partial agonist to a potent D_2 antagonist (e.g. first-generation antipsychotic, risperidone > 6 mg/d, olanzapine > 25 mg/d, etc.) could result in symptomatic worsening as the D_2 receptor antagonist is displaced with partial agonism [73]. Brexpiprazole was not widely available until recent years so no cases have been reported as yet, but it remains an important concern when any partial agonist antipsychotic is subsequently added in the context of significant D_2 antagonism.

There are multiple brexpiprazole PET studies and the range of EC_{50} values is quite broad, from 8.99 ng/ml to 52 ng/ml, with one investigator selecting 22 ng/ml as the value which fits the most parsimonious model based on a study in 12 adult schizophrenia patients imaged after 10 days on 1 mg/d or 4 mg/d [74, 72]. Using the logic presented above, a 12h trough brexpiprazole plasma level of 36 ng/ml (equal to 2 mg/d) would need to achieve 80% D_2 receptor occupancy to be effective (Figure 17.11). The EC_{50} most consistent with this relationship is the lowest value of 8.99 ng/ml; however, given the range of EC_{50} estimates, a therapeutic threshold derived from the clinical studies appears more easily justifiable.

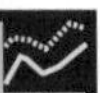

Figure 17.11 Fitted D_2 receptor occupancy curve for brexpiprazole [72]

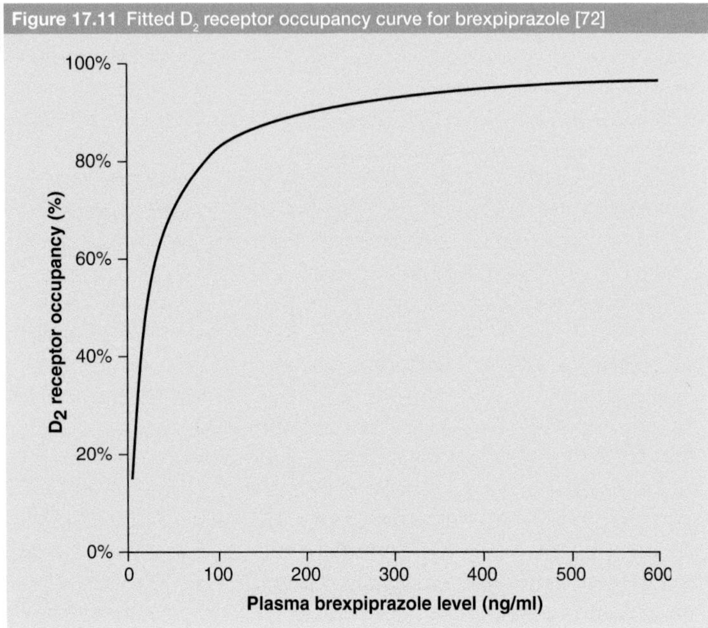

(Adapted from: R. R. Girgis, A. Forbes, A. Abi-Dargham, *et al.* [2020]. A positron emission tomography occupancy study of brexpiprazole at dopamine D2 and D3 and serotonin 5-HT_{1A} and 5-HT_{2A} receptors, and serotonin reuptake transporters in subjects with schizophrenia. *Neuropsychopharmacology*, 45, 786–792.)

Brexpiprazole is still under patent protection, so prescribing is limited by the licensed dose maximum of 4 mg. Discussions about the point of futility are an intellectual exercise, particularly given the absence of schizophrenia outcomes data for doses > 4 mg. As a partial agonist, the point of futility will be reached with 100% D_2 occupancy, but the large range of EC_{50} values makes these calculations problematic. The AGNP/ASCP consensus paper provides an upper limit for the therapeutic threshold of 140 ng/ml but the rationale for this choice is not known [42]. (The AGNP/ASCP laboratory alert level of 280 ng/ml is two times the upper limit.) The AGNP/ASCP upper limit of the therapeutic range of 140 ng/ml is a plasma level that might be seen with patients on 6 mg (an unapproved dose), or those on 4 mg who are CYP 2D6 intermediate or poor metabolizers [2]. Future studies examining schizophrenia response and tolerability for doses > 4 mg will prove useful in defining the point of futility.

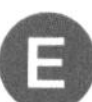

E Cariprazine

1 Oral Pharmacokinetic Information

Cariprazine is the third dopamine partial agonist antipsychotic, first approved in the US on September 17, 2015 for adult schizophrenia and for acute manic or mixed episodes in bipolar I, with a subsequent indication as monotherapy for bipolar I depression [13]. These are several interesting aspects of cariprazine's pharmacology that distinguish it from the other two partial agonists (aripiprazole and brexpiprazole). As noted in Table 17.1, cariprazine has a half-life ($T_{1/2}$) of 31.6–68.4 hours, and it has two active metabolites, desmethylcariprazine (DCAR) with $T_{1/2}$ 29.7–39.5 hours, and didesmethylcariprazine (DDCAR) with an extraordinarily long $T_{1/2}$ of 314–446 hours (13–18 days) [13]. Due to the long $T_{1/2}$ of DDCAR, it is the most prevalent molecule at steady state, and on 6 mg/d the relative proportions are: cariprazine 28%, DCAR 9%, and DDCAR 63% (Figure 17.12) [5]. Another result of the long $T_{1/2}$ is that mean DDCAR plasma levels decrease only 50% 1 week after discontinuation; importantly,

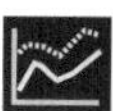

Figure 17.12 Kinetic profile of oral cariprazine (CAR) 6 mg/d showing the contributions of the two metabolites desmethylcariprazine (DCAR) and didesmethylcariprazine (DDCAR) [13]

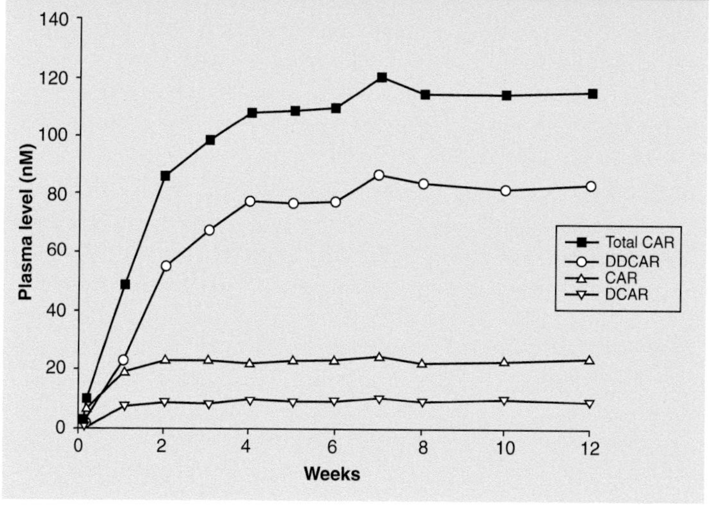

(Adapted from: Allergan USA Inc. [2019]. Vraylar package insert. Madison, NJ.)

this persistence of antipsychotic exposure has been shown to reduce relapse risk compared to other oral antipsychotics after abrupt cessation [13, 18]. The potential downside of DDCAR's 13–18-day $T_{1/2}$ is that certain neurological adverse effects may not appear until DDCAR reaches steady state many weeks after initiation or a dose increase [75]. The late appearance of adverse effects was more prominent at doses from 9 to 12 mg/d, and was one factor in limiting the maximum dose for schizophrenia and acute mania to 6 mg [75].

Another unusual aspect of cariprazine's pharmacology is the marked difference in intrinsic agonism between cariprazine and DDCAR. *In vitro* functional assays indicate that cariprazine has approximately 21% of the activity of dopamine, while DDCAR has only 11% [69]. Given their relative prevalence at steady state, the net effect is a partial agonist with postsynaptic activity in the range of 13%–15%, but this is only an estimate and cannot be verified by imaging studies since they quantify receptor binding and not the extent of agonist action. While cariprazine and DDCAR differ in their D_2 intrinsic activity, both metabolites and cariprazine have six times higher affinity for D_3 than for $D_{2,}$ and this higher affinity is evident in PET imaging studies that differentiate between D_3 and D_2 binding (Figure 17.13) [76]. Moreover, *in vitro* Ki values at the D_3 receptor for cariprazine and its metabolites are in the range of 0.038–0.085 nM, ten-fold higher than for aripiprazole or brexpiprazole [13, 77, 12]. Although cariprazine and its metabolites have intrinsic activity at the D_3 receptor, the net action at D_3 autoreceptors is to diminish feedback inhibition at striatal sites or cortical GABA interneurons [35]. This markedly higher affinity for D_3 may explain why cariprazine is effective for bipolar depression in a manner not seen with aripiprazole or brexpiprazole, and why cariprazine was superior to risperidone for treatment of the negative symptoms of schizophrenia [78, 79].

Using the abundant schizophrenia trials plasma level data, a concentration–dose conversion factor was generated from population kinetic models that predicts a mean active moiety level of 47 nmol/l at 3 mg/d, and 73 nmol/l at 4.5 mg/d [3]. Converting this active moiety level into a cariprazine level in units of ng/ml requires two steps: (a) multiplying the active moiety level by 28%, as cariprazine represents 28% of the active moiety at steady state; (b) dividing this result by 2.34 to obtain units in ng/ml. From these calculations, we expect mean cariprazine levels of 5.62 ng/ml for 3 mg, and 8.74 ng/ml for 4.5 mg. The conversion factors for these two doses are 1.87 and 1.94 respectively, with a mean of 1.91 (see InfoBox). Cariprazine plasma level monitoring is considered useful (level 3 recommendation) in the 2020 AGNP/ASCP consensus paper [42].

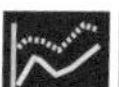

Figure 17.13 Fitted D_2 and D_3 receptor occupancy curve for cariprazine active moiety levels [76]

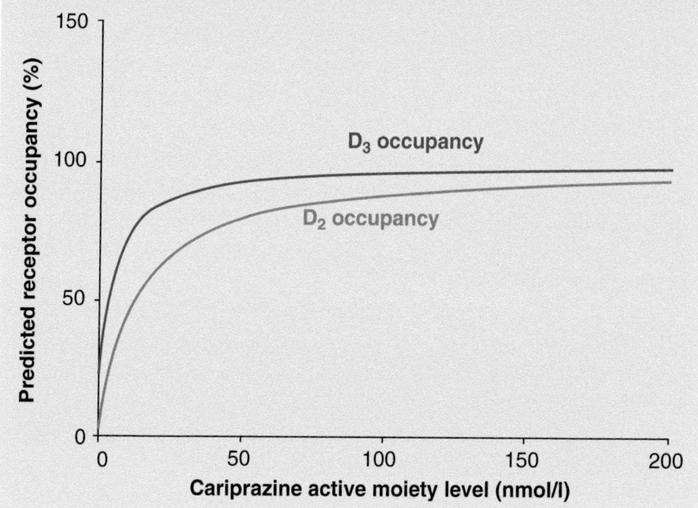

(Adapted from: R. R. Girgis, M. Slifstein, D. D'Souza, *et al.* [2016]. Preferential binding to dopamine D3 over D2 receptors by cariprazine in patients with schizophrenia using PET with the D3/D2 receptor ligand [(11)C]-(+)-PHNO. *Psychopharmacology (Berl)*, 233, 3503–3512.)

2 Therapeutic Threshold and Point of Futility

Cariprazine's recommended dosing was derived from an extensive clinical trials program for adults with an acute exacerbation of schizophrenia [64]. Although the package insert lists 1.5 mg as the minimum dose for schizophrenia, there is compelling data to indicate that differences from placebo only emerge in the range of 3–6 mg/d, with diminishing benefit for schizophrenia at doses > 6 mg/d [3]. This conclusion is not based on responder ROC curves, but on a pharmacokinetic/pharmacodynamic (PK/PD) population modeling analysis that examined longitudinal exposure and response relationships in the cariprazine schizophrenia trials [3]. Due to DDCAR's significant contribution to therapeutic response, the active moiety (referred to in the paper as the total cariprazine level) was used as the plasma level input for the model. The data set comprised 10,327 observations from 1756 patients, and the model accounted for the distinct contributions of placebo and drug effects to symptom response, with the latter quantified as change in the PANSS total score [3]. Based on the maximum drug effect (minus placebo effect) in the adult schizophrenia trials, the active moiety level associated with 50% of the maximal response (EC_{50}) was 55 nmol/l, slightly above the expected mean population active moiety level for 3 mg/d (47 nmol/l) [3]. When the predicted change in PANSS total score relative to placebo was analyzed, the independent effect of cariprazine started to become evident at 3 mg in those whose psychiatric response was at the upper end of the 90% confidence interval; moreover, cariprazine was superior to placebo at doses from 4.5 to 6 mg [3]. Cariprazine is 28% of the active moiety, so an active moiety level of 47 nmol/l represents a cariprazine level of 13.18 nmol/l. When converted to ng/ml units, this cariprazine level becomes 5.6 ng/ml, very close to the 5 ng/ml threshold level suggested in the 2020 AGNP/ASCP consensus paper (see InfoBox, footnote c) [42]. A 2019 PET study in schizophrenia patients calculated an EC_{50} for D_2 occupancy of 13.03 nmol/l for the active moiety [76]. Therefore, the mean active moiety level of 47 nmol/l for a dose of 3 mg/d translates to 78% D_2 occupancy, a value very consistent with the two other partial agonist antipsychotics, and well above the response threshold of 65% occupancy for D_2 antagonists. Due to cariprazine's high affinity for the D_2 receptor and the fact that it operates at extremely high levels of D_2 receptor occupancy, there is a significant risk for the types of situations described with aripiprazole in which addition of the partial agonist to a potent D_2 antagonist (e.g. first-generation antipsychotic, risperidone > 6 mg/d, olanzapine > 25 mg/d, etc.) could result in symptomatic worsening as the D_2 receptor antagonist is displaced with partial agonism [73].

As with other antipsychotics still under patent protection, most clinicians are limited to the licensed maximum dose of 6 mg/d, making discussions about the point of futility somewhat moot. The schizophrenia trials used doses up to 12 mg/d, but there are no responder analyses to help to estimate the point at which odds of response are < 5% even if tolerated. It should be noted that the PK/PD analysis found incremental improvement on the PANSS lessens significantly at doses > 9 mg/d, and 9 mg/d translates to a cariprazine level of 17 ng/ml [3]. The active moiety level for the maximum dose studied (12 mg/d) is close to 200 nmol/l, which equates to 94% D_2 receptor occupancy, and for which the plasma cariprazine level is 23 ng/ml. With the extensive data up to 12 mg/d, hopefully a future investigator will perform a responder analysis for this dose and its associated plasma level using a standard definition (e.g. 50% PANSS reduction). The AGNP/ASCP consensus paper provides a laboratory alert level of 40 ng/ml, but the logic underlying this choice is not known [42]. A cariprazine plasma level of 40 ng/ml obtained as a 12h trough would be expected for a dose of close to 20 mg, well beyond what is usually permissible.

Summary Points

a Amisulpride has a well-defined concentration–dose relationship, and moderate data to establish a therapeutic response threshold of 100 ng/ml. Despite the risk of hyperprolactinemia, it may have slight efficacy advantages over other antipsychotics, although it is not effective for resistant schizophrenia. Amisulpride's antidepressant properties derive from $5HT_7$ antagonism.

b Asenapine has both sublingual and transdermal formulations with marked differences in kinetic profiles, and which have differing trough levels despite equivalent drug exposure. While not available in most countries yet, the transdermal patch has a low peak–trough ratio of 1.5, and avoids twice daily dosing and the need to avoid water for several minutes after each sublingual dose. Both formulations have minimal drug–drug interactions. There is moderate evidence to support an asenapine therapeutic response threshold of 1.0 ng/ml.

c Lurasidone has indications for schizophrenia and bipolar I depression, and low risk for metabolic and endocrine adverse effects. Drug exposure is decreased by 50% if not ingested with a 350 kcal meal. The concentration–dose relationship is well established, and the biggest influence on trough plasma levels in routine practice is adherence to ingestion with food. Tolerability is significantly improved when dosed with an evening meal, so prescribing instructions should explicitly state "take within 30 minutes of dinner." There is moderate evidence to support a therapeutic response threshold of 7.2 ng/ml for adults with schizophrenia.

d Brexpiprazole is a dopamine partial agonist with 18% intrinsic activity at dopamine receptors, and with indications for schizophrenia and adjunctive use in major depression. The dosage range is 2–4 mg for adults with schizophrenia, but there is limited plasma level data from which to infer a response threshold, so the mean plasma level for 2 mg should be used (36 ng/ml). Very few laboratories have brexpiprazole assays at the present time, but the availability is increasing slowly.

e Cariprazine is also a dopamine partial agonist, with indications for schizophrenia, for acute manic/mixed episodes in bipolar I, and for bipolar I depression. It has an active metabolite DDCAR with a half-life of 13–18 days, and DDCAR is 63% of the active moiety at steady state, while cariprazine is 28%. Cariprazine has 21% intrinsic activity at dopamine receptors, but it is close to 11% for DDCAR, so the net effect is the sum of the two. Cariprazine and its metabolites have ten-fold higher D_3 affinity than the other partial agonists. This D_3 affinity is responsible for its antidepressant activities, and also for efficacy in the negative symptoms of schizophrenia. The dosage range with demonstrable efficacy is 3–6 mg for adults with schizophrenia. Very few laboratories have cariprazine assays and none reports metabolite levels, but the response threshold that can be used is 5.6 ng/ml, the mean cariprazine level for 3 mg/d.

References

1. **Sparshatt, A., Taylor, D., Patel, M. X., *et al.* (2009).** Amisulpride – dose, plasma concentration, occupancy and response: implications for therapeutic drug monitoring. *Acta Psychiatr Scand*, 120, 416–428.
2. **Ishigooka, J., Iwashita, S., Higashi, K., *et al.* (2018).** Pharmacokinetics and safety of brexpiprazole following multiple-dose administration to Japanese patients with schizophrenia. *J Clin Pharmacol*, 58, 74–80.
3. **Periclou, A., Willavize, S., Jaworowicz, D., *et al.* (2020).** Relationship between plasma concentrations and clinical effects of cariprazine in patients with schizophrenia or bipolar mania. *Clin Transl Sci*, 13, 362–371.
4. **Loebel, A., Silva, R., Goldman, R., *et al.* (2016).** Lurasidone dose escalation in early nonresponding patients with schizophrenia: a randomized, double-blind, placebo-controlled study. *J Clin Psychiatry*, 77, 1672–1680.
5. **FDA Center for Drug Evaluation and Research (2015).** Cariprazine pharmacology/toxicology NDA review and evaluation.
6. **Findling, R. L., Goldman, R., Chiu, Y. Y., *et al.* (2015).** Pharmacokinetics and tolerability of lurasidone in children and adolescents with psychiatric disorders. *Clin Ther*, 37, 2788–2797.
7. **Schmitt, U., Abou El-Ela, A., Guo, L. J., *et al.* (2006).** Cyclosporine A (CsA) affects the pharmacodynamics and pharmacokinetics of the atypical antipsychotic amisulpride probably via inhibition of P-glycoprotein (P-gp). *J Neural Transm (Vienna)*, 113, 787–801.
8. **O'Brien, F. E., Dinan, T. G., Griffin, B. T., *et al.* (2012).** Interactions between antidepressants and P-glycoprotein at the blood-brain barrier: clinical significance of in vitro and in vivo findings. *Br J Pharmacol*, 165, 289–312.
9. **Bartlett, J. A. and van der Voort Maarschalk, K. (2012).** Understanding the oral mucosal absorption and resulting clinical pharmacokinetics of asenapine. *AAPS PharmSciTech*, 13, 1110–1115.
10. **Allergan USA Inc. (2017).** Saphris package insert. Irvine, CA.
11. **Noven Therapeutics LLC (2020).** Secuado package insert. Miami, FL.
12. **Otsuka America Pharmaceutical Inc. (2020).** Rexulti package insert. Rockville, MD.
13. **Allergan USA Inc. (2019).** Vraylar package insert. Madison, NJ.
14. **Nakamura, T., Kubota, T., Iwakaji, A., *et al.* (2016).** Clinical pharmacology study of cariprazine (MP-214) in patients with schizophrenia (12-week treatment). *Drug Des Devel Ther*, 10, 327–338.
15. **Blier, P., Oquendo, M. A., and Kupfer, D. J. (2017).** Progress on the Neuroscience-Based Nomenclature (NbN) for Psychotropic Medications. *Neuropsychopharmacology*, 42, 1927–1928.
16. **Uchida, H. (2018).** Neuroscience-based Nomenclature: what is it, why is it needed, and what comes next? *Psychiatry Clin Neurosci*, 72, 50–51.
17. **Siafis, S., Davis, J. M., and Leucht, S. (2020).** Antipsychotic drugs: from 'major tranquilizers' to Neuroscience-based-Nomenclature. *Psychol Med*, 1–3.
18. **Correll, C. U., Jain, R., Meyer, J. M., *et al.* (2019).** Relationship between the timing of relapse and plasma drug levels following discontinuation of cariprazine treatment in patients with schizophrenia: indirect comparison with other second-generation antipsychotics after treatment discontinuation. *Neuropsychiatr Dis Treat*, 15, 2537–2550.
19. **Vanda Pharmaceuticals Inc. (2018).** Fanapt package insert. Washington, DC.
20. **Komossa, K., Rummel-Kluge, C., Hunger, H., *et al.* (2009).** Sertindole versus other atypical antipsychotics for schizophrenia. *Cochrane Database Syst Rev*, CD006752.
21. **Beedham, C., Miceli, J. J., and Obach, R. S. (2003).** Ziprasidone metabolism, aldehyde oxidase, and clinical implications. *J Clin Psychopharmacol*, 23, 229–232.

22. **Roerig Division of Pfizer Inc. (2020).** Geodon package insert. New York.
23. **Asmal, L., Flegar, S. J., Wang, J., *et al.* (2013).** Quetiapine versus other atypical antipsychotics for schizophrenia. *Cochrane Database Syst Rev*, CD006625.
24. **Vanasse, A., Blais, L., Courteau, J., *et al.* (2016).** Comparative effectiveness and safety of antipsychotic drugs in schizophrenia treatment: a real-world observational study. *Acta Psychiatr Scand*, 134, 374–384.
25. **Intra-Cellular Therapies Inc. (2019).** Caplyta package insert. New York.
26. **Vyas, P., Hwang, B. J., and Brasic, J. R. (2019).** An evaluation of lumateperone tosylate for the treatment of schizophrenia. *Expert Opin Pharmacother*, 30, 1–7.
27. **Meyer, J. M. (2020).** Lumateperone for schizophrenia. *Curr Psychiatr*, 19, 33–39.
28. **Huhn, M., Nikolakopoulou, A., Schneider-Thoma, J., *et al.* (2019).** Comparative efficacy and tolerability of 32 oral antipsychotics for the acute treatment of adults with multi-episode schizophrenia: a systematic review and network meta-analysis. *Lancet*, 394, 939–951.
29. **Kahn, R. S., Winter van Rossum, I., Leucht, S., *et al.* (2018).** Amisulpride and olanzapine followed by open-label treatment with clozapine in first-episode schizophrenia and schizophreniform disorder (OPTiMiSE): a three-phase switching study. *Lancet Psychiatry*, 5, 797–807.
30. **Delcker, A., Schoon, M. L., Oczkowski, B., *et al.* (1990).** Amisulpride versus haloperidol in treatment of schizophrenic patients – results of a double-blind study. *Pharmacopsychiatry*, 23, 125–130.
31. **Abbas, A. I., Hedlund, P. B., Huang, X.-P., *et al.* (2009).** Amisulpride is a potent 5-HT7 antagonist: relevance for antidepressant actions in vivo. *Psychopharmacology*, 205, 119–128.
32. **Meyer, J. M., Loebel, A. D., and Schweizer, E. (2009).** Lurasidone: a new drug in development for schizophrenia. *Expert Opin Investig Drugs*, 18, 1715–1726.
33. **Meyer, J. M. (2018).** Pharmacotherapy of psychosis and mania. In L. L. Brunton, R. Hilal-Dandan and B. C. Knollmann, eds., *Goodman & Gilman's The Pharmacological Basis of Therapeutics*, 13th edn. Chicago, IL: McGraw-Hill, pp. 279–302.
34. **Schoemaker, H., Claustre, Y., Fage, D., *et al.* (1997).** Neurochemical characteristics of amisulpride, an atypical dopamine D2/D3 receptor antagonist with both presynaptic and limbic selectivity. *J Pharmacol Exp Ther*, 280, 83–97.
35. **Stahl, S. M. (2017).** Drugs for psychosis and mood: unique actions at D3, D2, and D1 dopamine receptor subtypes. *CNS Spectr*, 22, 375–384.
36. **Kahn, R. S., Fleischhacker, W. W., Boter, H., *et al.* (2008).** Effectiveness of antipsychotic drugs in first-episode schizophrenia and schizophreniform disorder: an open randomised clinical trial. *Lancet*, 371, 1085–1097.
37. **Hartter, S., Huwel, S., Lohmann, T., *et al.* (2003).** How does the benzamide antipsychotic amisulpride get into the brain? – An in vitro approach comparing amisulpride with clozapine. *Neuropsychopharmacology*, 28, 1916–1922.
38. **Wang, R., Sun, X., Deng, Y. S., *et al.* (2018).** ABCB1 1199G > A polymorphism impacts transport ability of P-gp-mediated antipsychotics. *DNA Cell Biol*, 37, 325–329.
39. **Arrowtex Pharmaceuticals (2019).** Amisulpride package insert. Macquarie Park, NSW, Australia.
40. **Bergemann, N., Kopitz, J., Kress, K. R., *et al.* (2004).** Plasma amisulpride levels in schizophrenia or schizoaffective disorder. *Eur Neuropsychopharmacol*, 14, 245–250.
41. **Muller, M. J., Eich, F. X., Regenbogen, B., *et al.* (2009).** Amisulpride doses and plasma levels in different age groups of patients with schizophrenia or schizoaffective disorder. *J Psychopharmacol*, 23, 278–286.
42. **Schoretsanitis, G., Kane, J. M., Correll, C. U., *et al.* (2020).** Blood levels to optimize antipsychotic treatment in clinical practice: a joint consensus statement of the American Society of Clinical Psychopharmacology (ASCP) and the Therapeutic Drug Monitoring (TDM) Task Force of

the Arbeitsgemeinschaft für Neuropsychopharmakologie und Pharmakopsychiatrie (AGNP). *J Clin Psychiatry*, 81, https://doi.org/10.4088/JCP.4019cs13169.

43. **Puech, A., Fleurot, O., and Rein, W. (1998).** Amisulpride, and atypical antipsychotic, in the treatment of acute episodes of schizophrenia: a dose-ranging study vs. haloperidol. The Amisulpride Study Group. *Acta Psychiatr Scand*, 98, 65–72.
44. **Muller, M. J., Regenbogen, B., Hartter, S., *et al.* (2007).** Therapeutic drug monitoring for optimizing amisulpride therapy in patients with schizophrenia. *J Psychiatr Res*, 41, 673–679.
45. **Mota, N. E., Lima, M. S., and Soares, B. G. (2002).** Amisulpride for schizophrenia. *Cochrane Database Syst Rev*, 2002, CD001357.
46. **Linden, M., Scheel, T., and Xaver Eich, F. (2004).** Dosage finding and outcome in the treatment of schizophrenic inpatients with amisulpride: results of a drug utilization observation study. *Hum Psychopharmacol*, 19, 111–119.
47. **Shahid, M., Walker, G. B., Zorn, S. H., *et al.* (2009).** Asenapine: a novel psychopharmacologic agent with a unique human receptor signature. *J Psychopharmacol*, 23, 65–73.
48. **Citrome, L. (2014).** Asenapine review, part I: chemistry, receptor affinity profile, pharmacokinetics and metabolism. *Expert Opin Drug Metab Toxicol*, 10, 893–903.
49. **Vieta, E. and Montes, J. M. (2018).** A review of asenapine in the treatment of bipolar disorder. *Clin Drug Investig*, 38, 87–99.
50. **El-Mallakh, R. S., Nuss, S., Gao, D., *et al.* (2020).** Asenapine in the treatment of bipolar depression. *Psychopharmacol Bull*, 50, 8–18.
51. **Koytchev, R., Alken, R. G., McKay, G., *et al.* (1996).** Absolute bioavailability of oral immediate and slow release fluphenazine in healthy volunteers. *Eur J Clin Pharmacol*, 51, 183–187.
52. **Andree, B., Halldin, C., Vrijmoed-de Vries, M., *et al.* (1997).** Central 5-HT2A and D2 dopamine receptor occupancy after sublingual administration of ORG 5222 in healthy men. *Psychopharmacology*, 131, 339–345.
53. **Carrithers, B. and El-Mallakh, R. S. (2020).** Transdermal asenapine in schizophrenia: a systematic review. *Patient Prefer Adherence*, 14, 1541–1551.
54. **Seager, H. (1998).** Drug-delivery products and the Zydis fast-dissolving dosage form. *J Pharm Pharmacol*, 50, 375–382.
55. **Pillinger, T., McCutcheon, R. A., Vano, L., *et al.* (2020).** Comparative effects of 18 antipsychotics on metabolic function in patients with schizophrenia, predictors of metabolic dysregulation, and association with psychopathology: a systematic review and network meta-analysis. *Lancet Psychiatry*, 7, 64–77.
56. **Citrome, L. (2014).** Asenapine review, part II: clinical efficacy, safety and tolerability. *Expert Opin Drug Saf*, 13, 803–830.
57. **Dogterom, P., Riesenberg, R., de Greef, R., *et al.* (2018).** Asenapine pharmacokinetics and tolerability in a pediatric population. *Drug Des Develop Ther*, 12, 2677–2693.
58. **de Greef, R., Maloney, A., Olsson-Gisleskog, P., *et al.* (2011).** Dopamine D2 occupancy as a biomarker for antipsychotics: quantifying the relationship with efficacy and extrapyramidal symptoms. *AAPS Journal*, 13, 121–130.
59. **Food and Drug Administration Center for Drug Evaluation and Research (2009).** Asenapine medical review.
60. **Hiemke, C., Bergemann, N., Clement, H. W., *et al.* (2018).** Consensus guidelines for therapeutic drug monitoring in neuropsychopharmacology: update 2017. *Pharmacopsychiatry*, 51, 9–62.
61. **Chapel, S., Hutmacher, M. M., Haig, G., *et al.* (2009).** Exposure-response analysis in patients with schizophrenia to assess the effect of asenapine on QTc prolongation. *J Clin Pharmacol*, 49, 1297–1308.

62. **Ward, H. B., Yudkoff, B. L., and Fromson, J. A. (2019).** Lurasidone malabsorption following bariatric surgery: a case report. *J Psychiatr Pract*, 25, 313–317.
63. **Baldessarini, R. J., Tondo, L., and Vazquez, G. H. (2019).** Pharmacological treatment of adult bipolar disorder. *Mol Psychiatry*, 24, 198–217.
64. **Sunovion Pharmaceuticals Inc. (2019).** Latuda package insert. Marlborough, MA.
65. **Wong, D. F., Kuwabara, H., Brašić, J. R., *et al.* (2013).** Determination of dopamine D2 receptor occupancy by lurasidone using positron emission tomography in healthy male subjects. *Psychopharmacology*, 229, 245–252.
66. **Potkin, S. G., Keator, D. B., Kesler-West, M. L., *et al.* (2014).** D2 receptor occupancy following lurasidone treatment in patients with schizophrenia or schizoaffective disorder. *CNS Spectr*, 19, 176–181.
67. **Maeda, K., Lerdrup, L., Sugino, H., *et al.* (2014).** Brexpiprazole II: antipsychotic-like and procognitive effects of a novel serotonin–dopamine activity modulator. *J Pharmacol Exp Ther*, 350, 605–614.
68. **Maeda, K., Sugino, H., Akazawa, H., *et al.* (2014).** Brexpiprazole I: in vitro and in vivo characterization of a novel serotonin–dopamine activity modulator. *J Pharmacol Exp Ther*, 350, 589–604.
69. **Tadori, Y., Forbes, R. A., McQuade, R. D., *et al.* (2011).** In vitro pharmacology of aripiprazole, its metabolite and experimental dopamine partial agonists at human dopamine D2 and D3 receptors. *Eur J Pharmacol*, 668, 355–365.
70. **McEvoy, J. and Citrome, L. (2016).** Brexpiprazole for the treatment of schizophrenia: a review of this novel serotonin–dopamine activity modulator. *Clin Schizophr Relat Psychoses*, 9, 177–186.
71. **Ward, K. and Citrome, L. (2019).** Brexpiprazole for the maintenance treatment of adults with schizophrenia: an evidence-based review and place in therapy. *Neuropsychiatr Dis Treat*, 15, 247–257.
72. **Girgis, R. R., Forbes, A., Abi-Dargham, A., *et al.* (2020).** A positron emission tomography occupancy study of brexpiprazole at dopamine D2 and D3 and serotonin 5-HT_{1A} and 5-HT_{2A} receptors, and serotonin reuptake transporters in subjects with schizophrenia. *Neuropsychopharmacology*, 45, 786–792.
73. **Takeuchi, H. and Remington, G. (2013).** A systematic review of reported cases involving psychotic symptoms worsened by aripiprazole in schizophrenia or schizoaffective disorder. *Psychopharmacology (Berl)*, 228, 175–185.
74. **Wong, D. F., Malikaarjun, S., Raoufinia, A., *et al.* (2011).** 619. A phase I, open-label PET study of the pharmacokinetics, tolerability and D2/D3 striatal occupancy of single-dose oral OPC-34712 in healthy subjects. *Biol Psychiatry*, 69, 187s.
75. **Food and Drug Administration Center for Drug Evaluation and Research (2015).** Cariprazine pharmacology/toxicology NDA review and evaluation.
76. **Girgis, R. R., Slifstein, M., D'Souza, D., *et al.* (2016).** Preferential binding to dopamine D3 over D2 receptors by cariprazine in patients with schizophrenia using PET with the D3/D2 receptor ligand [(11)C]-(+)-PHNO. *Psychopharmacology (Berl)*, 233, 3503–3512.
77. **Otsuka America Pharmaceutical Inc. (2020).** Abilify package insert. Rockville, MD.
78. **Németh, G., Laszlovszky, I., Czobor, P., *et al.* (2017).** Cariprazine versus risperidone monotherapy for treatment of predominant negative symptoms in patients with schizophrenia: a randomised, double-blind, controlled trial. *Lancet*, 389, 1103–1113.
79. **Ragguett, R. M. and McIntyre, R. S. (2019).** Cariprazine for the treatment of bipolar depression: a review. *Expert Rev Neurother*, 19, 317–323.

APPENDIX
Therapeutic Threshold, Point of Futility, AGNP/ASCP Laboratory Alert Level, and Average Oral Concentration–Dose Relationships

Antipsychotic	Therapeutic threshold (ng/ml)	Point of futility (ng/ml)	AGNP/ASCP laboratory alert level (ng/ml)	Oral concentration–dose relationship[a]
Amisulpride	100	550–700	Not reported	Females: 0.60 Males: 0.46
Aripiprazole	110	500	1000	11.0
Asenapine (sublingual)	1.0	(Based on maximal licensed dose of 10 mg sublingual BID)	10	5 mg BID: 0.15 10 mg BID: 0.20
Asenapine (transdermal)[b]	1.0	(Based on maximal licensed dose of 7.8 mg/24 hours)	10	0.53
Brexpiprazole	36	(Based on maximal licensed dose of 4 mg QHS)	280	CYP 2D6 EM: 18 CYP 2D6 IM: 46
Cariprazine[c]	5.6	(Based on maximal licensed dose of 6 mg QHS)	40[c]	1.91
Chlorpromazine	3–30	100	600	0.06
Clozapine	350	1000	1000	Female Smoker: 0.80 Female Nonsmoker: 1.32 Male Smoker: 0.67 Male Nonsmoker: 1.08
Flupenthixol (*cis* isomer)	0.43	3.0	15	0.20
Fluphenazine	1.0	4.0	15	Smoker: 0.06 Nonsmoker: 0.08–0.10
Haloperidol	2.0	18	15	0.78
Loxapine	3.8	18.4	20	0.22

Antipsychotic	Therapeutic threshold (ng/ml)	Point of futility (ng/ml)	AGNP/ASCP laboratory alert level (ng/ml)	Oral concentration–dose relationship[a]
Lurasidone[d]	7.2	(Based on maximal licensed dose of 160 mg with an evening meal)	120	0.18
Olanzapine	23	150	100	Smoker: 1.43 Nonsmoker: 2.0
Paliperidone	20	90	120	4.09
Perphenazine	0.81	5.0	5	CYP 2D6 EM: 0.04 CYP 2D6 PM: 0.08
Risperidone (active moiety)[e]	15	112	120	7.0
Thiothixene	1.0	12	Not reported	Smoker: 0.04 Nonsmoker: 0.05
Trifluoperazine	1.0	2.3	Not reported	Unknown
Zuclopenthixol	2.0	9.0	Not reported	0.65

CYP: cytochrome P450; **EM:** extensive metabolizer; **IM:** intermediate metabolizer; **PM:** poor metabolizer

[a] Multiply by the conversion factor to obtain 12h trough levels in ng/ml for patients receiving all or most of their dose at bedtime. These mean values apply to patients not exposed to metabolic inhibitors or inducers, and who are extensive metabolizers for the relevant enzymes. Due to extensive population variation for most 12h trough levels, low levels may not reflect poor adherence. A second data point on the same dose will be of significant help in differentiating kinetic and adherence issues (see Chapter 4).

[b] Although the lowest transdermal formulation dose of 3.8 mg/24 hours provides equivalent asenapine exposure to the sublingual dose of 5 mg BID (as calculated by the AUC), the trough levels for the sublingual dose are lower due to higher peak–trough variation. This conversion factor of 0.53 is for the transdermal dose (per 24 hours). **Example:** 3.8 mg/24 hours x 0.53 = 2.0 ng/ml.

[c] The values provided for cariprazine do not include the metabolites. At steady state on 6 mg/d, the active moiety is: cariprazine 28%, DCAR 9%, and DDCAR 63% [1]. However, very few laboratories have cariprazine assays, and none reports the metabolites at present. Should this change, the active moiety values represented will be four-fold higher. For example, the steady state cariprazine level on 6 mg/d is 11.2 ng/ml, but the active moiety level will be approximately 40 ng/ml [2]. The rationale behind the AGNP/ASCP laboratory alert level of 40 ng/ml is not clearly delineated in the paper [3].

[d] The concentration–dose relationships for lurasidone are based on 12h trough values obtained at steady state (day 9 or later) and with lurasidone administered within 30 minutes of an evening meal of at least 350 kcal. This does not include the active metabolite ID-14283 (exohydroxylurasidone), which comprises 25% of the active moiety, but whose levels are not reported by commercial laboratories presently [4].

[e] The risperidone active moiety is the sum of risperidone + 9-OH risperidone levels.

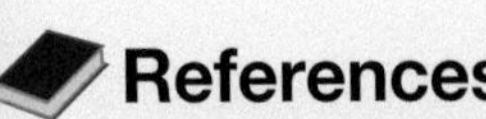

References

1. **FDA Center for Drug Evaluation and Research (2015).** Cariprazine pharmacology/toxicology NDA review and evaluation.
2. **Periclou, A., Willavize, S., Jaworowicz, D., *et al.* (2020).** Relationship between plasma concentrations and clinical effects of cariprazine in patients with schizophrenia or bipolar mania. *Clin Transl Sci*, 13, 362–371.
3. **Schoretsanitis, G., Kane, J. M., Correll, C. U., *et al.* (2020).** Blood levels to optimize antipsychotic treatment in clinical practice: a joint consensus statement of the American Society of Clinical Psychopharmacology (ASCP) and the Therapeutic Drug Monitoring (TDM) Task Force of the Arbeitsgemeinschaft für Neuropsychopharmakologie und Pharmakopsychiatrie (AGNP). *J Clin Psychiatry*, 81, https://doi.org/10.4088/JCP.4019cs13169.
4. **Findling, R. L., Goldman, R., Chiu, Y. Y., *et al.* (2015).** Pharmacokinetics and tolerability of lurasidone in children and adolescents with psychiatric disorders. *Clin Ther*, 37, 2788–2797.

Index